PERICARDIAL DISEASES
Clinical Diagnostic Imaging Atlas

DVD Table of Contents

Pericardial Diseases

CLINICAL DIAGNOSTIC IMAGING ATLAS

Pericardial Diseases

CLINICAL DIAGNOSTIC IMAGING ATLAS

Stuart J. Hutchison

MD, FRCPC, FACC, FAHA, FASE, FSCMR, FSCCT

Clinical Associate Professor of Medicine
University of Calgary
Foothills Medical Center
Stephenson Cardiac Magnetic
Resonance Imaging Center
Libin Cardiovascular Institute of Alberta
Calgary, Canada

Original artwork and animations by
Gail Rudakewich, Myra Rudakewich, and **Stuart J. Hutchison**

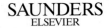

1600 John F. Kennedy Blvd.
Ste 1800
Philadelphia, PA 19103-2899

PERICARDIAL DISEASES: CLINICAL DIAGNOSTIC
IMAGING ATLAS

ISBN: 978-1-4160-5274-6

Notice

Knowledge and best practice in this field are constantly changing. As new research and experience broaden our knowledge, changes in practice, treatment, and drug therapy may become necessary or appropriate. Readers are advised to check the most current information provided (i) on procedures featured or (ii) by the manufacturer of each product to be administered, to verify the recommended dose or formula, the method and duration of administration, and contraindications. It is the responsibility of the practitioner, relying on his or her experience and knowledge of the patient, to make diagnoses, to determine dosages and the best treatment for each individual patient, and to take all appropriate safety precautions. To the fullest extent of the law, neither the Publisher nor the Author assumes any liability for any injury and/or damage to persons or property arising out of or related to any use of the material contained in this book.

The Publisher

Library of Congress Cataloging-in-Publication Data
Hutchison, Stuart J.
    Pericardial diseases : clinical diagnostic imaging atlas with DVD / Stuart J. Hutchison.—1st ed.
        p. ; cm.—(Cardiovascular emergencies : atlas and multimedia series)
    Includes bibliographical references.
    ISBN 978-1-4160-5274-6
    1. Pericardium—Diseases—Diagnosis—Atlases. 2. Heart—Imaging—Atlases. I. Title. II. Series.
    [DNLM: 1. Heart Diseases—diagnosis. 2. Pericardium—pathology. 3. Diagnostic Imaging.
WG 275 H978p 2009]
    RC685.P5H88 2009
    616.1′10754—dc22

2008018634

Executive Publisher: Natasha Andjelkovic
Publishing Services Manager: Frank Polizzano
Project Manager: Rachel Miller
Design Direction: Lou Forgione
Illustration Direction: Ceil Nuyianes
Multimedia Producer: Bruce Robison

To Noel Keith and Cindy Hutchison, for the immeasurable gifts of love and time.

To Bob Chisholm—an inspired and inspiring physician, colleague, and friend, a man of insuppressible alacrity, integrity, and loyalty, and the best cath lab director an echo lab director could ever hope to work with.

Foreword

Diseases of the pericardium represent one of the most intriguing yet demanding areas in clinical cardiology. Understanding the pathophysiology of pericardial disorders, their diagnostic uncertainties, and the associated dilemmas in their treatment continue to challenge all who study the cardiovascular system, from students to experienced cardiologists. Dr. Stuart Hutchison's masterful atlas provides a comprehensive, balanced, and authoritative source covering the full spectrum of diseases of the pericardium. Although the primary focus of *Pericardial Diseases* is the practical application and interpretation of cardiovascular imaging techniques in patients with pericardial disorders, the atlas is also a clinically relevant resource covering the full spectrum of this field, including thoughtful discussions of epidemiology, clinical presen-

tation, physical examination, diagnostic tools, and treatment. The imaging examples from 2-dimensional and Doppler echocardiography and the advanced fields of cardiac magnetic resonance and computed tomography are superbly presented. This scholarly work will be an essential resource for cardiovascular practitioners, cardiothoracic surgeons, researchers, and imaging subspecialists.

Robert O. Bonow, MD, MACC
Goldberg Distinguished Professor
Northwestern University Feinberg School of Medicine
Chief, Division of Cardiology
Northwestern Memorial Hospital
Chicago, Illinois

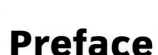

Preface

Pericardial diseases provide ongoing diagnostic and treatment challenges to clinicians. They comprise a considerable breadth of disorders that range from acute to chronic, insidious to fulminant, benign to malignant, self-limited to progressive, symptomatic-only to life-threatening, limited to systemic, consistent to variable, and straightforward to complex. Pericardial diseases are similarly encountered by a wide range of physicians, particularly emergency physicians, cardiologists, cardiac surgeons, trauma surgeons, nephrologists, rheumatologists, immunologists, oncologists, intensivists, and others.

The evaluation of pericardial diseases entails a broad-based approach that begins at the bedside and draws heavily on imaging assessment as well as hemodynamic assessment. The pericardial compressive disorders of constriction and tamponade and their variants involve complex, incompletely established and fascinating interactions of cardiac and pulmonary physiology. Proficiency with the underlying pathophysiology assists immeasurably in the clinical, imaging, and hemodynamic assessment, especially in atypical cases.

The advent of contemporary imaging modalities has brought a new era to the assessment of pericardial diseases that comple-

ments the traditional and often historic character of pericardial diseases and rounds out the medical sphere of knowledge of pericardial diseases. As with many classic diseases, learning and discussing the surgical and pathological findings in cases encountered are invaluable in gaining understanding and proficiency. I am indebted to my clinical colleagues, and especially to my surgical and pathology colleagues, for their feedback, knowledge, insights, and willingness to discuss cases and their wonderful collegiality.

My motivation in developing this book and its companion DVD was to integrate contemporary cardiovascular imaging with the overall assessment of pericardial diseases and to emphasize the pathophysiologic basis of the clinical, imaging, and hemodynamic signs and consequences of pericardial diseases. The book provides both traditional chapter presentations of the different pericardial diseases and cases that have been chosen to illustrate significant aspects of the diseases, including the difficulties encountered. The DVD includes dynamic image files to complement the static images within the book.

Stuart J. Hutchison, MD

Acknowledgments

My sincere appreciation and gratitude go to Inga Tomas; Simon Abrahmson, MD; Natasha Andjelkovic, PhD; Daniel Bonneau, MD; Robert O. Bonow, MD; Jagdish Butany, MD; John Burgess, MD; Jason Burstein, MD; Warren Cantor, MD; Kanu Chatterjee, MB; Robert Chisholm, MD; the CCU, cardiac ward, cardiac OR, and CVICU nurses; Patrick Disney, MD; Lee Errett, MD; Neil Fam, MD; Matthias Friedrich, MD; Michael Heffernan, MD; Majo Joseph, MD; David Latter, MD; Yves Leclerc, MD; Anne Lenehan; Mat Lotfi, MD; Danny Marcuzzi, MD; David Mazer, MD; Rachel Miller; Abdulelah Mobeirek, MD; Juan Carlos Monge, MD; Ashok Mukherjee, MD; Mark Peterson, MD, PhD; Susan Pioli; Bill Parmley, MD; Geoffrey Puley, MD; Michael Regan; Gail Rudakewich; Myra Rudakewich; Nazmi Said, RVT; Jan-Peter Smedema, MD; Jim Stewart, MD; Bradley Strauss, MD; Subodh Verma, MD; and Andrew Yan, MD.

Stuart J. Hutchison, MD

Abbreviations

Ao, aorta
AV, atrioventricular
BP, blood pressure
bpm, beats per minute
CAD, coronary artery disease
CHF, congestive heart failure
CMR, cardiac magnetic resonance
CO, cardiac output
COPD, chronic obstructive pulmonary disease
CP, constrictive pericarditis
CSPAMM, complementary spatial modulation of magnetization
CT, computed tomography
CVICU, cardiovascular intensive care unit
CVP, central venous pressure
CXR, chest radiography
ECG, electrocardiography; electrocardiogram
ESV, end-systolic volume
GFR, glomerular filtration rate
HR, heart rate
HIV, human immunodeficiency virus
ICD, implantable cardioverter-defibrillator
ICU, intensive care unit
INR, international normalized ratio
IPP, intrapericardial pressure
IRGE, inversion recovery gradient echo
IV, intravenous
IVC, inferior vena cava
IVS, interventricular septum
JVP, jugular venous pressure
LA, left atrium; left atrial
LAA, left atrial appendage
LAO, left anterior oblique
LLPV, left lower pulmonary vein
LUPV, left upper pulmonary vein
LV, left ventricle; left ventricular
LVDP, left ventricular diastolic pressure
LVH, left ventricular hypertrophy
LVOT, left ventricular outflow tract
LVSP, left ventricular systolic pressure
MAP, mean arterial pressure
MPA, main pulmonary artery

MR, magnetic resonance
MRI, magnetic resonance imaging
NPV, negative predictive value
NSAIDs, nonsteroidal anti-inflammatory drugs
NYHA, New York Heart Association
PA, pulmonary artery
PCI, percutaneous coronary intervention
PCR, polymerase chain reaction
PCWP, pulmonary capillary wedge pressure
PEEP, positive end-expiratory pressure
PI, pulmonary insufficiency
PPD, purified protein derivative
PPV, positive predictive value
PTP, pretest probability
RA, right atrium; right atrial
RAA, right atrial appendage
RAO, right anterior oblique
RAP, right atrial pressure
RCA, right coronary artery
RCM, restrictive cardiomyopathy
RLPV, right lower pulmonary vein
RPA, right pulmonary artery
RR, respiratory rate
RUPV, right upper pulmonary vein
RV, right ventricle; right ventricular
RVDP, right ventricular diastolic pressure
RVEDP, right ventricular end-diastolic pressure
RVH, right ventricular hypertrophy
RVOT, right ventricular outflow tract
RVSP, right ventricular systolic pressure
SEM, systolic ejection murmur
SLE, systemic lupus erythematosus
SPAMM, spatial modulation of magnetization
SSFP, steady-state free precession
SV, stroke volume
SVC, superior vena cava
TEE, transesophageal echocardiography
TR, tricuspid regurgitation
TTE, transthoracic echocardiography

Contents

CHAPTER 1

Anatomy and Physiology of the Pericardium

KEY POINTS

▸ Histologically, the pericardium contains both elastic and collagenous matrices that confer physical properties of compliance and stiffness, respectively. The interior layer of the pericardium is lined by serosal cells. The exterior layer of the pericardium is the predominantly fibrous parietal pericardium, which is 1 mm thick anatomically and 2 mm or less thick by imaging depiction (the limitation of contemporary imaging modalities is illustrated by their inability to depict true anatomic pericardial thickness).

▸ Anatomically, the pericardial sac surrounds the entire heart other than small areas behind the left atrium, extends up the great vessels and pulmonary veins, and is as simple anteriorly as it is complex posteriorly.

▸ Fluid accumulation (effusion) occurs in pericardial recesses. Absence of parietal pericardium allows lung tissue into otherwise excluded recesses, such as between the main pulmonary artery and the ascending aorta, under the left ventricle, and over the dome of the left diaphragm.

▸ Physiologically, the pericardium limits acute diastolic overfilling to maintain myocardial systolic function. The parietal pericardium imparts an important pressure : volume relationship.

▸ Pathophysiologically, the pericardium may confer high degrees of ventricular interdependence and may also be responsible for compression of the heart—tamponade, effuso-constriction, and constriction.

The anatomic and histologic features of the pericardium confer its physiologic properties and underlie both its resistance to and susceptibility to disease. Knowledge of pericardial anatomy assists greatly with interpretation of imaging findings and disease detection, and knowledge of pericardial physiology assists immeasurably with understanding of the pathophysiologic manifestations of pericardial diseases.

ANATOMIC COMPONENTS OF THE PERICARDIUM

The components of the pericardium (Fig. 1-1) are the following:

- Visceral (serosal) layer
- Parietal (fibrous) layer
- Pericardial fluid
- Pericardial space and pericardial reflections
- Pericardial attachments

Visceral (Serosal) Layer and the Epicardium

The visceral (serosal) layer of the pericardium is a monolayer of ciliated mesothelial cells that line the entirety of the inside (interior) of the pericardial space; that is, the serosal layer lines the back side of the parietal pericardium and the outside surface of the underlying cardiac chambers and great vessels (Fig. 1-2). It sits on a very thin fibrous layer and a layer of fat of variable thickness. The cilia of the visceral layer increase the surface area available for fluid transport[1] for both production and resorption, and the cilia also reduce friction between opposite layers of the pericardium (Figs. 1-3 and 1-4). The opposing pericardial surfaces move considerable distances over each other through the cardiac cycle. For example, at the atrioventricular groove the pericardial surfaces move 1.5 cm each way over each other through each cardiac cycle. At 105,000 cardiac cycles per day over an 80-year life span, this equates to 92,000 km of movement. In health, the serosal layer has only microscopic thickness and is not even remotely imageable by echocardiography, computed tomography (CT), or cardiac magnetic resonance (CMR) (Fig. 1-5).

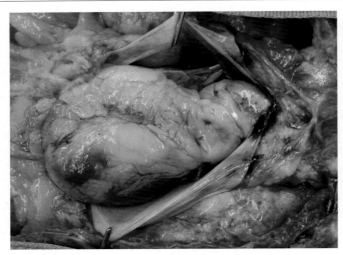

Figure 1-1. This autopsy photograph shows the thin and partially translucent nature of normal parietal pericardium; the invisible thinness of the normal serosal pericardium, whose only visual manifestation is a smooth sheen over the heart; and the epicardial and parietal pericardial fat layers. This view, slightly from the left side, demonstrates that there is less epicardial fat over the left ventricular free wall than there is over the anterior wall of the right ventricle. The parietal pericardial reflection can be seen extending well up the ascending aorta. (Courtesy of Jagdish Butany, MD, FRCPC, Toronto, Canada.)

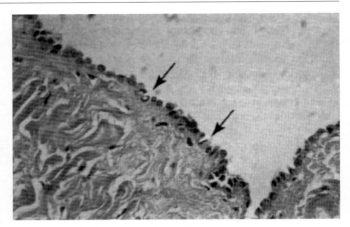

Figure 1-3. The monolayer of serosal cells that lines the entirety of the inside of the pericardial space. The thinness of the layer, in health, is obviously beneath the resolution of any imaging modality other than microscopy. (From Butany J, Woo A: The pericardium and its diseases. In Silver M, Gotlieb AI, Schoen F, eds: Cardiovascular Pathology. Philadelphia, Elsevier, 2001, figure 12-3. Copyright Elsevier, 2001.)

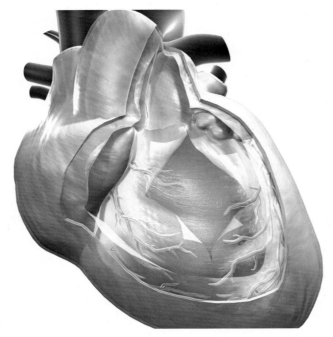

Figure 1-2. Representation of the serosal (visceral) and parietal (fibrous) pericardial layers. The outer thicker parietal pericardial layer extends over the heart chambers and proximal great vessels. The very thin serosal (visceral) layer lines the inside of the parietal layer and the outside of the epicardial layer of the heart, over epicardial coronary arteries and fat.

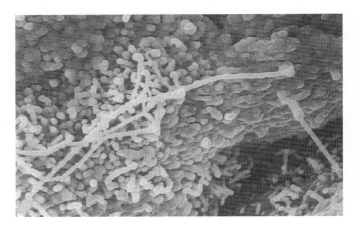

Figure 1-4. Scanning electron micrograph of the delicate multitudinous microvilli arising off of serosal cells. (From Butany J, Woo A: The pericardium and its diseases. In Silver M, Gotlieb AI, Schoen F, eds: Cardiovascular Pathology. Philadelphia, Elsevier, 2001, figure 12-4. Copyright Elsevier, 2001.)

Because the visceral reflection of the serosal layer lies over the epicardium, it is sometimes referred to as the epicardial layer, but the same layer of ciliated cells also lines the inside of the fibrous parietal pericardium. Epicardium is essentially that which overlies the myocardium up to the serosal layer of pericardium. Epicardium includes variable amounts of fat and is the layer

where the "epicardial" coronary arteries and their branches run (Fig. 1-6). Epicardial fat is an important facilitator of parietal pericardial imaging because it confers contrast to the inside surface of the parietal pericardium, which otherwise would be difficult to distinguish from myocardium by CMR, CT, and echocardiography. Most epicardial fat is distributed over the anterior right ventricle and also a short distance around the lateral wall of the left ventricle (Fig. 1-7). Because the presence of epicardial fat is needed to distinguish (contrast) parietal pericardium from myocardium and hence to assist in assessing its thickness, assessment of parietal pericardium over the lateral and posterior left ventricle is more difficult.

Innervation of the epicardium and the overlying serosal pericardium is through sympathetic afferent fibers. Therefore, inflammation of this layer may result in a vague midline visceral pain of anginal nature.

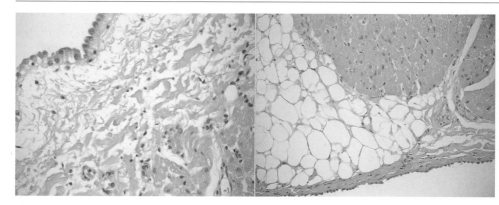

Figure 1-5. The serosal pericardium consists of a single monolayer of palisading cells (LEFT) that lie on a thin layer of connective tissue overlying the epicardial fat and epicardial coronary vessels (RIGHT). The distribution of epicardial fat is variable, as can be seen in the right image. In places, the serosal pericardium and its thin underlying layer of connective tissue lie against the myocardium. In other places, they are offset by fat. (Courtesy of Jagdish Butany, MD, FRCPC, Toronto, Canada.)

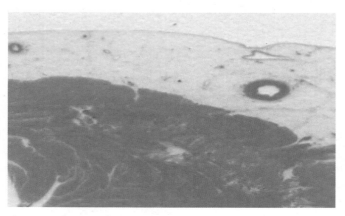

Figure 1-6. The epicardial tissue layer lies on the myocardium, extends up to the serosal pericardium layer, and comprises a highly variable thickness of fat. The epicardial coronary arteries run in this layer, usually nestled and cushioned in fat, as can be seen in this hematoxylin and eosin–stained low-power micrograph. (Courtesy of Gerald Prud'homme, MD, FRCPC, Toronto, Canada.)

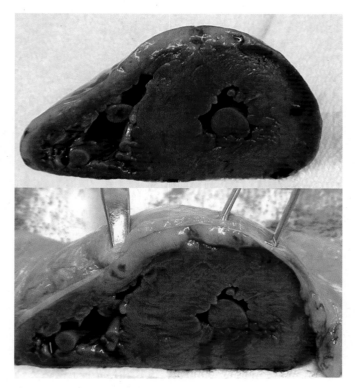

Figure 1-7. TOP, The parietal pericardium and its overlying fat have been removed. Epicardial fat is thick and continuous over the right ventricle and the anterior aspect of the left ventricle, but it has diminished considerably by the mid left ventricular lateral wall. BOTTOM, The parietal pericardium and its fat have been placed on the heart. The parietal pericardium is very thin in health. Fat on the outside of the parietal pericardium (pericardial fat versus epicardial fat) is thickest over the right ventricle and diminishes also over the left ventricular free wall. The outside (parietal) fat layer forms an apron at the diaphragm level. (Courtesy of Gerald Prud'homme, MD, FRCPC, Toronto, Canada.)

Parietal (Fibrous) Layer

The outer layer of pericardium, at the outer limit of the pericardial space, is the fibrous or parietal layer that itself consists of several layers. There are three collagen layers, the fibers of each of which are oriented approximately 120 degrees to each other.[1] The inner collagen layers are interwoven with a small amount of reticulum (elastin fibers). The final inside layer is the lining of mesothelial serosal cells, opposite those overlying the heart chambers and vessels. Because the parietal layer is predominantly collagen, it is tough, constitutes a physical barrier to disease, and has limited stretch (Fig. 1-8). Because it can stretch less than the myocardium, it therefore limits acute myocardial distention and preserves sarcomere architecture and function. The collagen component provides limitation to distention. The lesser elastin component confers only limited compliance to accommodate a finite pericardial volume reserve. The elastin fibers are arranged in a wavy pattern that straightens when stretched, allowing slight lengthening.[1]

The parietal layer is normally at most only about 1 mm thick (Fig. 1-9). Stated "normal" pericardial thickness by advanced imaging techniques depends on the imaging adequacy of the modality. Quite misleadingly, thickened parietal pericardium by CT or CMR was formerly defined as 4 mm or more, far greater than the true pericardial thickness and reflecting former limitations of imaging rather than true anatomic thickness. By modern gated cardiac CT imaging, representation of the thickness of the parietal pericardium is almost anatomically true.

Innervation of the parietal pericardium is achieved mainly from the phrenic nerves, which run over the parietal pericardium and generally generate a discrete, rapid, localized somatic pain—hence, the usual pleuritic nature of pericardial inflammatory diseases.

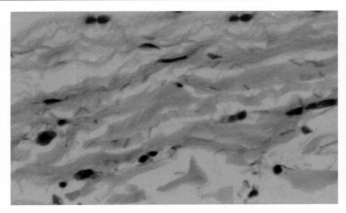

Figure 1-8. Mason trichrome stain of parietal pericardium. The collagen bundles run in planes. (Courtesy of Gerald Prud'homme, MD, FRCPC, Toronto, Canada.)

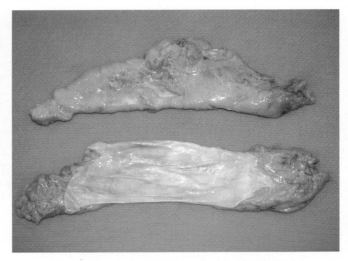

Figure 1-9. Normal parietal pericardium, viewed on its outside (TOP) and on its inside (BOTTOM). Pericardial fat covers much of the outside of the parietal pericardium in many patients. It is only loosely attached. The inside surface of the parietal pericardium is fat free and very smooth. Its thickness is only at most 1 mm. (Courtesy of Jagdish Butany, MD, FRCPC, Toronto, Canada.)

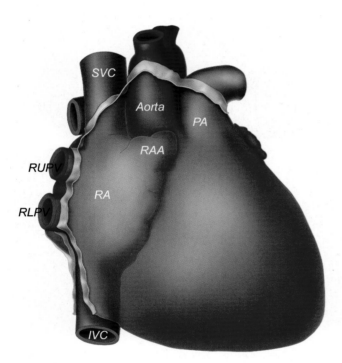

Figure 1-10. The pericardial space extends several centimeters up the great vessels; thus, rupture of the ascending aorta (as with acute dissection) will cause tamponade, and tamponade will compress the right atrium (RA), the right ventricle, and also the first several centimeters of the superior vena cava (SVC) and the inferior vena cava (IVC). PA, pulmonary artery; RAA, right atrial appendage; RLPV, right lower pulmonary vein; RUPV, right upper pulmonary vein.

Pericardial Fluid

Between the visceral and the parietal pericardium normally resides 15 to 50 mL of an ultrafiltrate "lubricating fluid," produced by the serosal cells, in both health and disease states. It is transparent and minimally "straw" colored. This amount of fluid is minimally visible by 2-dimensional echocardiography or appears as only a scant fluid layer, best seen in ventricular systole when reduction of ventricular volume and dimension allows separation of the pericardial layers and renders the appearance of the fluid layer more obvious. There is continuous flux of production and resorption of the fluid; therefore, the net amount reflects the

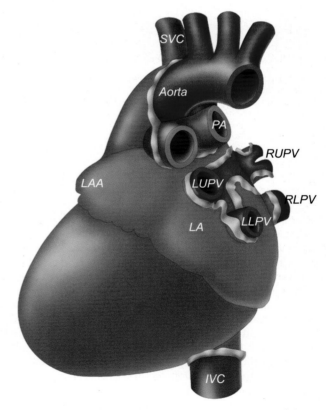

Figure 1-11. The pericardial space extends posteriorly over most of the left atrium (LA), other than between the upper pulmonary veins. Hence, fluid or clot may compress the left atrium or pulmonary veins. IVC, inferior vena cava; LAA, left atrial appendage; LLPV, left lower pulmonary vein; LUPV, left upper pulmonary vein; PA, pulmonary artery; RLPV, right lower pulmonary vein; RUPV, right upper pulmonary vein; SVC, superior vena cava.

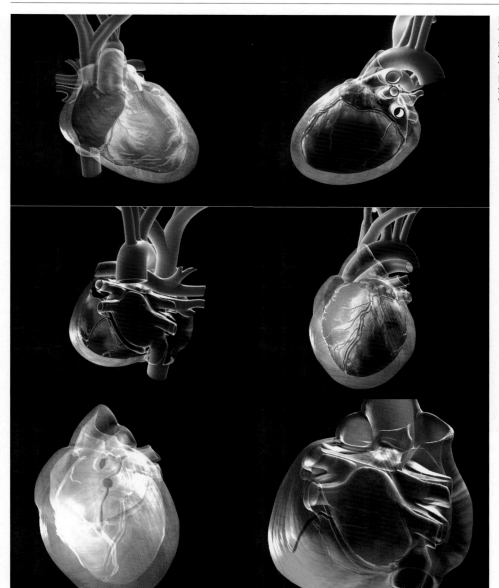

Figure 1-12. The pericardium is not a "round" container but one with a complex shape that envelops both cardiac chambers and all of the great vessels with "sleeves." The pericardial space, here exemplified by a pericardial effusion, is therefore complex in shape, especially in the posterior aspect of the heart.

balance of production and removal. In many states of increased production, such as pericarditis, there is no accumulation because removal is as rapid as fluid formation is. The composition of "normal" pericardial fluid is of less protein than serum but more albumin, as albumin is more readily transported than other larger proteins are. The fluid has a high phospholipid content, which is believed to confer the lubricant quality. The fluid equalizes pericardial pressure onto the underlying heart chambers.

Pericardial Space

The continuity of the pericardial layers (visceral and parietal) establishes the pericardial space, a space lined on its interior side (against the heart chambers and against the parietal pericardium of the outside) by the thin monolayer of serosal cells. On the outside, the same monolayer of serosal cells and also a restraining and protective layer of fibrous tissue (parietal pericardium) are present.

The parietal pericardium and space cover the proximal parts of all of the great vessels (Fig. 1-10) and all the cardiac chambers other than a limited part of the posterior left atrium (Fig. 1-11). Thus, rupture of the ascending aorta, as commonly occurs with type A aortic dissection, leads to pericardial tamponade, whereas rupture of the descending aorta, which is extrapericardial, generally leads to intrapleural exsanguination. The pericardial space is as complex posteriorly, where it runs up the venous and arterial sleeves, as it is simple anteriorly, where it covers the cardiac chambers (Fig. 1-12).

The *pericardial reflections*, where the visceral pericardium folds back on itself to line the outer fibrous pericardium, extend to the first arch branch vessel of the aorta, to the pulmonary artery bifurcation, up (and down) the cavae (Fig. 1-13) a few centimeters, and up the pulmonary veins a few centimeters (Figs. 1-14 to 1-16). The cohesion of the connective tissue at the sites of reflection is variable: the fibrous parietal pericardium is securely attached to the aorta and pulmonary arteries but imperfectly attached to the pulmonary veins. This fact underlies the extension

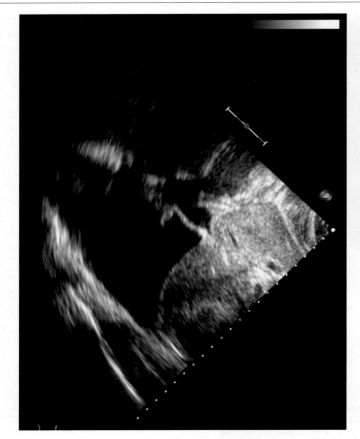

Figure 1-13. This transthoracic echocardiographic image reveals a large right pleural effusion over the liver and also the supradiaphragmatic portion of IVC as it enters into the right atrium. There is normally 2 or 3 cm of supradiaphragmatic IVC above the diaphragm. It is largely intrapericardial and occasionally is a site of localized compression. The supradiaphragmatic IVC, when visible on the lateral chest radiograph, is a useful yardstick to gauge posterior left ventricular dilation (the rule of Rigler).

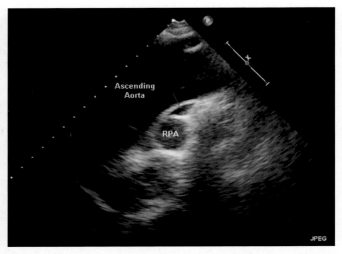

Figure 1-14. There is a small amount of pericardial fluid posterior to the ascending aorta *(arrow)* over the right pulmonary artery (RPA), at the most superior extent of the pericardial cavity recesses.

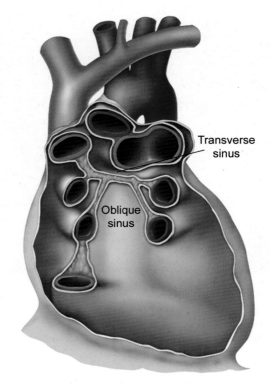

Figure 1-15. The posterior parietal pericardial anatomy is complex. The pericardial space does extend behind the left atrium and also along the pulmonary veins. The pericardial space also surrounds the proximal aorta and pulmonary artery. The cul-de-sac of pericardial space between the pulmonary veins is the oblique sinus; the passageway under the aorta and pulmonary artery is the transverse sinus, through which saphenous vein grafts to the circumflex territory are sometimes passed.

of mediastinal air into the pericardial space through the pulmonary venous reflections and the secondary indirect development of pneumopericardium (Fig. 1-17).

The parietal pericardium and space therefore cover a more extensive field than is usually anticipated. The sleeve-like extension of the parietal pericardium over the great arteries is significant for multiple reasons: the demise of type A dissection is usually rupture of the ascending aorta into the pericardial space, pericardial fluid collection can be anticipated to occur around the great vessels, and the parietal pericardium normally excludes lung parenchyma from anatomic recesses between the aorta and main pulmonary artery.

Pericardial Attachments

Ligamentous attachments of the parietal pericardium tether it, and the underlying heart, stably in place in the chest, which is important given the weight and inertia of the heart. Pericardial-sternal ligaments attaching to the sternum, pericardial-diaphragmatic ligaments attaching to the diaphragm (the most extensive ligaments), and pericardial-vertebral ligaments attaching to the vertebrae hold the heart in place when acceleration-deceleration forces occur within the chest (Fig. 1-18). The heart is well anchored by these ligaments within the chest and is moved little by anteroposterior acceleration forces. Conversely, the descending aorta is poorly anchored within the chest and is subject to motion and distortion by acceleration forces, and it is therefore subject to motion-related injury. Congenital deficiency

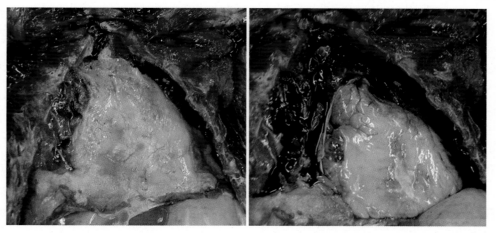

Figure 1-16. These autopsy photographs demonstrate the wider extent of pericardial coverage of the heart than is often appreciated. TOP, With the chest opened, there is abundant fat anterior and exterior to the parietal pericardium and the far superior extension of the pericardium well up the great vessels into the mediastinum. As well, there is a copious "skirt" of fat at the diaphragm level on either side of the heart, often visible on the posteroanterior chest radiograph. BOTTOM, After the anterior parietal pericardium had been excised, its free edge can be seen beside the right atrial appendage and across the ascending aorta. The free edge has folded over onto itself, making it look thicker than it truly is. The superior reflection of the parietal pericardium is higher than the location of the excision across the ascending aorta. The anterior epicardial fat over the right ventricle is obvious. Thus, anterior to the right ventricle, there is normally a fat plane beneath (epicardial fat) and exterior to (pericardial fat) the parietal pericardium. (Courtesy of Gerald Prud'homme, MD, FRCPC, Toronto, Canada.)

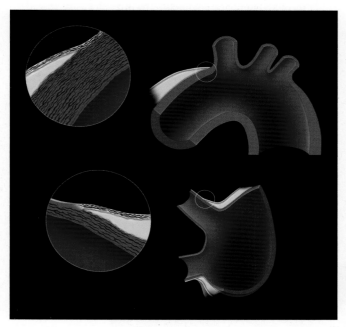

Figure 1-17. Pericardial reflections and connective tissue integrity. TOP, Pericardial reflection at the ascending aorta. BOTTOM, Pericardial reflection at the pulmonary veins. The reflection of the pericardium over the great vessels, such as the aorta, involves incorporation of the collagen connective tissue layers of the parietal pericardium into those of the aortic wall; hence, there is continuity of connective tissue and an effective barrier. The serosal layer of the inside of the parietal pericardium reflects back over the outside surface of the vessel. The reflection of the pericardium at the pulmonary veins occurs without interweaving of the collagen layers of the parietal pericardium with those of the pulmonary veins; hence, this represents a possible weak site of pericardial anatomy and a potential weakness of the barrier. In fact, air tracking along the intrapulmonary perivascular sheaths of pulmonary veins (that resulted from pneumomediastinum) can gain entry into the pericardial space at this site (resulting in pneumopericardium).

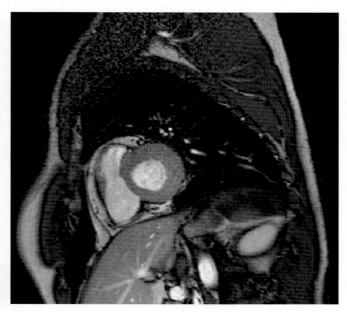

Figure 1-18. On this steady-state free precession CMR image, the fat planes over the right side of the heart (epicardial and pericardial) are sufficiently distinct for the insertion of the parietal pericardium into the diaphragm to be seen. There is little epicardial or pericardial (outside) fat over the left ventricular free wall.

(absence) of the pericardium removes restraining forces on the heart, and accordingly the heart shifts toward the defect. Because absence of the left pericardium is the most common variant of congenital absence, leftward shift of the heart is the usual. Absence of parietal pericardium allows lung tissue into otherwise excluded recesses, such as between the main pulmonary artery and the ascending aorta, under the left ventricle, and over the dome of the left diaphragm. These are reliable imaging details by chest radiography, CT, and CMR to detect the absence of pericardium.

Fat Planes

The parietal pericardium is difficult to image because its imaging characteristics (relaxation times on CMR, attenuation coefficient on CT scanning) are too similar to those of the underlying atrial and ventricular myocardium. It is the presence of adjacent fat planes on either side of the parietal pericardium (when both are present), which have very different CT and CMR characteristics and therefore appearance, that enables clear depiction of the parietal pericardium. Epicardial fat (under the parietal pericardium) and overlying (outside, parietal) fat are far more likely over the right ventricular free wall than over the left ventricular free wall or over either atrium. Adjacent fat planes that "sandwich" the parietal pericardium are requisite to imaging of the parietal pericardium (Fig. 1-19).

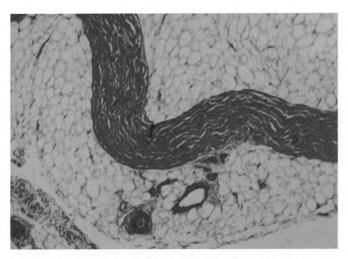

Figure 1-19. Hematoxylin and eosin–stained low-power micrograph. The collagenous parietal pericardium consists principally of bundles of collagen. In certain areas of the heart, particularly over the right ventricle, there is likely to be an underlying "epicardial" fat plane and an overlying parietal (outside) fat layer. The "fat sandwich" is required to image the pericardium by CMR and by CT scanning; otherwise, without the contrast with fat, the parietal pericardium cannot be distinguished from myocardium or adjacent exterior tissues. (Courtesy of Gerald Prud'homme, MD, FRCPC, Toronto, Canada.)

Other Anatomic and Physiologic Considerations

The internal thoracic arteries confer blood supply to most of the parietal pericardium, and their proximity to the pericardium (their avoidance) is relevant for percutaneous pericardial drainage procedures. The aorta supplies small branches to the posterior pericardium. The internal thoracic and azygos venous system confer the venous drainage to the pericardial space (Fig. 1-20). As the azygos vein drains into the superior vena cava, central venous pressure elevation increases the forces (hydrostatic pressure) that favor pericardial fluid accumulation.

The anterior mediastinal lymph nodes and the internal thoracic duct supply the lymphatic drainage but unfortunately also establish proximity and continuity of the lymph system to the pericardium. Therefore, malignant involvement of anterior mediastinal nodes is particularly likely to extend to the pericardium, either through lymphatic channels or by direct invasive spread.

Mechanical receptors and chemoreceptors use sympathetic afferent fibers to mediate reflexes and pain. The left and right phrenic nerves run over the lateral surface of the parietal pericardium; their presence is relevant to surgical procedures, particularly pericardiectomy, in which they must be left intact to preserve diaphragmatic function. Innervation of the pericardium also involves the left recurrent laryngeal nerve, the vagus nerve, and the esophageal plexus.[1]

A very important relation of the pericardial space, for imaging purposes, is the retrocardiac descending thoracic aorta. The pericardial space extends between the left atrium and the descending aorta, whereas the left pleural space does not extend between the descending aorta and the left atrium but rather extends posteriorly behind the descending aorta.

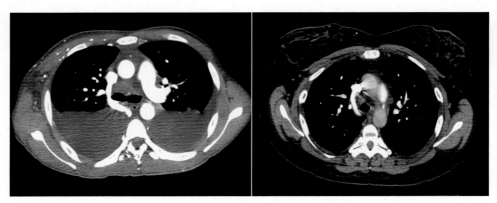

Figure 1-20. Azygos vein and pericardial disease. The azygos vein drains the pericardium, among many other structures, and empties into the SVC above the right pulmonary artery. Pericardial diseases that compress the heart, such as constriction or even tamponade, result in increased central venous pressure and dilation of the cavae and their branches. The left image (contrast-enhanced CT) depicts the dilated SVC and azygos vein of a patient with a severe case of pericardial constriction. The azygos vein is remarkably dilated, consistent with the central venous pressure of nearly 30 mm Hg. As the pleural cavities are drained by the azygos and hemiazygos veins, it is not surprising that there are bilateral pleural effusions due to the increased hydrostatic pressure. The right image, also a contrast-enhanced CT image, depicts a moderately dilated azygos vein in a patient with a case of moderate constriction but without pleural effusions.

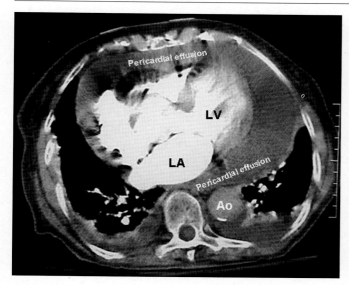

Figure 1-21. The large circumferential pericardial effusion extends lateral and posterolateral to the left ventricle (LV) and the left atrium (LA) and, importantly, between the LA and the descending thoracic aorta (Ao), that is, *anterior* to the descending aorta. There are small pleural effusions seen bilaterally. The left pleural effusion is *posterior* to the descending aorta.

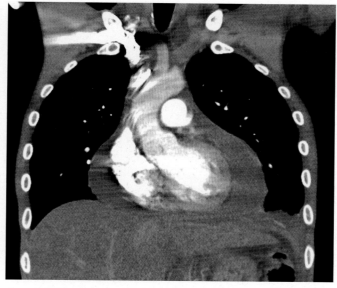

Figure 1-22. This contrast-enhanced CT scan of a patient with a large pericardial effusion demonstrates the extension of the pericardial space over and along the main pulmonary artery and the ascending aorta, to its first branch vessel.

Terminology of Pericardial Anatomy

The term *pericardium* is common and often confusing. There are many components, widely distributed, of the pericardium. Hence, *pericardium* is too unspecified and reductive a term to be useful in an era of high-resolution imaging and detailed knowledge of pathophysiologic processes. The term *epicardium* is also unclear and is often used to describe the visceral layer over the heart chambers or the visceral layer and underlying connective tissue and fat; however, the same serosal layer lines the inside of the fibrous parietal pericardium. The clearest terms that establish anatomic distinction of the inner and outer layers of the pericardium and that lend themselves to clinical understanding, to analysis of imaging findings, and to surgical procedures are *parietal and visceral layers of the pericardium* (Fig. 1-21).

The use of precise and reproducible terminology to describe pericardial anatomy is requisite to achieve an optimal and clear understanding and communication of pericardial diseases, pathophysiologic changes of pericardial disease, imaging findings, surgical findings, and surgical procedures. For example, in pericarditis, inflammation of the parietal pericardium may produce somatic-type pain, whereas inflammation of the visceral pericardium may produce visceral or angina-type pain. In pericardial constriction, either the parietal or visceral layer may compress the heart, or the two layers may fuse together into a single indistinguishable and compressive layer. To alleviate the disorder, the specific responsible layers would have to be resected. Furthermore, pathophysiologic states may involve combinations of visceral and parietal constriction and also of concurrent tamponade (effuso-constrictive pericarditis).

Imaging modalities such as cardiac CT and CMR currently have the resolution to depict pathologic abnormalities of the different components of the pericardium, such as thickening of the visceral pericardium, fluid or tissue within the pericardial space (Figs. 1-22 and 1-23), and thickening of the parietal pericardium (Figs. 1-24 to 1-26). The approach to analysis of imaging findings

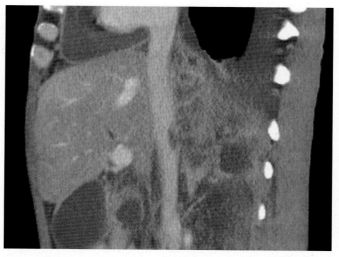

Figure 1-23. A few centimeters of the supradiaphragmatic portion of the IVC are located within the pericardial space, as is seen in this case of a patient with a pericardial effusion associated with pancreatitis.

should be to assess the multiple components of the pericardium, rather than to reduce all layers to "the pericardium," generally inferring the parietal layer alone. In some patients, the parietal pericardium is negligibly thickened, but the visceral layer is severely thickened, responsible for constrictive physiology and needing resection.

Surgical procedures are optimally understood by specific knowledge of the intervention on the particular anatomic component of the pericardium. A *pericardial window* is resection of the parietal layer to afford drainage of the pericardial cavity into the pleural cavity or to provide histologic material. Surgical *pericardiectomy* is simply resection of pericardial tissue, which may be the parietal pericardium (incomplete or complete) and also the visceral pericardium if it appears thickened and constrictive. Sur-

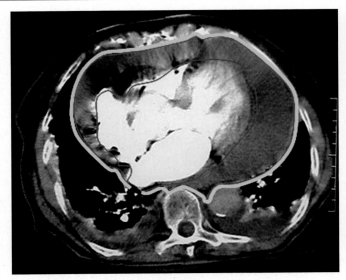

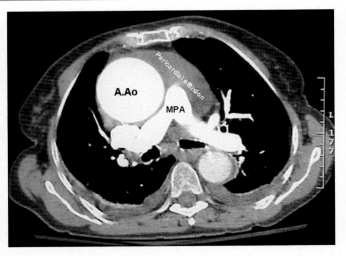

Figure 1-26. The pericardial effusion surrounds and extends up the ascending aorta (A.Ao) and the main pulmonary artery (MPA).

Figure 1-24. Contrast-enhanced CT scan of a heart surrounded by a large pericardial effusion. The parietal pericardium is marked in a yellow line. The inside of the pericardial space is lined throughout by a layer of serosal cells (marked by the red line), which is normally only of histologic thickness, that lies over the cardiac chambers and great vessels and also lines the inside of the parietal layer. The pericardial space resides between the descending aorta and the left atrium.

ROLE OF THE PERICARDIUM

The functions of the parietal pericardium are (1) to tether the heart securely in place within the chest; (2) to preserve myocyte function under stress and to limit acute distention of the heart chambers, which, if excessive, could place myocardial sarcomeres at disadvantageous length:tension relations; (3) to distribute hydrostatic forces over the heart; and (4) to exclude extracardiac intrathoracic disease from extension into the heart.

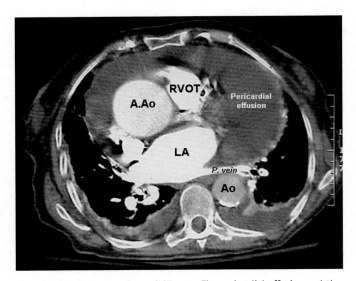

Figure 1-25. Contrast-enhanced CT scan. The pericardial effusion and the contrast-opacified right ventricular outflow tract (RVOT), aneurysmal ascending aorta (A.Ao), and left atrium (LA) are represented. The pericardial space-sac extends along the great vessels (seen easily around the ascending aorta) and also extends along the pulmonary veins—the left upper pulmonary vein is clearly seen running through several centimeters of pericardial effusion anterior to the descending aorta (Ao). The parietal pericardium extends well up onto the great vessels and also down the pulmonary veins and cavae.

Limitation of Cardiac Dilation by the Pericardium

Acute (excessive) dilation of myocardium may render myofibril overlap and their length:tension (stress:strain) relationships disadvantaged and may activate left ventricular mechanoreceptors to incite bradycardia and hypotension. The parietal pericardium is compliant (because of its elastic material) within the range of usual cardiac filling but can "stretch" only a limited further amount (the acute pericardial reserve volume, about 15% to 20%); beyond this, the collagenous properties dominate and limit distention. In patients undergoing cardiac surgery, the pericardium does constrain filling if the right atrium pressure is elevated higher than 6 mm Hg.[2] Beyond this, the pericardium no longer compliantly accommodates increases in volume without an increase in pressure, which occurs at an exponential rate, and limits filling. The pericardium thus contributes an important protective function to the myocardium by limiting acute volume distention of the heart and acute stretching of the myofibrils.[3]

Chronic Remodeling of the Pericardium

An increase in intrapericardial volume most commonly is due to dilation of cardiac chambers or to accumulation of pericardial fluid. Dilation of cardiac chambers may be advantageous for their function if, for example, the heart has to manage chronic volume overload lesions. Thus, remodeling of the pericardium to be more compliant at higher volumes is potentially adaptive. Chronic

gical pericardiectomy for recurrent debilitating inflammatory pericarditis may leave either residual pieces of parietal pericardium, which are still susceptible to inflammation and generate pain, or the visceral layer, which may continue to inflame and cause pain.

remodeling of the pericardium can occur during several months and is achieved by replacement of the connective tissue matrix of the fibrous pericardium with a new collagen matrix, affording a remodeling volume increase. The chronic pericardial reserve volume remains limited, conferring a similar steep slope to the far right of the pericardial pressure:volume relationship.

Similarly, an increase in intrapericardial volume may be due to chronic accumulation of a pericardial effusion (Figs. 1-27 and 1-28) and lead to remodeling of the pericardium, allowing accommodation of the additional volume without passively increasing filling pressure. The extent of remodeling of the pericardium determines its compliance and the physiologic consequence of the effusion. Thus, 200 mL of pericardial fluid accumulated rapidly may have the same effect on intracardiac pressure as 2 liters accumulated slowly. Most tamponade cases occur between these two ends of the spectrum. The compliance property of the pericardium is most easily understood by the passive pressure:volume relationship (stress:strain relationship) of the pericardium (Fig. 1-29). The compliance of the pericardium may be reduced by inflammation, causing constrictive pericarditis.

Intrapericardial Pressure

The anatomic complex (including fluid) of the pericardium distributes physical forces over the underlying heart chambers. The normal intrapericardial pressure is slightly negative (-3 mm Hg) and may normally vary slightly within the pericardial space according to underlying chamber volume. Intrapericardial pressure is affected by pleural pressure, intrapericardial volume, and intracavitary pressures. Intrapericardial pressure varies through the cardiac cycle, and as intracardiac volume falls briskly during ventricular systole, intrapericardial pressure falls during ventricular systole.

The intrapericardial pressure is an important determinant of the transmural (true) filling pressure of a cardiac chamber: transmural filling pressure = intracavitary pressure − intrapericardial pressure. As intrapericardial pressure elevates above zero, the recorded intracavitary pressure becomes less representative of the cavity's transmural filling pressure. For example, if the left ventricular diastolic pressure is 10 mm Hg (normal) but the intrapericardial pressure is 8 mm Hg, the left ventricular transmural filling pressure is significantly reduced, and the ventricle is underfilled. When the intrapericardial pressure exceeds the intracavitary pressure, the chamber wall compresses inward or collapses.

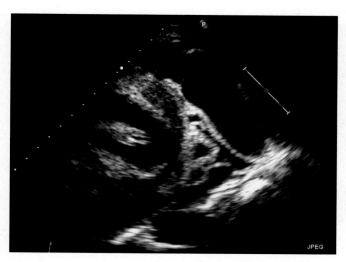

Figure 1-27. Complex distribution of pericardial effusion around superior and posterior cardiac structures. There is a pericardial effusion around several superior cardiac and vascular structures: anterior to the RVOT, anterior and posterior to the PA, around the left atrial appendage, and posterior to the LV.

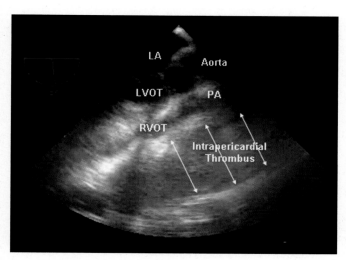

Figure 1-28. Transesophageal echocardiography vertical image showing a large intrapericardial thrombus anterior to the right ventricular outflow tract (RVOT) and pulmonary artery (PA), severely compressing both of them. There is as much compression above the pulmonary valve as there is beneath, illustrating the extent of the pericardial cavity above the heart and over the great vessels. LA, left atrium; LVOT, left ventricular outflow tract.

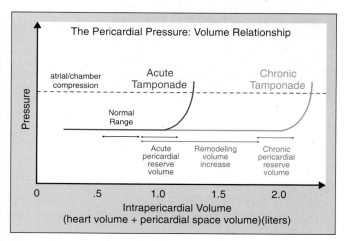

Figure 1-29. The passive pressure:volume relationship of the pericardium: normal cardiac volume occurs within the compliant range of the pericardium. Acute distention (>20%) of the pericardium that exceeds the acute pericardial reserve volume reveals the limited compliance of the pericardium, and the filling pressure rises very steeply, becoming vertical. Chronic progressive distention allows remodeling to occur such that the pericardium is much more compliant over an additional remodeling volume increase but then is subject to a similar chronic pericardial reserve volume that if exceeded reveals the limitations of compliance.

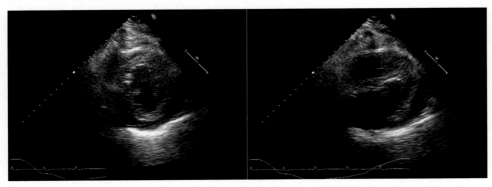

Figure 1-30. Ventricular interdependence in pericardial tamponade. Parasternal short-axis views during expiration (LEFT) and inspiration (RIGHT). With inspiration (note upward deflection of respirometry tracing), there is an abrupt shift of the septum from the right to the left side as inspiration augments RV filling, but ventricular interdependence results in transient reduced LV filling.

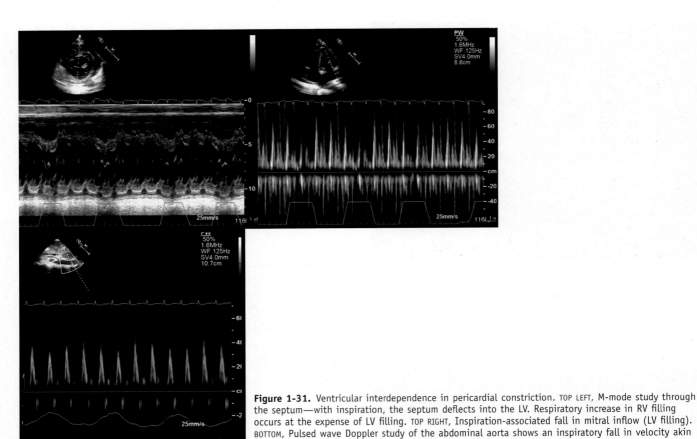

Figure 1-31. Ventricular interdependence in pericardial constriction. TOP LEFT, M-mode study through the septum—with inspiration, the septum deflects into the LV. Respiratory increase in RV filling occurs at the expense of LV filling. TOP RIGHT, Inspiration-associated fall in mitral inflow (LV filling). BOTTOM, Pulsed wave Doppler study of the abdominal aorta shows an inspiratory fall in velocity akin to pulsus paradoxus.

Ventricular Interdependence Imparted by the Pericardium

The parietal pericardium limits cardiac filling and distention. A consequence of this limitation of filling is that overfilling of one ventricle will reduce filling of the other ventricle because pericardial connective tissue properties confer a limited availability of maximal overall cardiac volume. At and beyond the point of maximal filling, overfilling of one ventricle will impair the filling of the other ventricle. This phenomenon of ventricular interaction is referred to as *ventricular interdependence* (Fig. 1-30).

Ventricular interdependence may be seen when the increase in total intrapericardial volume is due to chamber dilation, such as acute right ventricular dilation as a result of right ven-

tricular infarction; pericardial effusion or intrapericardial mass involvement; or reduced pericardial compliance, such as with the compressive syndromes of constrictive pericarditis and pericardial tamponade. Ventricular interdependence is seen in the following disease states:

- Constrictive pericarditis (noncompliant pericardium) (Figs. 1-31 to 1-33)
- Pericardial tamponade (Fig. 1-34)
- Effuso-constrictive pericarditis (noncompliant pericardium and fluid)
- Right ventricular infarction (severe acute dilation of the right ventricle) (Figs. 1-35 to 1-37)
- Tumor encasement of the heart (noncompliant tumor mass)

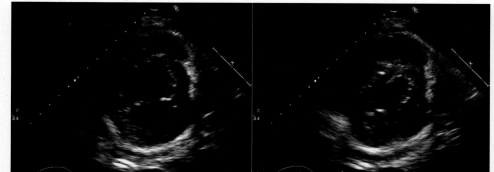

Figure 1-32. Ventricular interdependence in pericardial constriction. Parasternal short-axis views during expiration (LEFt) and inspiration (RIGHT). With inspiration (note upward deflection of respirometry tracing), there is an abrupt shift of the septum from the right to the left side as inspiration augments RV filling, but ventricular interdependence results in transient reduced LV filling.

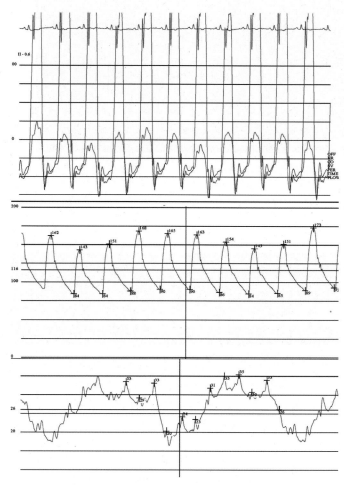

Figure 1-33. Hemodynamic tracings showing ventricular interdependence in pericardial constriction. TOP, Simultaneous left and right ventricular pressures. With the second cardiac cycle of inspiration, the right ventricular systolic pressure rises and the left ventricular systolic pressure falls. During inspiration, the increase in venous return cannot be accommodated by the right side of the heart because of noncompliant overlying constrictive pericardium; therefore, the right ventricular pressure rises in inspiration. The inspiratory increase in right ventricular volume and pressure competes with left ventricular filling, imparted by the pericardial constriction, resulting in reduced left ventricular filling and therefore reduced systolic pressure in inspiration. MIDDLE, Aortic pressure. There is a pulsus paradoxus (inspiratory fall in systolic pressure of more than 10 mm Hg), with lesser fall in diastolic pressure. The pulsus paradoxus is produced by a number of phenomena, including ventricular interdependence limiting left ventricular filling during inspiration. BOTTOM, Pulmonary capillary wedge pressure. With inspiration, there is a prominent (almost 50%) fall in pressure, as the pulmonary venous capacitance increases in inspiration because of increase in lung volume. The inspiratory decrease in driving force within the pulmonary veins to push blood into the left side of the heart is another factor diminishing the left ventricular filling in inspiration, contributing to interdependence findings and the pulsus paradoxus.

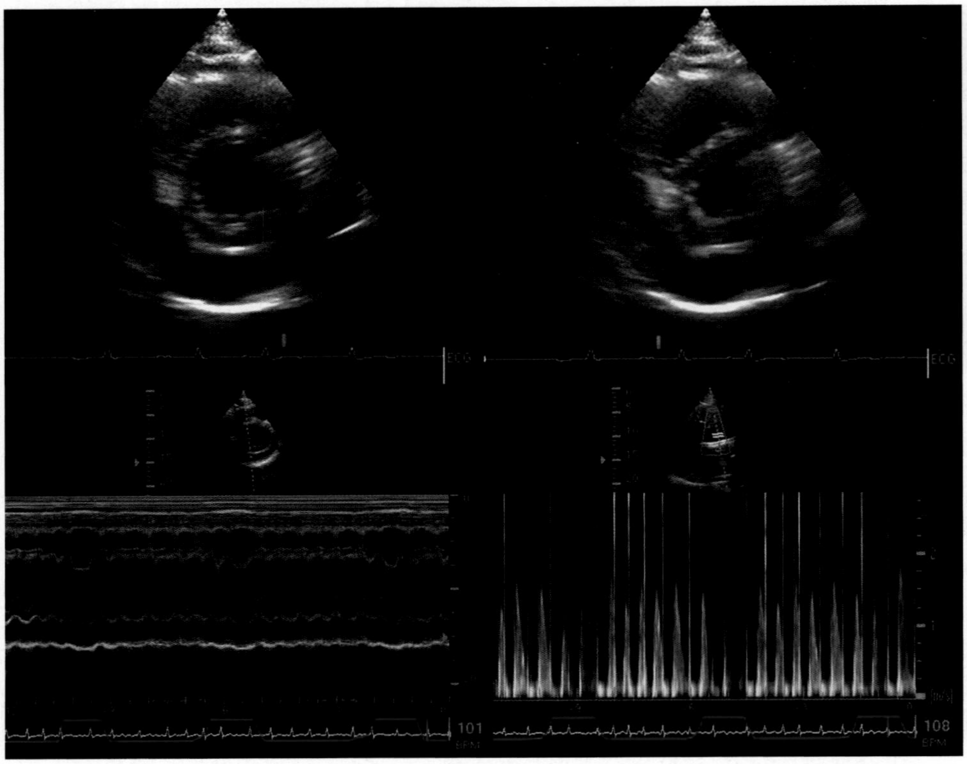

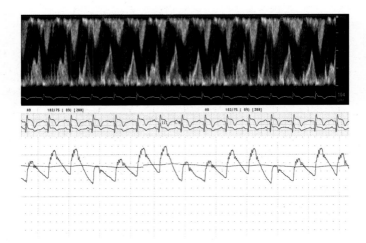

Figure 1-34. Ventricular interdependence in pericardial tamponade. TOP, Two-dimensional short-axis views of a patient with pericardial tamponade. TOP LEFT, The septal position and contour are normal, consistent with normal ventricular filling. TOP RIGHT, The septal position and contour are deflected into the LV cavity (during inspiration), consistent with reduced LV filling during inspiration. BOTTOM LEFT, M-mode study through the septum (note respirometry tracing on the bottom); with inspiration, the RV overfills and the LV underfills. BOTTOM RIGHT, LV inflow; with inspiration, there is an obvious fall in mitral inflow and LV filling.

Figure 1-35. Ventricular interdependence in acute RV infarction and dilation. TOP, Combined LVOT outflow and mitral inflow shows sinus rhythm and constant PR interval. Note the phasic variation of *early* diastolic velocities—in this case, the higher diastolic velocity is the *late* (atrial systolic) inflow. There is phasic variation of the *early* diastolic inflow velocity and the LVOT outflow velocity. BOTTOM, The lead III ECG tracing reveals current of injury (ST elevation) and a deep Q wave.

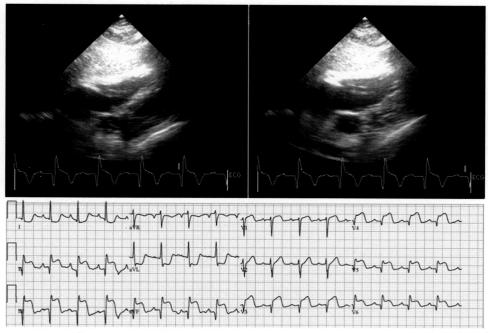

Figure 1-36. Ventricular interdependence in acute RV infarction and dilation. Subcostal long-axis views during expiration (LEFT) and inspiration (RIGHT). With inspiration, there is an abrupt shift of the septum from the right to the left side as inspiration augments RV filling, but ventricular interdependence results in transient reduced LV filling. The ECG records the ST elevation of the inferior wall and RV infarction. The infarction of the contiguous inferior septum may confer passivity to the septal motion, contributing to ventricular interdependence.

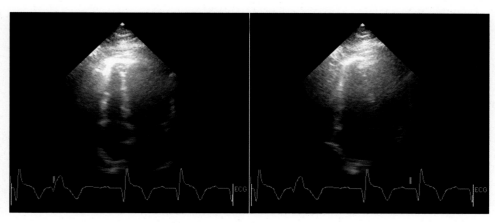

Figure 1-37. Apical 4-chamber views demonstrating ventricular interdependence in acute RV infarction and dilation. With inspiration, there is an abrupt shift of the septum from the right to the left side as inspiration augments RV filling, but ventricular interdependence results in transient reduced LV filling. The infarction of the contiguous inferior septum may confer passivity to the septal motion, contributing to ventricular interdependence.

Pericardium as a Barrier to Disease

The parietal pericardium is a barrier to disease, both in favorable and in unfavorable contexts. The parietal pericardium is a barrier to the spread of intrathoracic, initially extracardiac infections into the heart (e.g., most cases of empyema do not result in purulent pericarditis). Although the parietal pericardium appears to limit the spread of some intrathoracic (mediastinal) malignant neoplasms into the heart, it nonetheless remains the most common site for malignant involvement of the heart both by direct extension of the malignant disease and by hematogenous spread. Unfortunately, involvement of malignant disease within the intact pericardial space often leads to pericardial effusion that is limited by the pericardium and may accumulate under pressure, resulting in pericardial tamponade. Malignant involvement of the heart is 20 to 40 times more likely to be metastatic than primary cardiac. Thus, whether the pericardium is a barrier or a magnet to malignant disease varies, depending on chance alone.

References

1. Butany J, Woo A: The pericardium and its diseases. In Silver M, Gotlieb A, Schoen F, eds: Cardiovascular Pathology. New York, Churchill Livingstone, 2001.

2. Reynertson SI, Konstadt SN, Louie EK, et al: Alterations in transesophageal pulsed Doppler indexes of filling of the left ventricle after pericardiotomy. J Am Coll Cardiol 1991;18:1655-1660.

3. Lavine SJ, Campbell CA, Kloner RA, Gunther SJ: Diastolic filling in acute left ventricular dysfunction: role of the pericardium. J Am Coll Cardiol 1988;12:1326-1333.

CHAPTER 2

Physical Diagnosis of Pericardial Diseases

KEY POINTS

▶ Physical examination has a central role in the diagnosis of pericarditis, tamponade, and constriction. It is less useful for the assessment of atypical tamponade cases, cardiac compression from intrapericardial clots or masses, congenital absence of the pericardium, and pneumopericardium. Physical examination, except for its negative findings, is seldom useful for the assessment of pericardial cysts.

▶ Pulsus paradoxus is a fall in systolic pressure of more than 10 to 15 mm Hg during inspiration, typically with a fall in the pulse pressure amplitude (systolic fall greater than diastolic fall). The basis for pulsus paradoxus includes varying pulmonary venous capacitance, ventricular interdependence, and varying intrapleural pressure. Although it is a useful sign for the presence

of pericardial tamponade, there are significant and regular false-negative scenarios.

▶ The *x* descent is produced by atrial relaxation and descent of the tricuspid or mitral annulus. It is augmented in the compressive states of tamponade and constriction (and large right ventricular infarction) and lessened in atrial fibrillation and right atrial infarction.

▶ The *y* descent is produced by early ventricular filling and is augmented in constriction, diminished in tamponade, and not influenced by atrial fibrillation.

▶ The pericardial friction rub is usually triphasic (during sinus rhythm), is due to inflammation, and is a sound akin to friction rather than caused by friction.

Clinical acumen, important throughout the practice of cardiology, is particularly important in the recognition and assessment of pericardial diseases. Proficiency with bedside physical diagnostic skills is invaluable and imparts context and pretest probability to the results of subsequent testing. The presence and severity of pericardial diseases are reflected in arterial (pulse) waveforms, venous waveforms, and auscultation findings.

The basic physical diagnosis signs of pericardial diseases were well described hundreds of years ago, when pericardial diseases were prevalent. The early descriptions were so thorough that little has been added since, other than the clinical epidemiology and some unraveling of the responsible mechanisms of the signs. One enormously important point in particular was established through observation—that the manifestations of compressive cardiac syndromes are linked to the respiratory cycle.

PULSUS PARADOXUS

Pulsus paradoxus (also paradoxical pulse, pulsus respiratio, Kussmaul pulse) is a historic term acknowledging the paradox

of a fluctuating pulse volume despite regular heart sounds, with the fluctuations associated with the respiratory cycle. Gauchat's succinct and elegant 1924 definition of pulsus paradoxus is notable:

> ...a rhythmical pulse which diminishes perceptibly in amplitude or is totally obliterated during inspiration in all palpable arteries. It is a periodic waxing and waning of pulse amplitude, which from the standpoint of clinical interest must occur without conscious effort on the part of the patient to modify his breathing. This diminuation in pulse amplitude is always accompanied by a fall in systolic blood pressure.[1]

The term was first proposed in 1873 by the prolific and well-recognized German physician Adolf Kussmaul (1822-1902), initially of Heidelberg University, in his treatise *Über schwielge Mediastinopericarditis und den paradoxen Puls (On adhesive medi-astino-pericarditis and the paradoxical pulse)*, in which he described the findings of three individuals with constrictive pericarditis:

> A 34 year old unemployed servant girl, whose mother had died of pulmonary disease, had suffered for many years

each winter from a dry cough and for three years a constricting feeling which at times became dyspnea.... On admission, she appeared cachectic, with edema of the legs and ascites. The phenomenon of the arterial pulse with regular and constant action of the heart was observed at the initial examination. The pulse would become smaller with inspiration or would become totally impalpable on deep inspiration. On expiration it returned to its former amplitude.... The disappearance or diminution of the pulse during inspiration was manifest in all palpable arteries.

I suggest naming this pulse paradoxical, partly because of the conspicuous discrepancy between the cardiac action and the arterial pulse, partly because of the pulse, despite its irregularity, actually waxes and wanes in a regular fashion.... The interesting phenomenon which these three cases of mediastinopericarditis present is the pulse. In all three, it was rapid, almost always more than 100, the impulse of low amplitude, the tension soft, and the rhythm paradoxical in two ways: (1) despite continuing action of the heart, the pulse disappeared for short intervals at the palpating finger, one or two beats completely or almost completely and then returned immediately for two or more beats; (2) the apparent irregularity was in actuality only the difference associated with the phases of respiration.... This unique phenomenon was manifest in all palpable arteries.[2]

Kussmaul duly gave credit to Griesinger for having previously described the finding in 1854. In fact, Richard Lower (1631-1691), a brilliant but much less well known Cornish physician based at Oxford University, had recognized the finding of pulsus paradoxus two centuries earlier, but his treatise *De Corde* (1669) was less widely available and available only in Latin or French.

Pulsus paradoxus is currently defined as a fall in arterial systolic pressure of 10 mm Hg or more during *normal* inspiratory effort. Other definitions for pulsus paradoxus include 12 mm Hg, 15 mm Hg, or 9% inspiratory fall in arterial blood pressure. Pulsus paradoxus is detectable with particularly careful and *slow* sphygmomanometry, but it is most confidently and accurately established with direct arterial pressure recordings. Oximetry tracings often reveal the finding. Importantly, use of automated blood pressure cuffs will fail to detect pulsus paradoxus.

During normal inspiration, there is a slight fall in systolic blood pressure (<10 mm Hg) as venous return to the left ventricle decreases (because of increase in lung capacitance as lung volume increases) and as inspiratory negative intrapleural (intrathoracic) pressures are superimposed onto the aorta. It is classically emphasized that with pulsus paradoxus, the pulse pressure falls, but the diastolic pressure should fall less than does the systolic pressure (hence the pulse "weakening"). When the pulse pressure is no longer palpable or the pulse pressure is not recordable, "total pulsus paradoxus" is said to occur. Total pulsus paradoxus is most commonly seen in tamponade due to malignant disease or other chronic conditions.

Inspiration must be of normal effort. Patients with respiratory distress will nearly invariably have a phasic fall in blood pressure during inspiration because of large swings in pulmonary venous capacitance and intrapleural (intrathoracic) pressure, as increased respiratory muscle effort increases. Therefore, the sign of pulsus paradoxus is nonspecific for pericardial disease, as Kussmaul himself wrote: "the paradoxical pulse may also occur without pericarditis." The mechanism of pulsus paradoxus in tamponade and constriction classically also includes ventricular interdependence.

Pulsus paradoxus may be seen in cardiac disorders (pericardial tamponade and constriction; right ventricular infarction) or in any conditions with exaggerated inspiratory effort. Although originally described in constriction cases, pulsus paradoxus is seen in only a minority of constriction cases, whereas it is seen in a majority of pericardial tamponade cases. Pulsus paradoxus may also be seen in effuso-constrictive pericarditis. Other conditions with exaggerated inspiratory effort in which pulsus paradoxus may be observed include congestive heart failure (CHF), pulmonary diseases, large symptomatic pleural effusions, pulmonary embolism, and hypovolemic shock.

In the presence of tamponade, pulsus paradoxus may be absent when the following disease states are also present: CHF, aortic insufficiency, atrial septal defect, respiratory fatigue or failure, and mechanical ventilation with positive end-expiratory pressure (PEEP). CHF, aortic insufficiency, and atrial septal defect are all pathologic processes that normalize the degree of left ventricular filling by availing a volume load to the left ventricle such that it is not underloaded as a result of ventricular interdependence or varying pulmonary venous capacitance. PEEP regularizes venous return to the heart and renders pleural pressure positive, removing some of the forces that engender the pulsus paradoxus. Pulsus paradoxus is frequently absent when the heart is compressed by intrapericardial thrombus, rather than by fluid, and also when pericardial tamponade is localized (Fig. 2-1).

JUGULAR VENOUS PRESSURE

Normal central venous pressure is 0 to 8 mm Hg, or 4 or 5 cm above the manubrial-sternal angle (angle of Louis, Ludwig angle, angulus Ludovici, angulus sterni), which is, if the chest cage is normal and the viscera are situated normally, about 4 cm above the mid right atrium. Elevated central venous pressure is seen in right ventricular failure, tricuspid regurgitation, and volume overload and in several forms of pericardial diseases, such as pericardial tamponade, constrictive and effuso-constrictive pericarditis, and intrapericardial thrombus compressing the right atrium or right ventricle.

Concurrent volume depletion or contraction (e.g., from diuretic use, from bleeding, or from medical or surgical illness) may pseudonormalize the top of the jugular venous column or render it too low to be recognized, misleading the physician about the (concealed) presence of significant pericardial or right-sided heart disease. Conversely, volume overload will elevate the top of the venous column, exaggerating the findings of pericardial or right-sided heart disease, or may render it too high to be recognized, obscuring the presence of significant pericardial or right-sided heart disease.

During normal inspiration, the mean central venous pressure falls and the x and y descents deepen and therefore often become more obvious. With hypervolemia or volume loading, the mean central venous pressure increases, and the x and y descents proportionally increase.

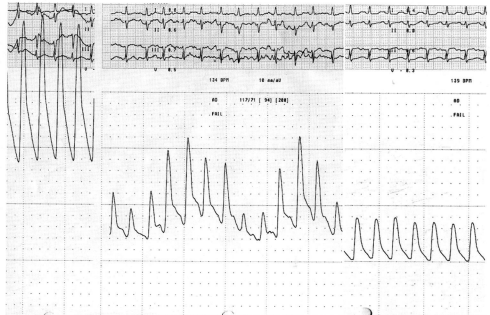

Figure 2-1. Tamponade from cardiac perforation: arterial pressure tracings. LEFT, Before perforation and tamponade, the patient is hypertensive. During normal spontaneous respiration, there is no pulsus paradoxus. MIDDLE, After perforation, tamponade has developed. There is hypotension and a striking pulsus paradoxus—a fall both in systolic blood pressure and in pulse pressure—with inspiration. The pattern is almost total pulsus paradoxus—almost complete disappearance of the pulse pressure in inspiration. RIGHT, After intubation and mechanical positive-pressure ventilation, the pulsus paradoxus is absent.

JUGULAR VENOUS CONTOURS

The *x* Descent

The *x* descent is produced in part by atrial relaxation but predominantly by the systolic descent of the atrioventricular plane from ventricular contraction. Hence, the *x* descent is present, but lessened, in the presence of atrial fibrillation. A steepened *x* descent may be seen in several disease states including pericardial tamponade, constrictive pericarditis, and restrictive cardiomyopathy. If the steepened *x* descent is seen without a steepened *y* descent and in the context of pressure elevation, pericardial tamponade or effuso-constriction is possible. In tamponade, the *x* descent is steep, as most venous emptying can, and does, occur only during ventricular systole. The steep *x* descent of tamponade is seen even in the presence of atrial fibrillation (Fig. 2-2).

An attenuated *x* descent is seen in many disease states, such as right ventricular systolic failure (less vigorous descent of the base of the heart) and tricuspid regurgitation (broad V wave fills in the *x* descent). It may also be seen in both congenital and surgical absence of the pericardium.

The *y* Descent

The *y* descent is produced by two factors that result in early ventricular filling and lowering of atrial venous pressure: passive early ventricular filling from atrial emptying (or "pushing") and active early ventricular filling (or "sucking") from myocardial recoil and pericardial recoil. A steepened *y* descent may be seen in several disease states, including constrictive pericarditis (Fig. 2-3) and restrictive cardiomyopathy. In constriction, the *y* descent is prominent because of two factors. The constrictive process around the right atrium renders it noncompliant, and thus, with the tricuspid valve closed during systole, the right atrial pressure

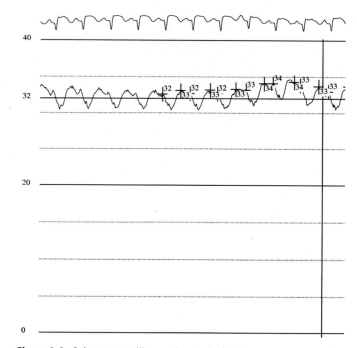

Figure 2-2. Pulmonary capillary wedge tracing during severe tamponade. The mean pressure is markedly elevated, and the contour is abnormal. As can be seen from the ECG tracing, there is a P wave that is shortly followed on the wedge tracing by an A wave. The *x* descent that follows is far greater than is the *y* descent, typical of tamponade physiology. The pattern is similar to that within the central veins in tamponade.

rises considerably (forms a large V wave). Also, the early diastolic rapid recoil outward of the fibrotic pericardium facilitates atrial emptying and ventricular filling. Thus, the *y* descents originate from an elevated level and are also rapid; therefore, they are prominent and usually dominant in cases of constriction.

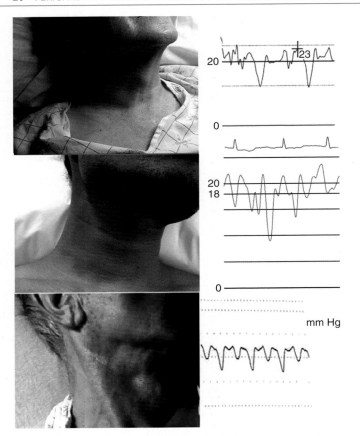

Figure 2-3. Three cases of constrictive pericarditis. LEFT IMAGES, Jugular venous distention (fullness in the neck). RIGHT IMAGES, Prominent *y* descents (concavity in the neck) and right atrial pressure tracings. The mean right atrial pressures are approximately 20 mm Hg in each of the cases. Given the height of the venous column, the *y* descent is the only waveform that comes into view in the neck. The *y* descent of the middle case increases with inspiration.

There is an attenuated *y* descent in tamponade. This attenuation is due to the compression (applied positive pressure) by pericardial fluid onto the right side of the heart throughout the cardiac cycle, including during early diastole—attenuating the magnitude of the *y* descent.

M or W Patterns

In constriction, the *y* descent is usually dominant; in tamponade, the *x* descent is dominant; and in effuso-constriction, the contours are the summation of the constrictive and tamponade effects. The *x* and *y* descents are therefore usually similar even though the *x* descent may be dominant when the effusion (tamponade) aspect is greater.

When both *x* and *y* descents are prominent, an M or W pattern in right atrial tracings and venous pressures is produced. These patterns are not specific for constrictive pericarditis and effuso-constrictive pericarditis but are also seen in heart failure from restrictive cardiomyopathy and right ventricular (± right atrial) infarction.

Kussmaul Sign

Kussmaul sign is most commonly defined as an inspiratory increase in central venous (or right atrial) pressure (Figs. 2-4 and 2-5). Normally, venous pressure falls as intrathoracic pressure falls during spontaneous inspiration. Inability of the pressure to fall denotes restricted filling of the right side of the heart due to either pericardial compressive states or intrinsic stiffness of the right ventricle (infarction, hypertrophy, cardiomyopathy). Another less commonly used definition for Kussmaul sign is a failure of the central venous pressure to fall with inspiration (Fig. 2-6). Kussmaul sign was first described in patients with constrictive pericarditis, but it is seen in only a minority (20%) of cases of constrictive pericarditis. The sign may be seen in pericardial

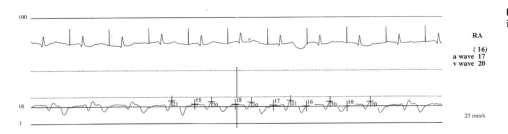

Figure 2-4. Kussmaul sign. There is no fall in right atrial pressure with inspiration.

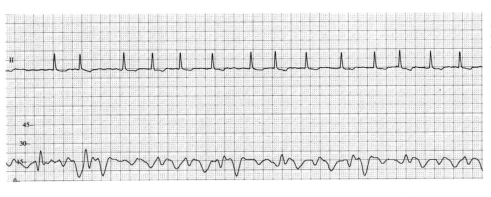

Figure 2-5. Kussmaul sign. There is no fall in right atrial pressure with inspiration. The *y* descents are deeper with inspiration. The presence of atrial fibrillation may contribute to the lesser *x* descents.

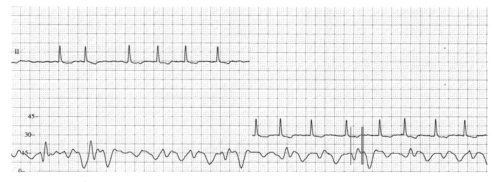

Figure 2-6. It is far easier to recognize the *x* and *y* descents when the ECG tracing, against which the waveforms are read, is brought close enough to associate timing. This is particularly true when the rhythm is atrial fibrillation, as in this case of constrictive pericarditis. There is inevitably a small time delay when fluid-filled catheters are used. Despite the rhythm being atrial fibrillation, there are *x* descents. The intermittent deepening of the *y* descents is probably the result of inspiration, although without a respirometry tracing, this is only speculative.

tamponade, restrictive cardiomyopathy, and virtually any cause or nature of right ventricular failure. Hemodynamic tracings should be annotated to describe whether they were recorded with normal spontaneous respiration, with exaggerated inspiratory effort, with apnea, or during mechanical ventilation.

PRECORDIAL FINDINGS IN PERICARDIAL DISEASE

Apical (and right parasternal) systolic retractions may occur in some cases of constrictive pericarditis. The apical impulse is left laterally displaced in cases of congenital absence of the pericardium—partial left sided, complete left sided, and complete absence, all of which allow the heart to be displaced laterally and to rotate posteriorly. In tamponade, the apical impulse may still be present.

The Pericardial Knock

The rapid early diastolic filling of the ventricles that is abruptly arrested by the noncompliant pericardium of constrictive pericarditis may produce an early diastolic sound—an S_3, which in the context of the diagnosis of constrictive pericarditis is popularly referred to as a pericardial knock, although it is similar to other S_3 early diastolic filling sounds.

A knock is heard in only a minority of cases of constriction and is the subject of considerable interphysician variation. Knocks and steep *y* descents are manifestations of exaggerated early diastolic filling and tend to be noted concurrently. The knock is temporally associated with the onset of the "plateau" of diastolic filling that follows the *y* descent and is absent in cases that do not have a well-defined plateau, establishing that the violent arresting of rapid filling is the origin of the sound.[3] Pericardial knocks are a sign of later stage constriction (higher filling pressures result in louder early diastolic filling sounds) (Fig. 2-7).

A knock is not present in tamponade, in which there is severely reduced early diastolic filling. Other early diastolic sounds include the opening snap of mitral stenosis (higher frequency), the near-mythical "tumor plop" of a small number of

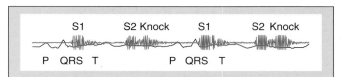

Figure 2-7. Phonocardiogram. The phonocardiogram tracing is superimposed on the ECG. In this case of transient severe pericardial constriction, a pericardial knock of equal intensity (amplitude) to the first and second heart hounds is present. The knock occurs in early diastole, concurrent with the abrupt cessation of rapid filling.

atrial myxomas, and S_3 sounds from disease (elevated atrial filling pressures—CHF) or health (childhood, athleticism).

Pericardial Friction Rubs

High-frequency discontinuous sounds due to pericardial inflammation are referred to as friction rubs. The term *friction rub* is potentially misleading; although the sound emulates friction of two surfaces, a rub may occur in the presence of an effusion or tamponade that would separate at least the majority of the pericardial surfaces. Rubs are typically triphasic, as a heart in sinus rhythm exhibits three motions per cardiac cycle—during ventricular systole, early diastole, and late diastole. The systolic component is usually the loudest as the cardiac motion is greatest in systole. Pericardial rubs may be evanescent, and repeated examinations are often necessary to detect them. Rubs are best heard at the lower left sternal border where the pericardium contacts the chest wall directly and through pericardiosternal ligaments. Maneuvers that increase contact of the heart with the chest wall (leaning forward, expiration) may facilitate recognition of a rub. Pericardial rubs are heard *per cardiac cycle* and pleural rubs are heard *per respiratory cycle*. Some pericardial rubs are accentuated during inspiration as right-sided heart volume increases.

Pleural diseases, particularly pleurisy but also pneumothoraces, may produce a rub, although it is phased with the respiratory, not cardiac, cycle. The bruit de moulin described by Bricketeau[4] in 1844 (watermill sound or mill wheel sound) is a rare sign of both air and fluid within the heart and may also be heard with massive air embolism into the heart cavities, or hydropneumopericardium. Pneumopericardium, pneumomediastinum, and pneumothorax may also produce rubs.

References

1. Gauchat H, Katz LN: Observations on pulsus paradoxus. Arch Intern Med 1924;33:371-393.

2. Woo H, Fung C: http://www.priory.com/homol/pulsus.htm

3. Tyberg TI: Genesis of pericardial knock in constrictive pericarditis. Am J Cardiol 1980;46:570-575.

4. Bricketeau M: Observation d'hydropneumopéricarde accompagné d'un bruit de fluctuation perceptible a l'oreille. Arch Gen Med 1844;4: 334-339.

Imaging of the Pericardium

KEY POINTS

▸ Chest radiography, fluoroscopy, transthoracic and transesophageal echocardiography, chest and cardiac CT, and cardiac MR each offer the ability to assess some aspects of pericardial diseases.

▸ Chest radiography is indispensable for its overview of lung and pleural disease involvement.

▸ Echocardiography is enormously useful to assess pericardial fluid and thrombus, to establish the physiologic consequences of pericardial fluid, and to guide drainage decisions. Echocardiography is also useful to assess the physiologic consequences of constriction, but it is limited in its extent of pericardial anatomic imaging and even more limited in chest imaging.

▸ Chest CT and cardiac CT are workhorses that offer good anatomic detail of the pericardium and excellent anatomic detail of the chest. CT is the most sensitive test for the identification of pericardial calcification, although pericardial calcification should not be viewed as synonymous with constriction physiology. CT lacks the means by which to assess most physiologic changes consistent with cardiac compression from tamponade or constriction.

▸ CMR is a valuable adjunct to the assessment of pericardial diseases and has the ability in most cases to offer the best delineation of pericardial layers. It has excellent ability to confirm fluid within the pericardium or suspected pericardial cysts.

Numerous modalities are available to image the pericardium:

- Chest radiography
- Fluoroscopy
- Echocardiography
  - Transthoracic echocardiography
  - Transesophageal echocardiography
- Computed tomography (CT)
- Cardiac magnetic resonance (CMR)
- Surgical inspection

CHEST RADIOGRAPHY

Plain film chest radiography has almost no means by which to image normal pericardium and only limited means to visualize abnormalities of the pericardium. A pericardial "fat stripe" seen on the lateral radiograph, which indicates fat-fluid-fat interfaces, is seen in some cases of pericardial effusion, although fluoroscopy is more adept at capturing this finding because the tower can be positioned to optimally (tangentially) depict these layers, whereas imaging of a fat stripe on the lateral chest radiograph depends on chance alone. A flask-like cardiopericardial silhouette is consistent with the presence of at least a moderate-sized pericardial effusion and differs from the somewhat similar globular appear-

ance of dilated cardiomyopathy in that the superior aspect of the cardiopericardial silhouette is tapered in the case of effusion (Fig. 3-1) but not in dilated cardiomyopathy. Gross calcification of the pericardium is evident by chest radiography, but precise localization of it is almost impossible because the soft tissue structures of the heart and the cavities are not directly depicted and can only be inferred (Figs. 3-2 to 3-4). A pericardial cyst is usually evident by chest radiography as a rounded opacity beside a midline structure (Figs. 3-5 and 3-6), usually located at a cardiophrenic angle (right:left = 3:1), with 5% located in the middle and 5% in the superior mediastinum.

Chest radiography depicts associated lesions relevant to pericardial diseases, such as pleural effusions and pleural plaques. Dilation of the azygos vein, consistent with elevated central venous pressure, may be evident by chest radiography (Figs. 3-7 to 3-12), as is dilation of the aorta.

FLUOROSCOPY

Fluoroscopy is not a primary diagnostic test for pericardial diseases. However, it is able to depict pericardial calcification (Figs. 3-13 and 3-14) and the pericardial fat stripe from pericardial fluid:fat interfaces (Figs. 3-15 and 3-16).

Text continued on p. 30.

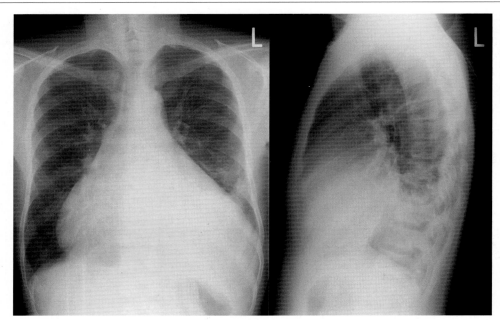

Figure 3-1. Pericardial effusion and tamponade from renal failure. Prominent cardiomegaly with a flask-like shape tapers from superior to inferior as the fluid settles dependently. The pulmonary vascular markings are increased because of raised pressure. There are no pleural effusions or obvious lung masses.

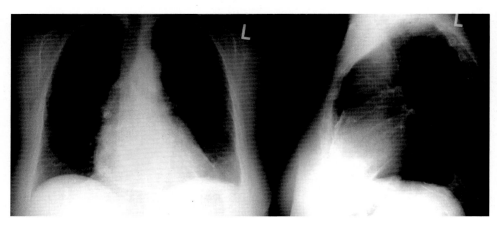

Figure 3-2. Constrictive pericarditis. There is cardiomegaly, but more striking is the thick pericardial calcification seen both on the anteroposterior film along the diaphragmatic surface and on the lateral film anterior to the right ventricle. Clear lung fields. Blunting of the left pleural costodiaphragmatic recess is present.

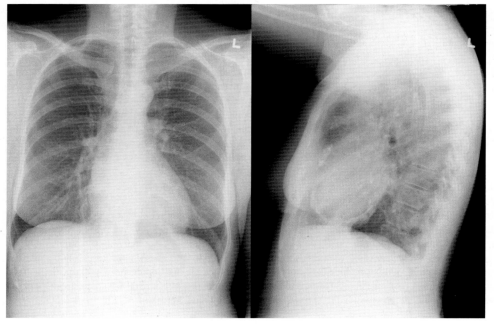

Figure 3-3. Pericardial calcification without constrictive physiology, proven by cardiac catheterization. There is no cardiomegaly or gross abnormality to the cardiac contour, but there is striking pericardial calcification seen best on the lateral radiograph along both the diaphragmatic and anterior surfaces of the heart. Normal pulmonary vascular markings. No pleural effusions.

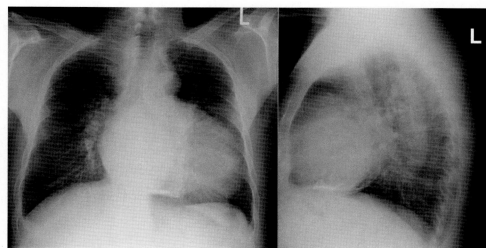

Figure 3-4. Cardiomegaly, left-sided heart failure, sternal wires, and a mass of calcification on the diaphragmatic aspect of the heart. Although it is usual to describe calcification in such locations as being pericardial, this patient had in fact undergone pericardiectomy for tuberculous constrictive disease and was without parietal pericardium over at least the anterior aspects of the heart. The calcified mass was presumed to be an organized paracardiac hematoma arising from remote perioperative bleeding, an organized hematoma within a segment of nonresected pericardium, or a residual calcific nonresected pericardium of prominent thickness.

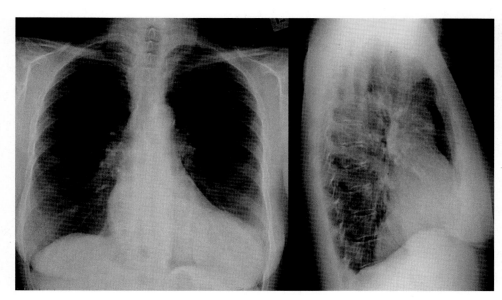

Figure 3-5. Pericardial cyst. Normal pulmonary vascular markings. No pleural effusions, no cardiomegaly, no pericardial calcification. Large rounded mass at the left cardiodiaphragmatic angle.

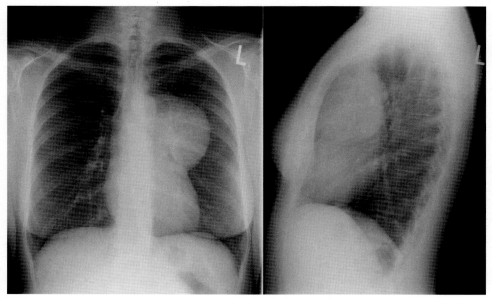

Figure 3-6. Pericardial cyst. Normal pulmonary vascular markings. No pleural effusions, no cardiomegaly, no pericardial calcification. Large rounded mass over the left hilum and left pulmonary artery.

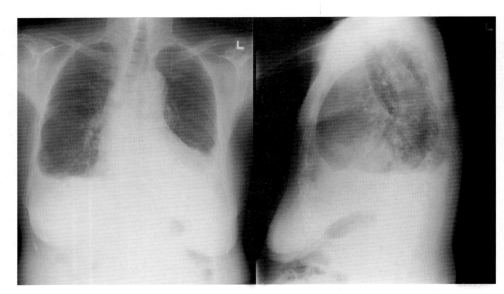

Figure 3-7. Constrictive pericarditis. Interstitial pulmonary edema due to high pulmonary venous pressure. Large bilateral pleural effusions due to high central venous pressure. There appears to be cardiomegaly, but the pleural effusions obfuscate assessment of both the heart shadow and the presence of calcification.

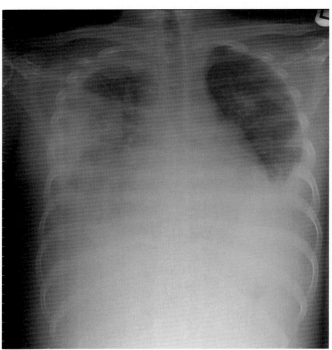

Figure 3-8. Florid acute constrictive pericarditis. Interstitial and airspace pulmonary edema. Large bilateral pleural effusions. There appears to be cardiomegaly, but the pleural effusions obfuscate assessment of the heart shadow. No pericardial calcification.

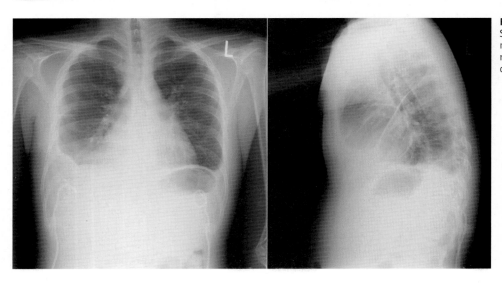

Figure 3-9. Constrictive pericarditis. Slightly increased pulmonary vascular markings. Bilateral pleural drains and small residual pleural effusions. Mild cardiomegaly. No pericardial calcification.

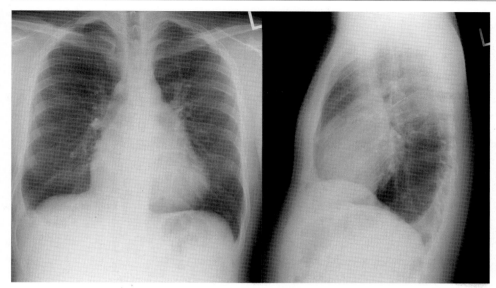

Figure 3-10. Constrictive pericarditis. Slightly increased pulmonary vascular markings. Prominent azygos vein due to elevated central venous pressure. Small right pleural effusion. Mild cardiomegaly. No pericardial calcification. Possible distortion of the lateral left ventricular border by the constrictive process.

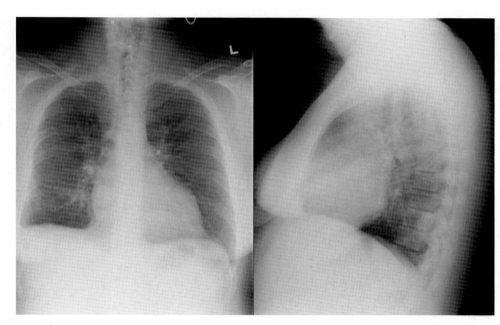

Figure 3-11. Constrictive pericarditis. Increased pulmonary vascular markings. Prominent azygos vein. Small left pleural effusion. Borderline cardiomegaly, with prominence of the left atrial posterior wall seen on the lateral radiograph. No calcification.

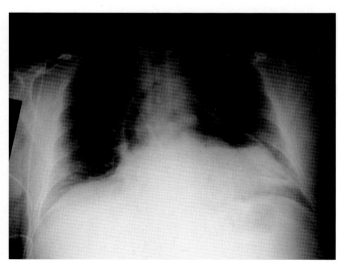

Figure 3-12. Pneumopericardium and effusion. Air-fluid level within the pericardial cavity, with silhouetting of the lateral wall of the ascending aorta and clear delineation of the pericardium by the air.

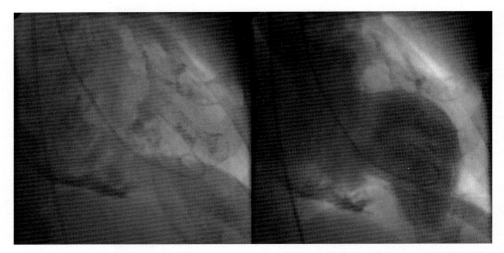

Figure 3-13. Fluoroscopy and contrast ventriculography. Calcification of the pericardium, especially the diaphragmatic surface. Marked distortion of the left ventricular cavity along the long axis by the compression of the left ventricle by the pericardial constriction process.

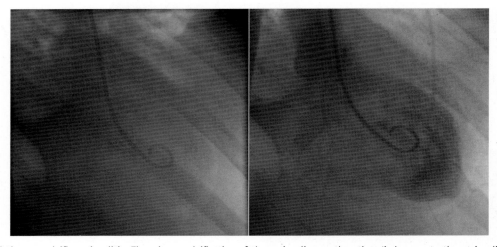

Figure 3-14. Constrictive noncalcific pericarditis. There is no calcification of the pericardium; rather, there is lucency to the pericardium in this case, seen over the anterior and apical walls.

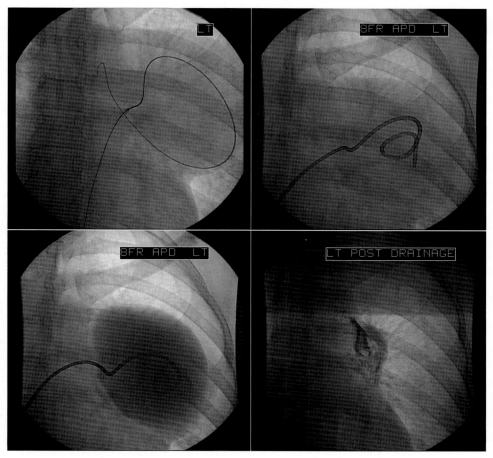

Figure 3-15. Fluoroscopy is a traditional and useful means to guide drainage procedures. Here, a pericardial cyst is drained by fluoroscopic guidance. TOP LEFT, Wire entered into the cyst. TOP RIGHT, Drainage catheter entered into the cyst. BOTTOM, Contrast dye opacification of the cyst before (LEFT) and after (RIGHT) drainage.

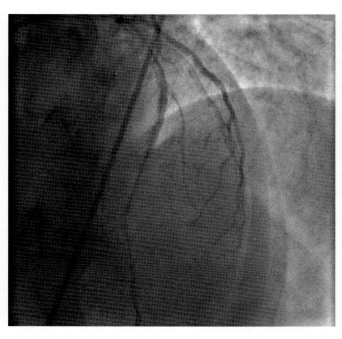

Figure 3-16. Fluoroscopic view during coronary angiography and percutaneous coronary intervention (LAO projection). A pericardial effusion (darker stripe) is evident. Two lucent layers are also apparent: one at the epicardial layer, resulting from epicardial fat; and the other one over the pericardial layer, resulting from pericardial fat. The lesser attenuation of radiation by fat tissue renders the fat layers lucent by comparison to the underlying myocardium and also to the effusion. The key to the image is the tangential alignment through sufficient fat to reveal the layers. The angiographic delineation of the obtuse marginal branches confirms the location of the epicardial layer of the heart and its fat layer, which lies over the arteries. The pericardial effusion is more radiopaque in this case, likely because of extravasation of contrast dye into the pericardial space due to transient coronary rupture caused by percutaneous coronary intervention.

ECHOCARDIOGRAPHY

Echocardiography is one of the most useful tests to evaluate pericardial diseases but has significant limitations. Echocardiography is a reliable test to identify pericardial fluid and to identify the compressive physiologic consequences of fluid (tamponade) and of constriction (Figs. 3-17 to 3-19). A significant attribute of echocardiography is its ease of portability for bedside studies and ease of guidance of pericardial fluid drainage. The probe may be kept sterile by placing it within a sterile sheath. Echocardiography is one of the best tests to distinguish pericardial fluid from intrapericardial blood clot (Fig. 3-20). In some cases, transesophageal echocardiography is needed to distinguish pericardial fluid from clot.

The echocardiographic delineation of pericardial anatomic details is limited by the lesser field of view compared with those of CT and CMR. Although pericardial thickening can be identified by echocardiography (particularly transesophageal echocardiography), this is true only for thickening in certain locations, and CT scanning and CMR imaging are far more robust in delineating pericardial thickening. Pericardial cysts that do not abut the chest wall are very difficult to image by transthoracic echocardiography; transesophageal echocardiography offers incremental yield, as do subcostal transthoracic views. Pericarditis commonly occurs without pericardial effusion; therefore, echocardiography is not as useful as is commonly believed to substantiate or to refute a clinically suspected diagnosis of pericarditis (Figs. 3-21 to 3-28). A significant asset of echocardiography for the assessment of pericardial diseases is the ability to depict cardiorespiratory phenomena that have predictive value of compressive syndromes.

The best uses of echocardiography for the evaluation of pericardial diseases include the following:

- Identification of pericardial fluid
- Identification of the physiologic (tamponade compressive) consequences of pericardial fluid
- Identification of intrapericardial clot
- Identification of the physiologic changes due to compression from constrictive pericardium
- Establishment that myocardial systolic and diastolic dysfunction (cardiomyopathy) does not underlie heart failure states

Potential limitations of the use of echocardiography for the evaluation of suspected pericardial diseases include the following:

- Limited field of view
- Limited ability to identify or to refute pericardial thickening
- Physiologic changes due to compressive syndrome become obscured by mechanical ventilation and are also affected by hypopnea and hyperpnea.
- Inability to image a pericardial abnormality unless there is a direct acoustic window to it

COMPUTED TOMOGRAPHY

CT scanning is a robust test to assess pericardial diseases and associated intrathoracic disease processes. Routine chest CT scanning is not electrocardiography (ECG) gated and has less temporal resolution than does ECG-gated cardiac CT. ECG gating improves the temporal resolution of cardiac imaging and is an effective means to address some of the motion-related problems of cardiac imaging. CT technology can offer optimal delineation of either chest disease (chest CT) or cardiac disease (ECG-gated cardiac CT), but not both at the present time. The resolution of CT is variable, depending on several parameters. Chest CT necessitates a large field of view, with some loss of resolution, particularly temporal resolution. Conversely, cardiac (ECG-gated) CT achieves excellent cardiac temporal and spatial resolution, but as the field of view is intentionally limited to the heart to contain radiation dosage, ECG-gated cardiac CT offers incomplete

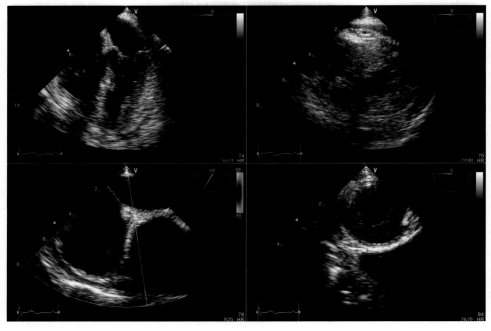

Figure 3-17. Terminal constrictive pericarditis. TOP LEFT, Apical 4-chamber view shows a bright layer of material (brighter than the myocardium) along the entire lateral wall of the left ventricle. TOP RIGHT, Transgastric short-axis view shows a small left ventricular cavity, and there is left ventricular hypertrophy. There is a layer of material posterior and lateral to the left ventricle. BOTTOM LEFT, There is a layer of material lateral to the right atrial wall. BOTTOM RIGHT, Short-axis view of the thoracic aorta shows that there is prominent spontaneous echo contrast, consistent with low flow.

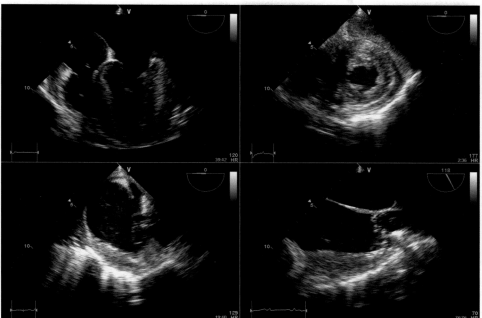

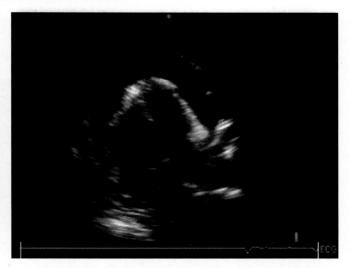

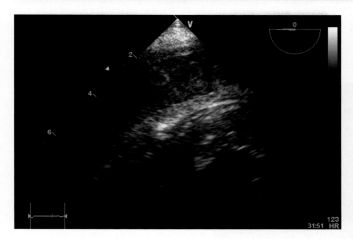

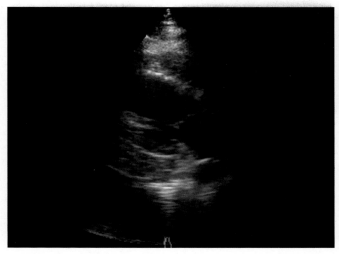

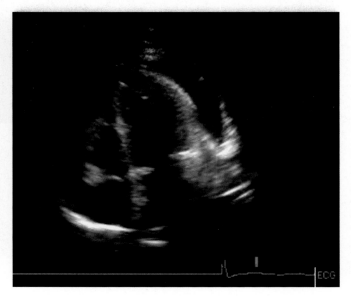

Figure 3-18. Constrictive pericarditis. TOP LEFT, Apical 4-chamber view shows a layer of material along the entire lateral wall of the left ventricle. TOP RIGHT, Transgastric short-axis view shows a layer of material lateral to the left ventricle. BOTTOM LEFT, There is a thick layer of material lateral to the right atrial wall. BOTTOM RIGHT, The thick layer of material lateral to the right atrium extends along its entire height.

Figure 3-19. Purulent bacterial and constrictive pericarditis. Transgastric short-axis view shows a thick layer of fluid with specular echoes and peculiar material within it, including a rounded entity.

Figure 3-21. Pericardial effusion and tamponade. Apical 4-chamber view shows a large pericardial effusion (echo-free space over the heart cavities).

Figure 3-20. Intrapericardial thrombus. There is a thick layer of material posterior to the left ventricular posterior wall. The material has the prominent specular texture typical of blood clot.

Figure 3-22. Pericardial effusion and tamponade. Apical 4-chamber view shows a moderate-sized pericardial effusion (echo-free space over the heart cavities); the right atrial cavity is entirely collapsed (inverted inward).

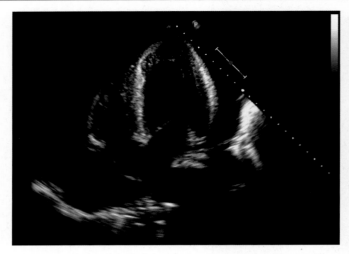

Figure 3-23. Pericardial effusion without tamponade. Apical 4-chamber view shows a large pericardial effusion (echo-free space over the heart cavities) but no chamber collapse.

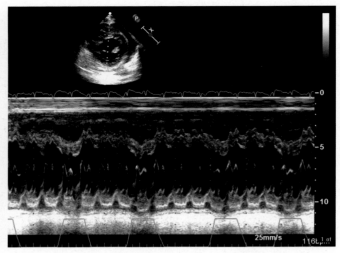

Figure 3-25. Pericardial constriction with signs of ventricular interdependence. M-mode study of the interventricular septum: with inspiration, there is increase in the right ventricular dimension and decrease in the left ventricular dimension. There is also an early diastolic dip.

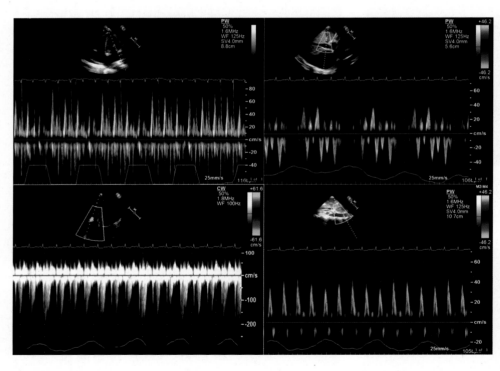

Figure 3-24. Pericardial constriction with signs of ventricular interdependence. TOP LEFT, Spectral profiles of left ventricular inflow. There is a significant fall in early diastolic inflow velocity with inspiration (which is denoted by the respirometry tracing at the bottom of the image). TOP RIGHT, Spectral profiles of hepatic venous flow. There is expiratory and end-inspiratory augmentation of diastolic flow reversal. BOTTOM LEFT, Spectral profiles of tricuspid insufficiency. There is increase in the tricuspid regurgitation velocity with inspiration and increase in the right ventricular systolic pressure with inspiration. BOTTOM RIGHT, Spectral profile of abdominal aortic flow. There is inspiratory decrease in flow velocity.

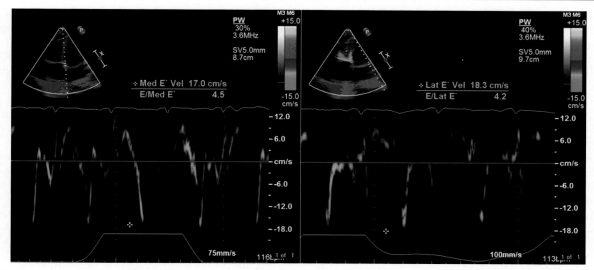

Figure 3-26. Pericardial constriction with normal myocardial properties. Tissue Doppler spectral recordings of the medial and lateral mitral annulus. The early diastolic (E′) velocities are more than 10 cm/s (normal), consistent with normal left ventricular myocardium.

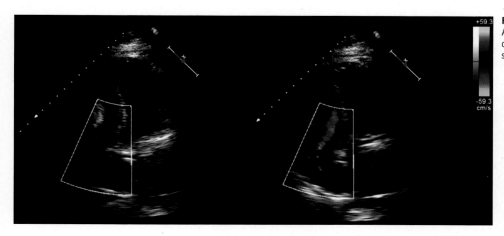

Figure 3-27. Constrictive pericarditis. Apical 4-chamber view shows marked distortion of the right ventricular cavity shape with indentation of the lateral wall.

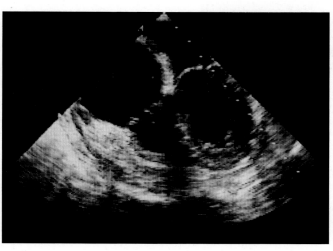

Figure 3-28. Constrictive pericarditis. On transesophageal echocardiography apical 4-chamber view, there is marked thickening of the pericardium, which is best seen over the right ventricular free wall. The right atrium is dilated and the interatrial septum deviates toward the left side, consistent with the right atrial pressure being greater than the left atrial pressure.

assessment of the remainder of the thorax. Therefore, CT technology remains somewhat dichotomized as offering excellent detail of the thorax (chest CT) or of the heart (ECG-gated cardiac CT). The evaluation of pericardial disease often requires both cardiac and chest imaging, though (Fig. 3-29).

CT is not as reliable as CMR for delineating anatomically complex pericardial disease that consists of both fluid and thickening.

As with CMR, a fundamental difficulty in determining the thickness of pericardium is the achievement of sufficient contrast of the margins of the pericardium, in particular to distinguish the myocardial:pericardial interface, as myocardium and pericardium have similar attenuation coefficients. The use of CT contrast agents assists only with delineation of the endocardial:myocardial interface and therefore does not facilitate delineation of the myocardial:pericardial interface (Fig. 3-30). Contrast in the right heart cavities may engender streak artifact that confounds imaging of the pericardium over the right heart (see Fig. 3-29). As with CMR, the ability to depict the parietal pericardial thickness is dependent on having sufficient fat planes overlying the myocardium (epicardial fat) and overlying the parietal pericardium (pericardial fat), which is a matter of chance. Fat has a lesser attenuation coefficient (appears darker) than does parietal pericardium and myocardium, and therefore it delineates, when it is present, the border of the parietal pericardium. This "fat sandwich" of the parietal pericardium is the basis of establishing parietal pericardial thickness by both CT scanning and CMR imaging. Depiction of true pericardial thickness by ECG-gated CT scanning is still challenging. Normal pericardium may appear up to a few millimeters thick; therefore, less than 3 mm is not necessarily abnormal, depending on the scanner and the protocol. A cautious "cutoff" of 3 mm to dichotomize normal and thickened fails to detect many cases of mild thickening (Fig. 3-31).

CT is exquisitely sensitive to the presence of calcification, including pericardial calcification. Calcification of the pericardium establishes pathologic involvement of the pericardium and is suggestive of constrictive pericarditis, although this association remains based on chronic tuberculous pericarditis and is less strong for nontuberculous cases of constriction and for acute constrictive syndromes (Figs. 3-32 to 3-36).

A prominent asset of CT scanning for the evaluation of suspected pericardial disease is its ability to provide comprehensive imaging evaluation of the entire thorax. CT scanning is able to superbly evaluate pleural effusions and plaques, adenopathy, masses, pneumothoraces or pneumomediastinum and pneumothorax, and a range of other findings relevant to suspected pericardial diseases. Whereas CMR is performed substantially at the expense of imaging the remainder of the thorax, chest CT offers both fairly good cardiac detail and superb chest detail.

The best uses of CT for the evaluation of pericardial diseases include the following:

- Detection of pericardial calcification
- Detection of pericardial cysts (T2-weighted spin echo CMR sequences are thought better suited to establish that the content is fluid filled.)
- Attempt to determine pericardial thickening (CMR is probably better to delineate the myocardial:pericardial plane.)

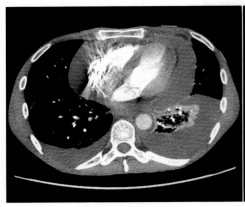
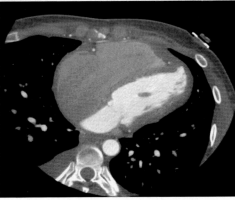

Figure 3-29. Contrast-enhanced chest CT (LEFT) and ECG-gated cardiac CT (RIGHT), different patients. Chest CT and cardiac CT are not synonymous techniques. Chest CT yields an abundance of relevant noncardiac detail, at some expense of cardiac spatial and temporal resolution (detail) and artifacts from high contrast within the right side of the heart. ECG gating, optimal bolus tracking, saline "chaser," and reduced field of view improve detail of the left and right sides of the heart, improve vessel visualization, and offer significantly improved resolution, at the expense of noncardiac disease detail.

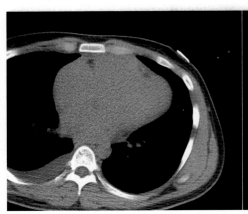
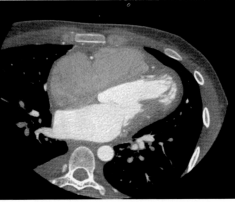

Figure 3-30. Severe constrictive pericarditis. Non–contrast-enhanced (LEFT) and contrast-enhanced (RIGHT) ECG-gated cardiac CT. A saline chaser bolus results in less contrast in the right ventricle. No pericardial calcification is present on this reconstructed slice. On neither image is the delineation of the myocardium from the parietal pericardium clear; hence, determination of pericardial thickness is still difficult. The patient was cachectic and with strikingly low body fat.

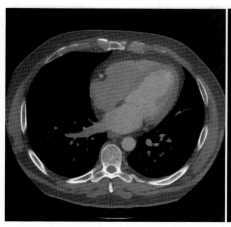

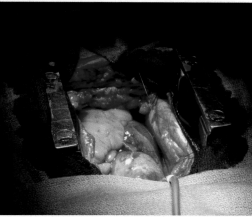

Figure 3-31. This patient underwent surgery of the ascending aorta. LEFT, Preoperative contrast-enhanced axial CT scan. The parietal pericardial layer is revealed wherever there is sufficient epicardial fat underneath it and parietal pericardial fat over it. Typically, this occurs over the right ventricular free wall and the atrioventricular grooves and not over the mid left ventricular free wall. Measurement of the pericardium on this image yields a thickness of 1 to 3 mm. RIGHT, Intraoperative photograph with the anterior pericardium incised. The pericardium is entirely normal in thickness and appearance; it is only minimally thicker than the sutures and is 1 mm or less in thickness.

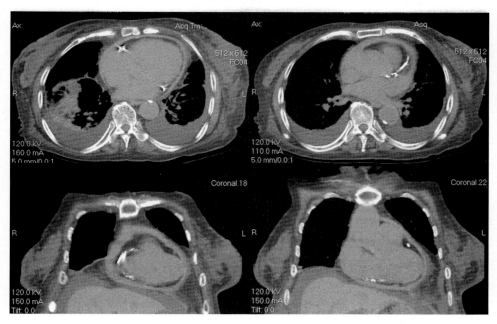

Figure 3-32. Constrictive pericarditis. Non–contrast-enhanced chest CT. There is a layer of epicardial fat over most of this heart (low attenuation similar to the subcutaneous fat) that allows delineation of the inside of the thickened pericardium. The calcification is coronary, not pericardial. There are pleural effusions and ascites.

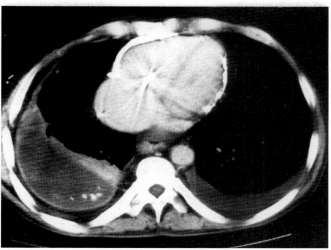

Figure 3-33. Contrast-enhanced chest CT. Despite affording much less resolution, this older generation CT image is able to demonstrate the markedly thickened and calcified pericardium over both the right and left ventricular free walls. The depicted thickness of the pericardial calcification may exceed that of its true thickness due to the partial volume averaging effect/artifact.

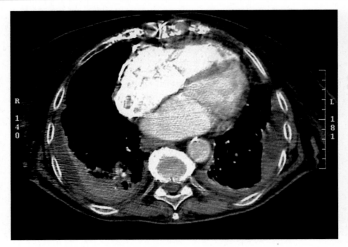

Figure 3-34. Constrictive pericarditis. Contrast-enhanced chest CT. There is pericardial calcification seen lateral to the right atrial lateral wall. There are bilateral pleural effusions.

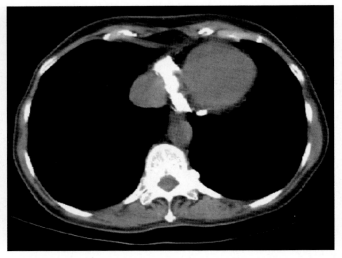

Figure 3-36. Calcified pericardium without constrictive physiology. Non–contrast-enhanced chest CT. A striking band of calcification is present in the atrioventricular groove.

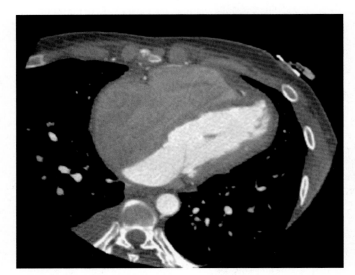

Figure 3-35. Constrictive pericarditis, noncalcified. Contrast-enhanced ECG-gated cardiac CT. The spatial resolution of ECG-gated cardiac CT imaging, versus that of chest CT imaging, is superior for cardiac detail. However, as this image demonstrates, pericardial thickening may have the same attenuation coefficient as does myocardium and may be difficult to resolve with confidence.

- Assessment of related intrathoracic disease, such as pleural effusions, masses, lymph nodes, and pulmonary lesions

   Potential limitations to the use of CT for the evaluation of suspected pericardial diseases include the following:

- The scenario of constriction with normal pericardial thickness (20% of constriction cases), in which rigid and thin (rather than rigid and thickened) pericardium has resulted in constrictive or compressive physiology (Figs. 3-37 to 3-40). The elastic properties of the pericardium are simply unpredictable according to the thickness of the pericardium.
- The distinction of intrapericardial clot from blood by CT is difficult because of their inherently similar attenuation coefficients. Other limitations of CT for the evaluation of suspected pericardial diseases include the requirement of transport,

which may be inadvisable in cases of critically reduced cardiac output, and the potential of contrast nephropathy and allergy.
- The lack of Doppler or other modality to depict physiology changes
- Potential radiation-associated risks.

CARDIAC MAGNETIC RESONANCE IMAGING

CMR is a powerful adjunct to echocardiography and CT scanning. The ability of CMR to delineate the layers of the peri-cardium is predicated on the fortuitously different relaxation properties of myocardium, epicardial fat (Figs. 3-41 to 3-43), pericardial fluid, and parietal pericardium, which makes CMR probably the best test to evaluate pericardial anatomic detail but, as with CT scanning, is dependent on the presence of sufficient fat under and over the parietal pericardium. To assess parietal pericardial thickness, it is essential to have fat planes underlying and overlying the parietal pericardium. There is seldom an underlying epicardial fat plane over the mid left ventricular lateral wall; epicardial fat predominates over the right ventricular free wall and beside the atrioventricular and interventricular grooves, and this is therefore generally where measurements are made (Figs. 3-44 and 3-45).

   Popular recent CMR developments, such as steady-state free precession (SSFP) sequences, offer an excellent overview of pericardial anatomy and reveal pericardial effusions, pericardial thickening, some of the septal motions consistent with constriction, and the free wall collapse signs of tamponade. SSFP imaging contends with susceptibility artifacts that are common at the epicardial:pericardial level, particularly if there is fluid (Figs. 3-46 to 3-49). An attribute of SSFP sequences is the ability to assess the heart through the cardiac cycle; this may reveal septal motions consistent with constrictive pericardial compression and free wall collapse consistent with pericardial fluid (tamponade) compression. With cine SSFP imaging, the parietal pericardium becomes

Text continued on p. 41.

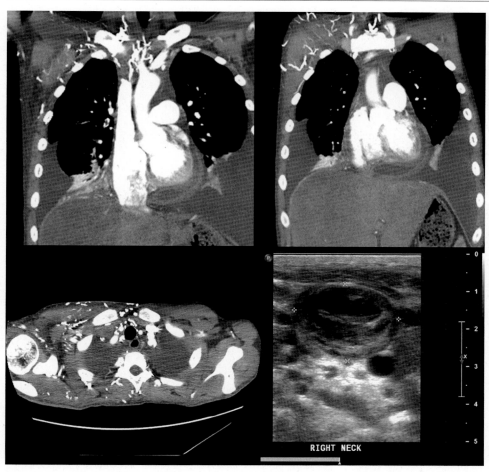

Figure 3-37. Constrictive pericarditis. Contrast-enhanced chest CT. The pericardium is thickened, and there is a layer of low attenuation and high attenuation. There is soft tissue (thrombus) within the upper superior vena cava, and there are extensive venous collaterals through the right shoulder. At the bottom right is an ultrasound view of the right internal jugular vein, which is completely thrombosed.

RIGHT NECK

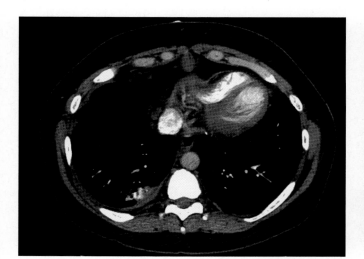

Figure 3-38. Constrictive pericarditis. Contrast-enhanced chest CT. The right ventricular lateral wall is indented (distorted) by regional compression from pericardial thickening. There is as well reflux of contrast material into the upper inferior vena cava, which is dilated.

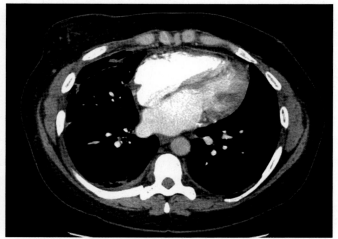

Figure 3-39. Contrast-enhanced chest CT scan of constrictive pericarditis shows normal pericardial thickness, although mild pericardial thickening was described at surgery. The pericardium is well seen over the right ventricular free wall, offset by epicardial and pericardial fat layers. The right ventricle is not distorted.

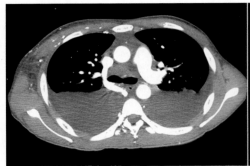
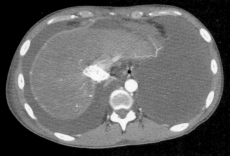

Figure 3-40. Constrictive pericarditis with markedly elevated central venous pressures imaged by contrast-enhanced chest CT. LEFT, At the level of the azygos vein, which is very dilated from an elevated distending pressure, there are bilateral pleural effusions. RIGHT, At the level of the upper abdomen, there is ascites and reflux of contrast material into the upper inferior vena cava.

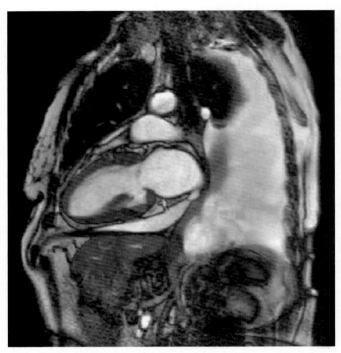

Figure 3-41. CMR SSFP sequence of early transient effuso-constriction after aortic valve replacement. The pericardial and pleural effusions are readily seen by SSFP imaging by their high signal, as are all the blood-containing cavities and vessels. The distribution of the pericardial effusion is also apparent, as is the lack of left atrial chamber collapse. There are prominent susceptibility artifacts at the fluid:epicardial fat interfaces and also the myocardial:epicardial fat interfaces. The anterior and superior aspects of the right ventricle are adherent to the parietal pericardium and do not exhibit slippage between the visceral and parietal layers when viewed as a cine image.

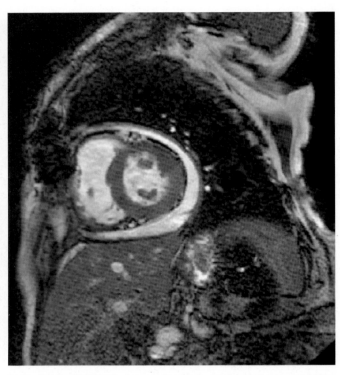

Figure 3-42. CMR SSFP sequence of an early transient effuso-constriction after aortic valve replacement. There is a pericardial effusion over the left and posterior aspects of the heart but not the right side. There are prominent susceptibility artifacts at the fluid:epicardial fat interface. The anterior and superior aspects of the right ventricle are adherent to the parietal pericardium and do not exhibit slippage between the visceral and parietal layers.

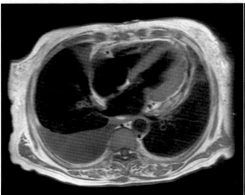
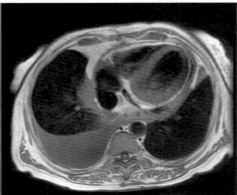

Figure 3-43. CMR T1-weighted black blood images. The parietal pericardium is seen as a low signal plane between the high signal pericardial and epicardial fat layers. The parietal pericardium is better seen over the right ventricular free wall, often, as seen on the right, slightly lower than in the 4-chamber view, at the level of the coronary sinus.

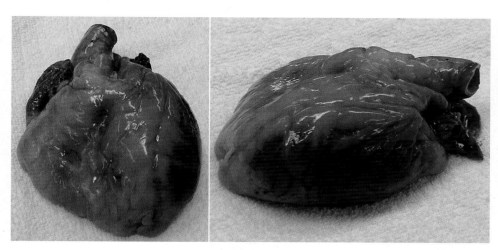

Figure 3-44. Left anterior oblique and left lateral perspective of the heart (parietal pericardium removed). There is an abundance of fat over the right ventricle and within and beside the atrioventricular and interventricular grooves. The left lateral aspect of the heart, though, is largely devoid of epicardial fat.

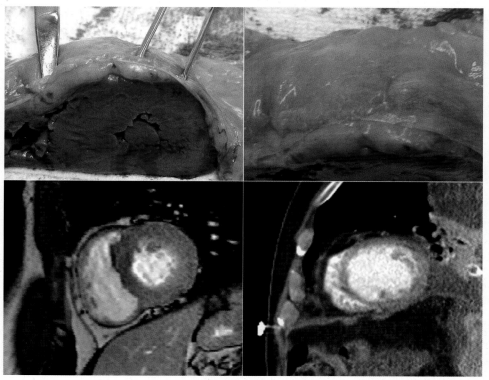

Figure 3-45. TOP ROW, Heart at autopsy, cut in short axis. The forceps and scissors are holding the parietal pericardium and its adherent fat in place. The parietal pericardium is thin (1 mm or less) and nearly translucent. The overlying parietal pericardial (outside) fat layer is more prominent over the right ventricle than the left ventricle, as is the epicardial fat layer. BOTTOM ROW, CMR SSFP (LEFT) and nongated CT (RIGHT) images. The parietal pericardium over the right ventricle is well depicted by the CMR image, between epicardial and outside fat layers of higher signal. The CT image is less clear.

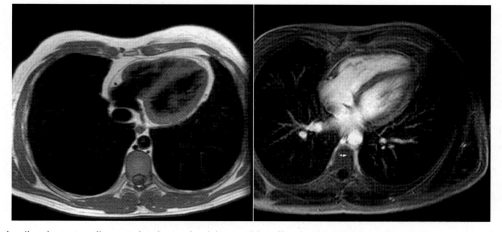

Figure 3-46. The pericardium is most easily appreciated over the right ventricle, offset by epicardial fat underneath and pericardial fat over it. Black blood (T1-weighted) techniques offer better anatomic detail, such as parietal pericardial thickness, than does SSFP bright blood technique. The pericardial fat and the parietal pericardium appear entirely different on CMR imaging according to the modality and sequence used. Without adjacent fat planes, ascertaining the parietal pericardial layer is vexing, as its appearance cannot be clearly distinguished from myocardium. Hence, over the left ventricular free wall in many patients (where there is less epicardial fat), defining the parietal pericardium, or its absence, is challenging or impossible.

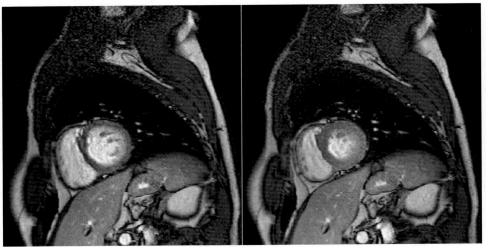

Figure 3-47. The parietal pericardium is seen surrounding the right ventricle. What is seen as well is a susceptibility artifact over the same area, which arises from the epicardium:epicardial tissue boundary. The systolic image reveals the usual separation of the parietal pericardium from the epicardium, and the parietal pericardium is now well seen anterior to the right ventricle, including its insertion into the diaphragm. The black line caused by the susceptibility artifact is now distinct and is seen to have been responsible for what appears to be pericardium. Note as well the inability to image or to depict normal parietal pericardium over much of the right ventricular free wall.

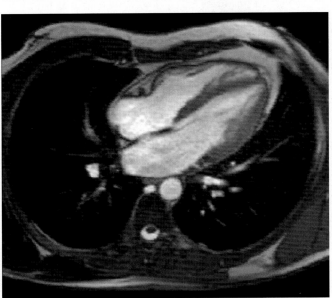

Figure 3-48. CMR SSFP imaging has achieved a central role in cardiac imaging because of its versatility and breadth of imaging. SSFP sequences are able to depict pericardial effusions and the abnormal cardiac chamber structure and motion of constriction. This image, taken in a healthy person, depicts part of the parietal pericardium where it is offset by fat (by the right atrioventricular groove).

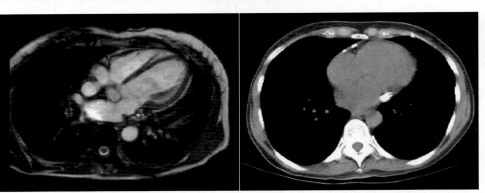

Figure 3-49. The CMR SSFP image and the non–contrast-enhanced CT image are from the same patient and are approximately commensurate. The considerable calcification in the atrioventricular groove is fairly inapparent by CMR imaging but strikingly obvious by CT scanning.

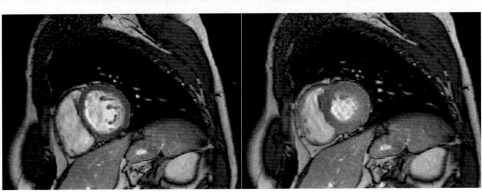

Figure 3-50. CMR SSFP short-axis images in diastole (LEFT) and systole (RIGHT). In systole, myopericardial separation occurs, projecting the parietal pericardium more distinctly away from the myocardium.

more obvious in systole, as myopericardial separation occurs (Fig. 3-50).

The traditional CMR techniques to assess pericardial thickness are T1-weighted spin echo black blood sequences. It is unknown what the contribution of gadolinium delayed contrast enhancement is to the evaluation of pericarditis and constrictive pericarditis (Fig. 3-51). Real-time imaging may be used to image changes in cardiac motion that depend on respiration, although with loss of resolution.

CMR is best used for the assessment of pericardial diseases in the following:

- Determination of the presence of pericardial fluid when it is unclear by echocardiography (Figs. 3-52 to 3-56)
- Characterization of pericardial cysts. CMR appears to be as good as echocardiography, and far better than CT, to establish that the content of the cyst is fluid-filled.
- Determination of pericardial thickness. CMR is probably the best test in existence to determine pericardial thickness, although it remains dependent on the presence of fat planes. The delineation of the myocardial:pericardial plane is more regularly feasible by CMR than by CT (Figs. 3-57 to 3-62).

Text continued on p. 47.

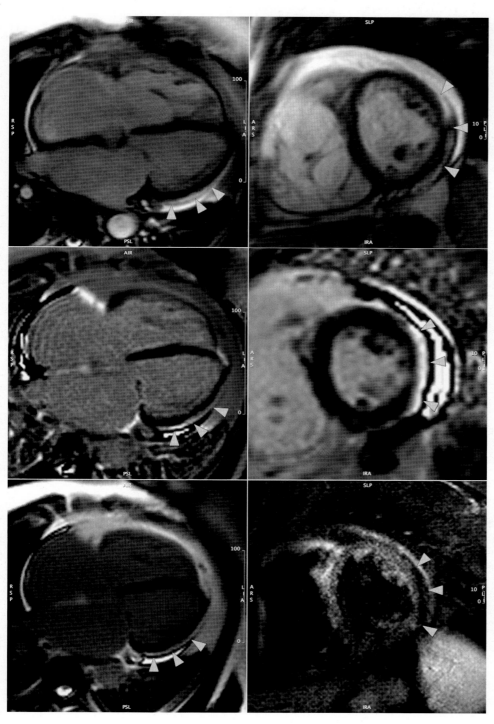

Figure 3-51. Regional pericarditis and a small pericardial effusion. TOP, SSFP 4-chamber (LEFT) and short-axis (RIGHT) views reveal a small pericardial effusion and epicardial thickening over the left ventricular free wall. MIDDLE AND BOTTOM LEFT, Late gadolinium enhancement of the epicardial thickening over the left ventricular free wall. BOTTOM RIGHT, T2 weighting reveals high signal from the same area, consistent with high water content and inflammation. (Courtesy of Matthias Friedrich, MD, Calgary, Canada.)

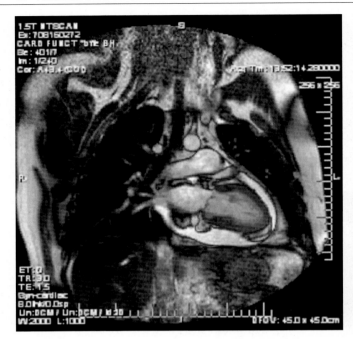

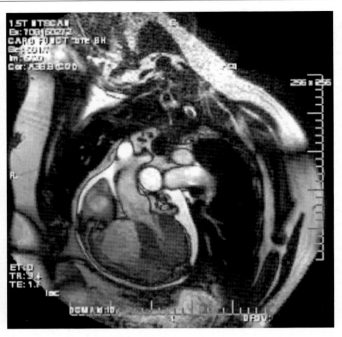

Figure 3-52. CMR SSFP sequence. The extent and distribution of pericardial fluid are apparent, as is the lack of right atrial or right ventricular chamber collapse. Susceptibility artifacts are located at many interfaces, especially the pericardial fluid : pericardial interfaces.

Figure 3-53. CMR SSFP sequence. The extent and distribution of pericardial fluid are apparent, as is the lack of right atrial or right ventricular chamber collapse. Susceptibility artifacts are located at many interfaces, especially the pericardial fluid : pericardial interfaces.

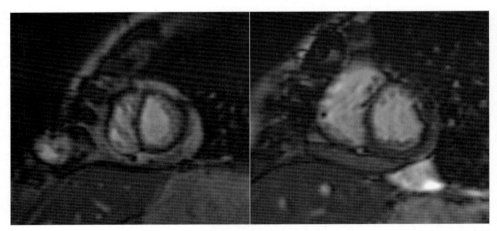

Figure 3-54. CMR SSFP sequence. The right and left ventricular cavities are normal sized. There is prominent pericardial thickening, which is circumferential and uniform at the mid left ventricle (LEFT) but greater inferiorly and nonuniform inferiorly at the base (RIGHT). There is no pericardial fluid, but there is a left pleural effusion under the posterior wall of the heart, seen on the right image.

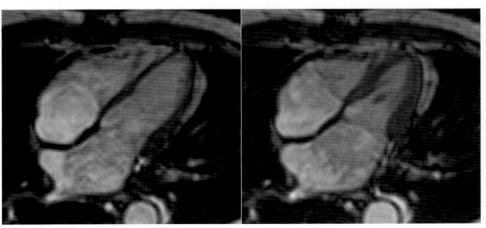

Figure 3-55. CMR SSFP sequence of constrictive pericarditis after aortocoronary bypass. Susceptibility artifacts are seen over the right ventricular and atrial and free walls, and there is artifact as well from sternal wiring. Note how the black band artifact seen in diastole (LEFT) near the right ventricular apex is absent in systole (RIGHT). Note as well the substantial dilation of the right atrium and the deviation of the interatrial septum toward the left side. The ventricular systolic function is normal. There is no pericardial fluid.

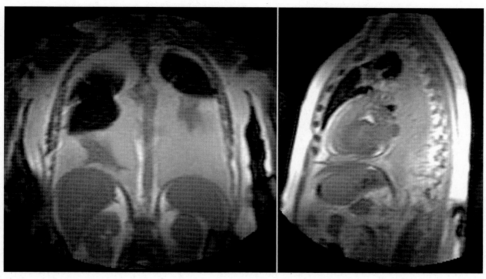

Figure 3-56. CMR is able to identify the presence of fluid with the same confidence as by ultrasonography but far more comprehensively. T2 weighting of contrast results in high signal from fluid and a bright image. This patient has large pleural effusions as well as a pericardial effusion.

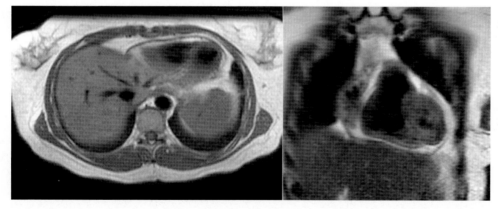

Figure 3-57. These T1-weighted spin echo black blood images are examples of how pericardial thickness is probably most convincingly assessed by CMR. The parietal pericardium lends itself to assessment where it is offset by overlying pericardial fat on the outside and epicardial fat on the inside. Delineation of the visceral pericardial thickness may be more difficult as the distinction of the myocardial:thickened epicardial border may be difficult.

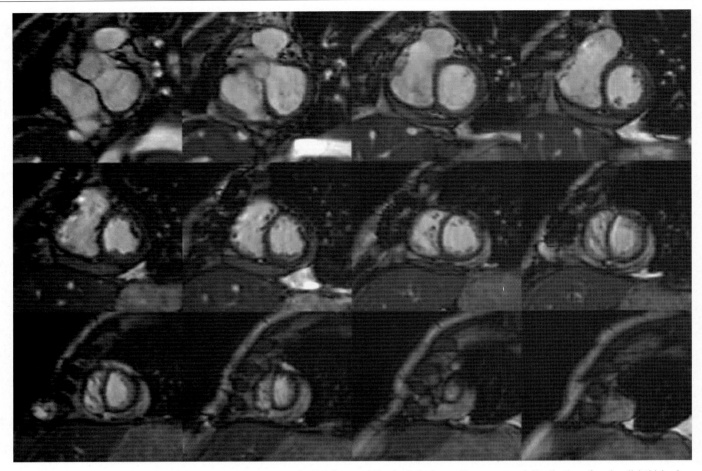

Figure 3-58. CMR cardiac cycle synchronized composite short-axis SSFP images (slices) of the heart. The extent and distribution of pericardial thickening are apparent. Several midventricular views demonstrate the abnormal early diastolic dip motion of the septum, which is not seen at all levels of the septum.

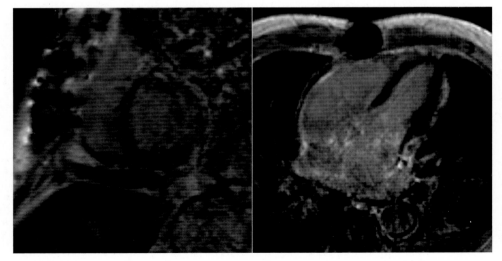

Figure 3-59. Post–aortocoronary bypass constrictive pericarditis. LEFT, CMR inversion recovery gradient echo gadolinium contrast enhancement, short axis. RIGHT, Apical 4-chamber view. Pericardial thickening exhibits complex delayed enhancement with gadolinium contrast, presumably due to tissue heterogeneity. The thickest area on the left image (posteriorly) does not enhance, but the visceral pericardium appears to enhance on both the short-axis and apical 4-chamber view images. There are prominent sternal wire artifacts that confound imaging of the anterior pericardium.

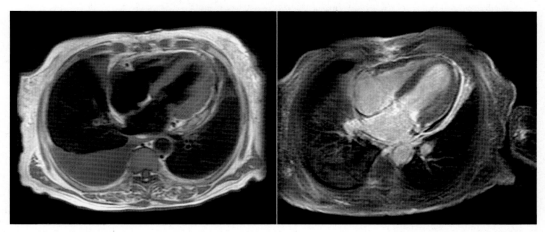

Figure 3-60. These CMR images are from the same patient with pericarditis after aortic valve replacement. The T1-weighted black blood image does not depict thickening of the parietal pericardium over the right side of the heart, where it is most easily measured. There is thickening of the pericardium or material within the pericardial space lateral to the basal left ventricle. The right image (inversion recovery gradient echo) depicts delayed enhancement of the visceral pericardial layer over the right and left ventricles and the left atrium.

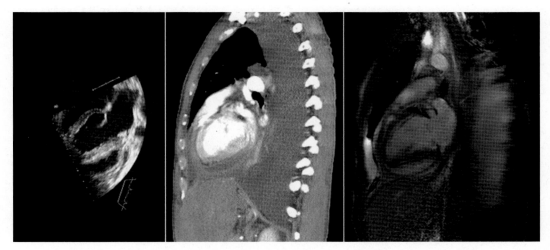

Figure 3-61. Each of these images depicts the heart cavities, the left pleural effusion, and the pericardial thickening. By transthoracic echocardiography (LEFT), inferiorly there is obvious echolucency, consistent with pericardial fluid. As well, the parietal pericardium is thickened, as is the visceral pericardium. The CT image (MIDDLE) shows layered pericardial thickening and suggests pericardial fluid, as one layer of the thickening has the same appearance as the pleural effusion. The CMR SSFP image (RIGHT) is quite convincing that there is pericardial fluid inferiorly and has delineated the pericardial layers nicely. The field of view of the echocardiographic image is very limited, but the cardiac detail is good.

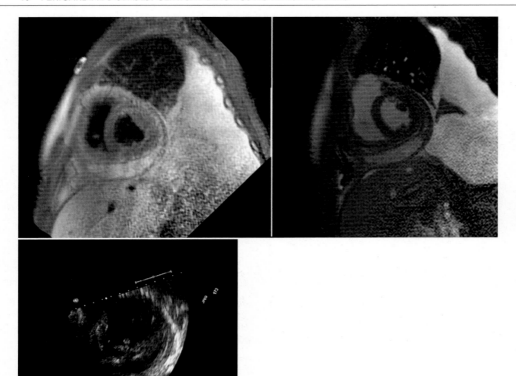

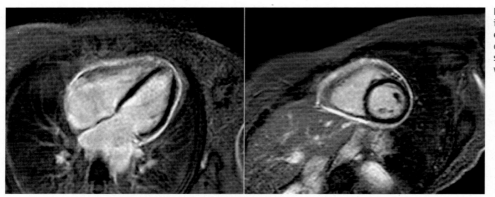

Figure 3-62. The CMR images (TOP) clearly depict the pericardial fluid inferiorly and the parietal pericardial thickening. The echocardiographic image, rotated to have the same perspective (BOTTOM), does reveal the pericardial fluid but much less detail about the pericardial layers and the rest of the thorax.

Figure 3-63. Acute pericarditis. CMR inversion recovery gadolinium delayed enhancement sequence images. Gadolinium contrast enhancement is resulting in high signal and contrast from the pericardium, which is thickened.

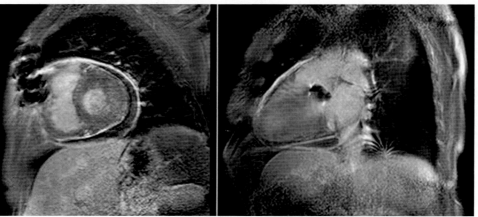

Figure 3-64. CMR inversion recovery gadolinium delayed enhancement sequence images from a patient with pericarditis after aortic valve replacement. There is delayed enhancement of both the visceral and parietal pericardial layers. As well, there is non–contrast-enhancing material within the pericardial space over the left lateral and under the posterior aspects of the heart. The pericardium over the anterior right ventricle is difficult to assess given the overlying artifacts from the sternal wires.

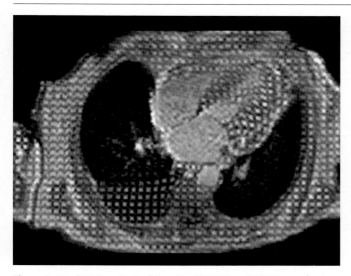

Figure 3-65. CMR "tagging" of the slice (SPAMM or CSPAMM sequence) confers a grid-like depiction that assists with determination of whether the pericardium is fused together (without slippage) or allowing normal slippage of the parietal and visceral layers, which would distort the grid pattern. In this heart, there is no slippage of the pericardial layers over the right ventricle, but there is over the left ventricular free wall. This was consistent with the overall impression of effuso-constriction, with the fluid only on the left side and frank constriction over the right side.

- Imaging of pericardial anatomy. CMR images pericardial anatomy far more comprehensively than does echocardiography and is extremely useful to further evaluate cases unsolved by echocardiography, particularly when CT scanning should be avoided, as with renal insufficiency (Figs. 3-63 to 3-66).

CMR has some important limitations for assessment of pericardial diseases:

- Constriction may occur with normal pericardial thickness.
- The depiction of epicardial thickening. Because the relaxation times of myocardium and epicardial thickening are usually similar, the determination of epicardial thickening is a challenge, as it is by CT scanning.
- CMR is insensitive to the presence of calcification.
- The requisite patient factors of being able to lie flat, to breath-hold, to tolerate claustrophobia, and to remain hemodynamically stable are significant exclusions to some CMR studies. As with CT, CMR imaging requires transport of the patient. Monitoring of the patient is more indirect for CMR than for CT.

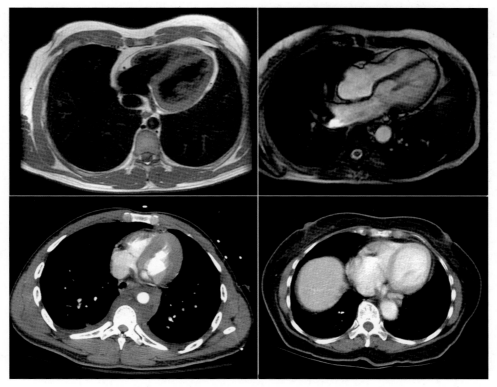

Figure 3-66. TOP LEFT, T1-weighted spin echo CMR image with black blood technique. The parietal pericardium is best seen between sandwiching epicardial and outside fat layers. TOP RIGHT, CMR SSFP sequence in the same patient. The parietal pericardium is evident although less well seen than by T1-weighted black blood imaging. BOTTOM IMAGES, CT. Epicardial and outside pericardial fat is dark (lesser attenuation coefficient as with subcutaneous fat). Depiction of parietal pericardium is more difficult by CT scanning than it is by CMR, but possible.

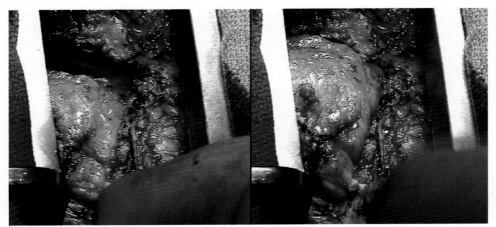

Figure 3-67. Constrictive pericarditis. The anterior pericardium has been partially resected. Systolic image (LEFT) and diastolic image (RIGHT). The right ventricle herniates outward in diastole because the right ventricular diastolic pressure is so strikingly elevated.

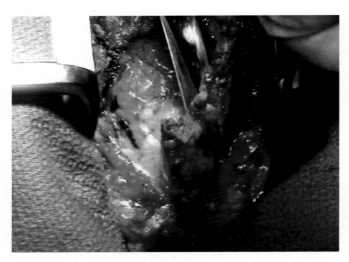

Figure 3-68. Constrictive pericarditis. The anterior pericardium is thickened, irregular, and clearly very stiff.

SURGICAL INSPECTION OF THE PERICARDIUM

Direct surgical inspection of the pericardium should be recalled as the ultimate form of pericardial imaging. It can readily provide fluid and tissue for immediate Gram staining and surgical pathologic and histologic examination, and it can be converted into a repair or drainage procedure. Surgical inspection of the pericardium may be warranted in cases of penetrating traumatic injury with tamponade or other suspected cardiac injury and in unresolved cases of constriction versus myocardial restriction, as surgery allows pericardial inspection and pericardial and myocardial biopsy (Figs. 3-67 and 3-68).

Acute Pericarditis

KEY POINTS

▸ Pericarditis is a syndrome arising from an inflammatory or infectious condition of the pericardium that may have a serious underlying cause.

▸ Knowledge of the many causes of pericarditis is essential to identifying an underlying disorder that may be more life-threatening than the pericarditis itself.

▸ The diagnostic pursuit of underlying causes should be driven by clinical suspicion.

▸ Most cases respond to analgesics and NSAIDs.

▸ Steroids are effective, but their chronic use may trigger relapses.

▸ Colchicine may have a role in treating recurrent pericarditis.

DEFINITION OF ACUTE PERICARDITIS

Acute pericarditis is a syndrome arising from an inflammatory or an infectious disease or an inflammatory state that follows an infection. Acute pericarditis may be an isolated disorder, a manifestation of another disease process, or a complication of drug use. Some cases of pericarditis develop complications (effusions, tamponade and compressive physiology, recurrences or relapses, or constrictive-compressive physiology).

Pericarditis and pericardial effusion are not synonymous. Some cases of acute pericarditis do not accumulate an effusion (because removal of fluid is as fast as production), and some cases of effusion do not have a clinical or significant histologic inflammatory component (Fig. 4-1). In acute pericarditis, there is thickening of both the parietal and serosal pericardium and rough irregularity of their surfaces (Fig. 4-2). The classic clinical triad of pericarditis is that of chest pain, pericardial friction rub, and appropriate serial electrocardiographic (ECG) changes; two of the three criteria are needed for a diagnosis.

CAUSES OF ACUTE PERICARDITIS

Idiopathic Pericarditis

Most investigations for a specific etiology, including viral investigations, will be inconclusive; thus, "idiopathic" is the single most common cause of acute pericarditis (Table 4-1). The likelihood of a case being classified as idiopathic is realistically influenced by the vigor of the attempt to identify an underlying cause.

Viral Pericarditis

After idiopathic pericarditis, viral pericarditis is believed to be the second most common form of pericarditis (Fig. 4-3). The most common specific viral causes include coxsackievirus, echovirus, adenovirus, mumps virus, varicella-zoster virus, and Epstein-Barr virus. A diagnosis is made by establishing significant difference between acute and convalescent neutralizing antibodies, although viral isolation from pericardial fluid and in situ hybridization techniques is possible. Although these techniques exist, they are not widely used. Because viral cases are generally managed similarly to idiopathic cases, viral serology testing is often omitted, effectively equating many cases of idiopathic and postviral forms of pericarditis.

Bacterial Purulent Pericarditis

The bacteria that are most commonly responsible for purulent pericarditis include streptococci, staphylococci, pneumococci, gram-negative rods, *Haemophilus influenzae, Mycoplasma, Legionella,* and others. Risk factors for the development of purulent pericarditis most commonly include pneumonia, empyema, after open chest surgery (particularly if there is mediastinitis), and immunocompromised state (particularly in children). Anaerobic bacteria generally gain access to the pericardium from fistulization from the esophagus or gut.

Surprisingly, bacterial pericarditis often lacks all the typical features of pericarditis and may therefore be recognized late or unfortunately only post mortem. A high degree of clinical suspicion is therefore needed. The exuberant inflammatory response to bacterial pericarditis commonly progresses to effusion and tamponade.[1]

The management of bacterial infection includes establishing a prompt diagnosis, prescribing appropriate intravenous antibiotics, and considering early drainage, which may prevent early tamponade and late constriction.[1]

Tuberculous Pericarditis

Tuberculosis is now a rare cause of pericarditis at most centers in North America (formerly 4%, now less than 0.5% of all patients affected with pericarditis), but it remains an important cause of pericarditis, particularly in underdeveloped countries and in some immigrant populations. The Transkei region in South Africa remains highly affected by tuberculous disease, rendering tuberculosis one of the most common forms of heart disease in that region ("Transkei heart").

Approximately 1% to 2% of patients with tuberculous pulmonary infection have cardiac involvement. Tuberculous pericarditis may occur secondary to hematogenous spread or erosion of parabronchial or mediastinal lymph nodes into the pericardium.

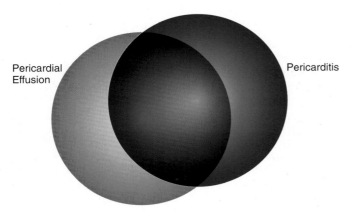

Figure 4-1. Pericarditis and pericardial effusion are *not* synonymous. Some cases of acute pericarditis do not accumulate an effusion (because removal of fluid is as fast as production), and some cases of effusion do not have a clinical or significant histologic inflammatory component.

Pericardial Effusion

Pericarditis

Tuberculous pericarditis appears not to occur without extracardiac foci, although the extracardiac foci may be clinically less prominent than cardiac involvement or clinically silent. Increase in human immunodeficiency virus (HIV) coinfection is leading to increases in tuberculosis and tuberculous pericarditis cases. The optimal management of tuberculous heart disease alone (with respect to the permutations of usage of steroids, early drainage, and early pericardiectomy to avoid late constriction) has never been established; many studies, although helpful, did not yield consistent observations or offer consistent conclusions. The optimal management of tuberculous pericardial disease with HIV coinfection is even less established.[2]

The presentations of tuberculous pericardial disease are sufficiently vague as to prompt consideration "in all instances of pericarditis without a rapidly self-limiting course."[3] Cardiac-specific presentations include pericarditis, pericardial effusion, pericardial tamponade, effuso-constrictive pericarditis, and constrictive pericarditis (Table 4-2). Concurrent myocardial involvement may also occur. The course of tuberculous pericardial disease is particularly difficult to predict once it begins: which effusions progress to tamponade, which tamponade cases recur, which pericarditis cases progress to constriction, which effuso-constrictive cases subside, or which cases eventually evolve to calcific constriction. The therapeutic effect of antimicrobial therapy is prominently beneficial (Figs. 4-4 and 4-5), irrespective of the controversial benefits from either steroid use or early open surgical drainage.

Standard four-drug regimen of antituberculous antimicrobial chemotherapy is indicated for 6 months. Drainage or stripping is considered on the basis of the presentation and is variably performed, depending on the medical center's practice and experience. Drainage of an effusion may offer a diagnosis of tuberculosis if it is not already established. Drainage of an effusion-producing tamponade (percutaneous or surgical) is therapeutic and may be diagnostic if a diagnosis has not already been established. Some cases of acute tuberculosis-related constriction are initially transient; the proportion is unclear. Surgical stripping of constrictive pericardium is therapeutic but entails risk. The optimal timing of surgery is also unclear. In many experienced centers, most cases of noncalcified tuberculous constriction proceed to surgical pericardiectomy after 4 to 8 weeks of antituberculous therapy and medical optimization.

The rate of progression of early tuberculous effusions to tamponade is substantial but unpredictable. Pericardiocentesis, although low risk, is not without risk, and open surgical drainage

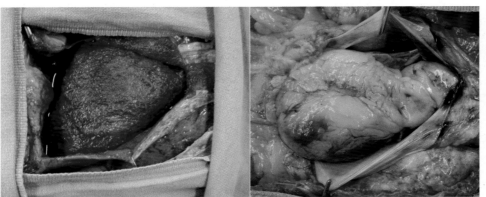

Figure 4-2. The surgical photograph (LEFT) reveals findings of acute pericarditis—thickening of both the parietal (retracted backward in the superior field of the image) and serosal pericardium over the heart and rough irregularity of their surfaces. The serosal layer is clearly thickened and now opaque, as the heart cannot be seen under it. RIGHT, For purposes of comparison, a normal heart (at autopsy) is shown. (Courtesy of Jagdish Butany, MD, Toronto, Canada.)

Table 4-1. Causes of Acute Pericarditis

Idiopathic, presumed postviral

Infectious

  Viral

  Fungal

  Tuberculous

  Protozoal

  Human immunodeficiency virus (HIV)

  Rickettsia

  Lyme disease

  Bacterial

Metabolic

  Uremia

  Dialysis related

  Myxedema

  Amyloidosis

Drugs

  Hydralazine, procainamide, isoniazid, minoxidil, methysergide

  Anticoagulants

Iatrogenic

  Drug related

  Catheter related

  Intervention related

  Pacemaker or ICD related

Inflammatory

  Systemic lupus erythematosus, rheumatoid arthritis

  Familial Mediterranean fever, Whipple disease, polyarteritis nodosa, Wegener granulomatosis

  Sarcoidosis, Reiter syndrome, Behçet syndrome, ankylosing spondylitis, dermatomyositis

  Postpericardiotomy syndrome

  Late post–myocardial infarction (Dressler syndrome)

  Acute myocardial infarction

  Post-traumatic

Traumatic

  Blunt

  Penetrating

    Aortic dissection

    Ruptured sinus of Valsalva

ICD, implantable cardioverter defibrillator.

Table 4-2. Management of Tuberculous Pericardial Disease According to Complication and Presentation

Effusion

  Antimicrobial therapy

  Drainage (usually as part of a diagnostic effort)

Tamponade

  Drainage

  Antimicrobial therapy

  Steroids commonly

Effusion-constriction

  Antimicrobial therapy

  Drainage. Many centers recommend pericardiectomy for tuberculous effuso-constrictive pericarditis to obviate late-state fibrocalcific constrictive pericarditis.

  Steroids commonly

Constriction

  Antimicrobial therapy

  Steroids commonly

  Pericardiectomy

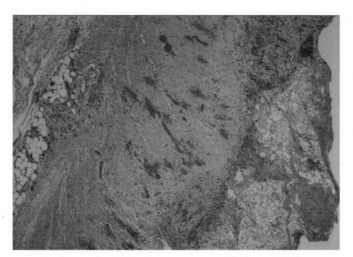

Figure 4-3. Viral pericarditis with ongoing nonspecific inflammation. Fat planes of variable thickness are present on either side of the parietal pericardium (the basis of CMR and CT imaging of the pericardium). (Courtesy of Geoffrey Gardiner, MD, Toronto, Canada.)

is also not without risk. Pericardiocentesis is performed in most cases of pericardial effusions that are undiagnosed when tuberculosis is suspected, as fluid evaluation and culture may be diagnostic. Overt tuberculous disease with a pericardial effusion but without tamponade does not necessitate pericardiocentesis; many experts suggest an early drainage procedure to obviate this complication. In cases without proven but with suspected tuberculosis, consideration of surgical drainage offers tissue for staining and culture for diagnosis as well. Early open surgical drainage

eliminates the need for pericardiocentesis but does not appear to reduce mortality from pericarditis or need for pericardiectomy to alleviate constriction.[4] The progression rate to constriction requiring pericardiectomy is variable in different published reports: 0%,[5] 8% steroid treated and 12% non–steroid treated,[4] or 57%.[3] Recommendations of prophylactic pericardiectomy also range widely. In general, prophylactic pericardiectomy is not recommended.[6]

    Pericardial fluid cultures are positive in only one third to two thirds of cases of tuberculous pericarditis but take weeks to yield a diagnosis. Tuberculous pericardial fluid is usually an exudate with elevated protein concentration and lymphocyte-monocyte predominance after the second week (polymorphonuclear cells may predominate in the first 2 weeks). Tuberculous

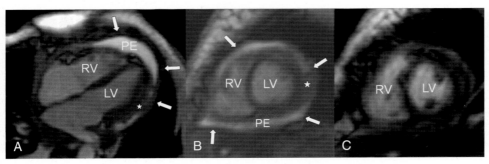

Figure 4-4. Steady-state free precession (SSFP) CMR imaging. End-diastolic 4-chamber (**A**) and short-axis (**B**) views demonstrate the presence of a pericardial effusion (PE), with epicardial fibrin strands *(asterisk)* and pericardial thickening *(arrows)* at presentation. Follow-up after 3 months of antituberculous chemotherapy shows resolution of the pericardial effusion (**C**). RV, right ventricle; LV, left ventricle. (Courtesy of Jan-Peter Smedema, MD, Capetown, South Africa.)

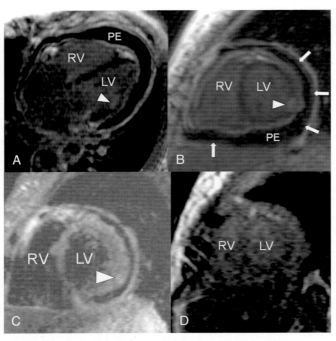

Figure 4-5. Inversion recovery gradient echo CMR imaging 10 minutes after the administration of 0.1 mmol/kg gadolinium-DTPA (**A**, **B**, and **D**) and T2-weighted short T1 inversion recovery sequence (**C**) demonstrate the presence of a protein-rich pericardial effusion (PE), pericardial thickening *(arrows)*, and a myocardial tuberculoma in the posterolateral left ventricular wall *(triangle)* at presentation. Follow-up after 3 months of antituberculous chemotherapy shows resolution of the pericardial effusion and myocardial tuberculoma (**D**). RV, right ventricle; LV, left ventricle. (Courtesy of Jan-Peter Smedema, MD, Capetown, South Africa.)

Table 4-3. Pericardial Fluid Levels of Adenosine Deaminase and Interferon-γ in Different Diseases

	Komsuoglu[8]	Burgess[9]	
	ADA (U/L)	ADA (U/L)	Interferon-γ (pg/L)
Tuberculous	126 ± 17	72 [10-304]	>1000
Idiopathic	29 ± 9		
Neoplastic	27 ± 7	27 [1-260]	20 ± 15
Purulent	30 ± 13		
Radiotherapy	26		
Nontuberculous infections		41 [15-166]	20 ± 10
Effusions of unclear etiology		15 [1-103]	

ADA, adenosine deaminase.

Table 4-4.[7-10] Cutoff Levels for the Detection of Tuberculous Disease

	ADA Cutoff		Interferon-γ Cutoff (200 pg/L)
	40 U/L	30 U/L	
Sensitivity	93%	94%	100%
Specificity	97%	68%	100%

ADA, adenosine deaminase.

pericardial fluid is blood stained in the majority of cases, frankly sanguineous in some, and often with shaggy fibrinous stranding.[6]

The low retrieval rate of tuberculous bacilli from pericardial fluid engendered the development of other assays. Elevated lymphocyte levels in tuberculous pericardial effusions confer high fluid levels of lymphocyte-produced substances, such as the purine metabolite adenosine deaminase, interferon-γ, and lysozyme (Table 4-3).[7-9] Proposed diagnostic "cutoff" levels for adenosine deaminase are inconsistent (30 to 70 U/L), and adenosine deaminase appears to be elevated in rheumatoid arthritis and sarcoidosis cases as well as in some empyemas (Table 4-4).[7-10] Polymerase chain reaction is a rapid, very specific, and fairly sensitive assay for the detection of tuberculous infection. Its sensitivity is similar to that of adenosine deaminase assay, but it appears to be more specific (Table 4-5).[10]

Some aspects of tuberculous disease overlap with inflammatory granulomatous disease (Figs. 4-6 and 4-7). The presence of tissue granulomas without bacilli is helpful but not specific for tuberculosis; it may also be seen with rheumatoid arthritis and sarcoidosis. Lymphocytosis, low glucose concentration, and elevated adenosine deaminase level may also be seen in rheumatoid arthritis and sarcoidosis. It remains unestablished how long it takes for tubercles to form, what proportion of cases develop them, and how their time course is affected by antimicrobial treatment and steroids.[4]

A presumptive diagnosis of pericardial tuberculosis is made when there is proof of tuberculosis elsewhere in the patient, positive contact history in addition to PPD conversion, lymphocytic pericardial exudate with positive adenosine deaminase levels or polymerase chain reaction, or appropriate response to antituberculous agents.[11] A definite or final diagnosis of tubercu-

Table 4-5. Pericardial Fluid Testing in Tuberculous, Malignant, and Idiopathic Effusions[10]

	Tuberculous	**Malignant**	**Idiopathic**
Lymphocytes	68 ± 25	22 ± 26	46 ± 33
White blood cells (/mm³)	45 ± 3500	2500 ± 2200	2000 ± 2500
Red blood cells	77,000 ± 150,000	1,150,000 ± 1,300,000	3000 ± 8000
Protein (g/dL)	5.1 ± 0.9	4.9 ± 1.4	4.9 ± 0.9
Glucose (g/dL)	48 ± 37	65 ± 73	130 ± 90
LDH (mg/dL)	3200 ± 2000	5000 ± 5400	1900 ± 3400
ADA (U/L)	95 ± 57	27 ± 15	32 ± 32
	PCR	**ADA > 40 U/L**	
Sensitivity	75%	83%	
Specificity	100%	78%	
Positive predictive value	100%	46%	
Negative predictive value	95%	79%	

ADA, adenosine deaminase; LDH, lactate dehydrogenase; PCR, polymerase chain reaction.

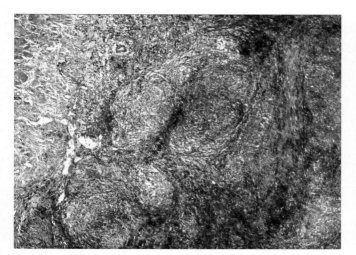

Figure 4-6. Tuberculous constrictive pericarditis. Large granuloma with giant cells, central necrotic debris, and lymphocytic infiltration. (Courtesy of Ashok Mukherjee, MD, Scarborough, Canada.)

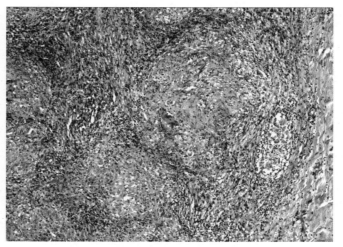

Figure 4-7. Tuberculous constrictive pericarditis. Higher magnification view: granuloma with giant cells, lymphocytic infiltration, and central necrotic debris. (Courtesy of Ashok Mukherjee, MD, Scarborough, Canada.)

lous pericardial disease is made with positive staining for tubercle bacilli or positive culture of either pericardial fluid or pericardial tissue.

The use of steroids remains controversial. In the largest and best placebo-controlled trial, 143 patients treated with four antituberculous agents (isoniazid, streptomycin, rifampin, and pyrazinamide) were randomized to placebo versus 30 to 60 mg of prednisolone tapering during 11 weeks, yielding some evidence of faster improvement (Table 4-6).[4] Studies have yielded inconsistent results of steroid use on the rate of pericardial fluid resorption. Some centers include a course of steroids in the acute phase of tuberculous pericarditis because there is some appearance of mortality reduction, and need for repeated drainage or pericardiectomy, although this has not been clearly proven.

Fungal Pericarditis

Fungal pericarditis may be caused by histoplasmosis, blastomycosis, aspergillosis, or candidiasis. Histoplasmosis pericarditis resembles tuberculous pericarditis other than that it seldom incites late calcific constrictive pericarditis. Serologic testing for histoplasmosis is useful other than in an endemic area, such as the Ohio River and St. Lawrence River valleys.

Blastomycosis, aspergillosis, and candidiasis of the pericardium are generally subacute disorders and nearly invariably progress to constriction. Fungal infections are more commonly seen in the immunocompromised population.

Table 4-6. Glucocorticoid Steroid Use in Acute Tuberculous Pericardial Disease[4]

	Steroid Treated	Placebo
Recovery (HR, JVP, and physical activity) significantly faster		
Acute-phase mortality	4%	11%
Adverse events during 24 months		
Death due to pericarditis	3%	14%
Pericardiectomy	8%	12%
Repeated pericardiocentesis	9%	23%
Open surgical drainage	4%	9%
With more than 1 event	22%	46%
Status at 24 months		
Total favorable	96%	84%
Favorable after pericardiocentesis, open drainage, or pericardiectomy	16%	30%
Alive but with ≥2 factors abnormal	1%	3%

HR, heart rate; JVP, jugular venous pressure.

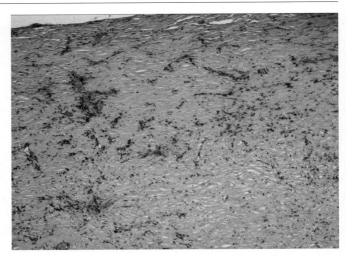

Figure 4-8. Dressler syndrome. Pericardial biopsy specimen shows increased connective tissue and lymphocytic infiltration. (Courtesy of Geoffrey Gardiner, MD, Toronto, Canada.)

Rheumatoid Pericarditis

Pericarditis associated with rheumatoid arthritis is generally mild and is seen in several percent of cases clinically and 50% at autopsy. Pericardial involvement is more common with nodular disease. Serology is diagnostic for rheumatoid arthritis. Rarely, rheumatoid arthritis causes *cholesterol pericarditis*. Pericardial fluid typically has low glucose and complement concentrations. The pathologic distinction of rheumatoid arthritis granulomas or nodules from tuberculosis granulomas may be difficult. Progression to tamponade is less common than with systemic lupus erythematosus (SLE). Late constriction may occur. Pericardial involvement may occur in both rheumatoid arthritis and juvenile rheumatoid arthritis.

Systemic Lupus Erythematosus Pericarditis

Pericarditis is a prominent aspect of SLE. Pericarditis is the most common form of cardiac disease encountered by SLE patients; it is the presentation in 40%, and it occurs in most patients at some time. Effusions and recurrences are common, and tamponade may occur. Late constriction is also possible. Pericardial fluid typically contains LE cells. Acute pericarditis may occur in both classic SLE and drug-induced lupus.

Scleroderma Pericarditis

Acute pericarditis is seen in about 10% of cases. Concurrent pulmonary hypertension, with right ventricular and atrial hypertrophy, and higher right-sided diastolic pressures complicate the assessment of pericardial tamponade. Late constriction may occur.

Postinfarction Pericarditis

Postinfarction pericarditis may occur early (episternopericarditis), late (delayed postinfarction pericarditis, or Dressler syndrome), or in association with procedures or subacute myocardial rupture.

Early Postinfarction Pericarditis (Episternopericarditis)

Early pericarditis may develop in approximately 10% of cases of transmural infarction, typically on the second or third day after infarction. Inflammation from necrosis of the epicardium is believed to underlie early pericarditis. Most cases are asymptomatic. Early postinfarction pericarditis is unlikely to progress to tamponade. The ECG is more difficult to interpret for pericarditic changes when the baseline morphology is already abnormal from the infarction. Atypical T-wave evolution may be a superior sign to ST elevation in postinfarction patients. The risk:benefit ratio of anticoagulation needs careful assessment in cases of pericarditis because hemorrhagic conversion rates appear higher. Some cases of early pericarditis reflect complications of associated interventional procedures or pacemakers. Leaking false aneurysms and subacute free wall rupture may also present with pericarditis.

Delayed Postinfarction Pericarditis (Dressler Syndrome)

Pericarditis occurring more than 2 weeks after infarction is usually an inflammatory disorder (Dressler syndrome) (Fig. 4-8), although it may also occasionally be due to a slowly leaking false aneurysm. Dressler syndrome may be recurrent or may lead to tamponade or late constriction. The erythrocyte sedimentation rate is elevated. Distinguishing of pericarditic pains after myocardial infarction from ischemic pains after myocardial infarction may be difficult in some cases. The management of postinfarction pericarditis is similar to that of early epvisternopericarditis.

Iatrogenic Pericarditis

The most common causes of iatrogenic pericarditis are the following:

- Drugs
  - Hydralazine, procainamide, isoniazid, minoxidil, methysergide
  - Anticoagulants, fibrinolytics
  - High-dose cyclophosphamide
- Coronary interventional procedures
- Insertion of pacemaker and implantable cardioverter defibrillator leads
- Esophageal sclerotherapy
- Pericarditis is seen in 5% to 30% of cases after open heart surgery and may progress to tamponade or late constriction.
- Pericarditis secondary to radiotherapy is due to the radiotherapy itself or lysis of tumor; it may be associated with tamponade, late constriction, and concurrent myocardial fibrosis.

Metabolic Pericarditis

Uremic pericarditis is encountered in a third of uremic patients. The associated mortality is high. Dialysis-related pericarditis is common and occurs often without typical features of acute pericarditis. Associated effusions with some cases of tamponade and late cases of constriction are seen. Myxedema is associated in about a third of cases with pericarditis but more often with effusions alone. Myxedema-related effusions may have cholesterol particles. Effusions regress when a euthyroid state is re-established. Amyloidosis is usually associated with small pericardial effusions, with a low likelihood of tamponade. Late constriction has been described.

CLINICAL PRESENTATION OF ACUTE PERICARDITIS

Chest Pain

Somatic-type pain is seen in the large majority of cases of pericarditis: sharp in nature and aggravated by deeper inspiration and by assuming a recumbent position. Pericarditic pains are often precordial; some run from the trapezius ridge down the left arm. A visceral-type pain is seen in a minority of cases of pericarditis: dull, pressure-like, and midline substernal or epigastric pains may be difficult to distinguish from myocardial ischemia or abdominal disease. In some cases, especially after open heart surgery or with dialysis, there is no pain or very little.

Although many cases of pericarditis are straightforward, in others there are many potentially confusing aspects of overlap of pericarditis and ischemic pains. Pericarditis with visceral-type pain in the substernal location is readily confused with ischemic pain. Exertional pains are common in pericarditis because breathing deepens with exertion. Pericarditic pains may improve with nitroglycerin because nitroglycerin reduces the heart volumes and may lessen pericardial friction and pain. However, the extent of improvement with nitroglycerin is less with pericarditis than with angina. Pericardial friction rubs are easily missed if there are concurrent murmurs. Cardiac biomarkers (e.g., troponins) are often elevated in pericarditis but are not adverse prognosticators. ECG manifestations of pericarditis and ischemia overlap. Distinguishing the ECG patterns of juvenile repolarization pattern and

pericarditis may be very difficult.[12] The time course of pericarditis is hours, days, or even a week, whereas ischemic pains last minutes or a few hours. This distinguishing feature is not helpful early in the presentation of either disorder. Some patients with infarctions have stuttering pains for days.[13]

Pericardial "Friction" Rubs

The pericardial rub sounds like friction but is not clearly due to friction—a rub may be present even when a pericardial effusion is present that separates most of the visceral and parietal layers. Notably, there is poor correlation of rubs with the amount of pericardial fluid.[14] It is possible that some pericardial reflections remain with contact of the pericardium in spite of separation of pericardial layers by fluid in most places. A "friction" rub is pathognomonic of pericarditis, although imperfectly sensitive for the diagnosis and with imperfect interphysician correlation. Rubs "squeak" like old leather or "crunch" like walking on dry snow or "scratch" like fingernails on the scalp. Rubs are typically transient; thus, repeated examination is needed to detect them. The rub has several phases that correspond to the motion of the heart—systolic motion, early diastolic filling motion, and late diastolic atrial contraction and filling motion (when in sinus rhythm). Most rubs are triphasic or biphasic (ventricular systole and atrial systole). Monophasic rubs have the least predictive value because they are readily confused with systolic murmurs.

Optimal positioning of the patient and bedside examination technique increase detection:

- Supine position of the patient
- Rolling the patient into the left lateral position
- Sitting, leaning the patient forward
- Lying the patient supine with arms raised over the head
- Listening at end-expiration
- Use of the diaphragm to hear high-frequency components
- Pericardial rubs are associated with the cardiac cycle; pleural rubs are associated with the respiratory cycle.

DIAGNOSIS OF ACUTE PERICARDITIS

The Role of Electrocardiography

ECG abnormalities are present in 90% of cases (Figs. 4-9 and 4-10). All four stages are seen in only 50% of cases, and only if the underlying ECG is normal. Stage one may be diagnostic: ST elevation *concave upward* and usually less than 5 mm. Sinus tachycardia is common when pain is severe. Atrial fibrillation is seen in about 5% of cases. The differential diagnosis of ST elevation includes infarction or ischemia, early repolarization, left ventricular aneurysm, bundle branch block, paced rhythm, and metabolic disturbances.

Potential Problems in the Electrocardiographic Assessment

The slow evolution of ECG changes of pericarditis (compared with ischemic or infarction changes) supports the diagnosis of

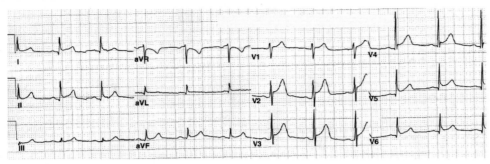

Figure 4-9. ECG of a 25-year-old student with pleuritic chest pains and a pericardial friction rub shows a widespread concave upward ST elevation (<5 mm) and PR elevation in lead aVR. This case of idiopathic pericarditis resolved with NSAIDs and analgesia, and there were no recurrences during 4 years.

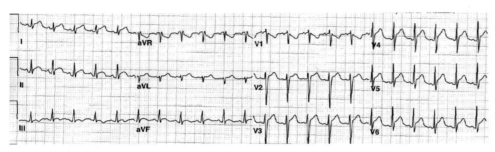

Figure 4-10. A 63-year-old man with several types of chest pains, including pleuritic pains, after an aortocoronary bypass. There was a loud pericardial friction rub. The ECG reveals widespread concave upward ST elevation, and PR deviation-elevation in lead aVR. This case of early postoperative pericarditis resolved with NSAIDs and analgesia in 3 days, and there was no associated tamponade.

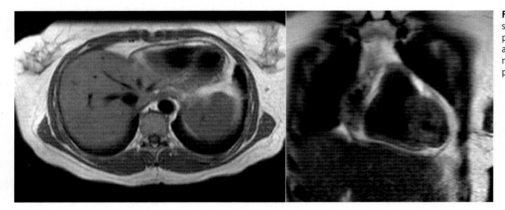

Figure 4-11. CMR T1-weighted black blood spin echo sequences. The parietal pericardium is well seen between epicardial and pericardial fat layers. The thickness is not increased. (Clinical diagnosis of acute pericarditis.)

pericarditis in retrospect. Baseline ECG abnormalities render it much less sensitive and specific for the detection of pericarditis. The presence of atrial fibrillation will confound the search for PR depression. Some patients have postinfarction or acute infarction-related pericarditis, and in such cases ECG changes of pericarditis are superimposed on those of infarction, frequently resulting in nondiagnostic changes.

The Role of Echocardiography

Echocardiography is not required to make a diagnosis of pericarditis. Most cases of pericarditis do not develop significant effusions; hence, echocardiography lacks specificity and sensitivity for the diagnosis of pericarditis. It is common practice to perform echocardiography in suspected cases of pericarditis to assist with the diagnosis, but the contribution is unclear. Echocardiography is useful to assess for *complications of pericarditis,* such as effusions and tamponade, and underlying causes of pericarditis, such as infarction and aortic dissection.

The Role of Chest Radiography

Posteroanterior and lateral chest radiographs are indicated in all cases of pericarditis to assess whether there are obvious signs of pleural disease, adjacent pulmonary parenchymal disease, cardiomegaly (possible effusion), or aortic disease.

The Role of Cardiac Magnetic Resonance

The role of cardiac magnetic resonance (CMR) in routine evaluation of pericarditis is unknown. CMR is able to depict some findings consistent with acute pericarditis: pericardial thickening and delayed gadolinium hyperenhancement. Pericardial thickening, though, is seen in some but not all cases of pericarditis and is not specific for acute pericarditis. The sensitivity and specificity of delayed hyperenhancement for the diagnosis of acute pericarditis are unknown (Figs. 4-11 to 4-14).

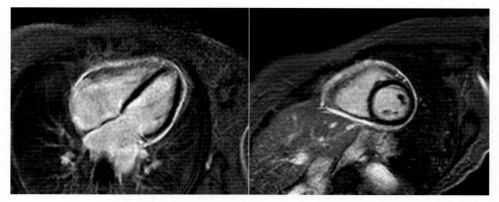

Figure 4-12. Inversion recovery gradient echo CMR imaging. The pericardium over the ventricular surfaces exhibits prominent delayed hyperenhancement (high signal). The hyperenhanced pericardium is most easily seen when the adjacent tissue has low signal (such as ventricular myocardium). A thick layer of adjacent myocardium more clearly confers the impression of hyperenhancement as the contrast of the two is obvious. Conversely, if the adjacent myocardium is thin (RV or atria) the degree of hyperenhancement of the pericardium is less clearly depicted. (Courtesy of Jan-Peter Smedema, MD, Capetown, South Africa.)

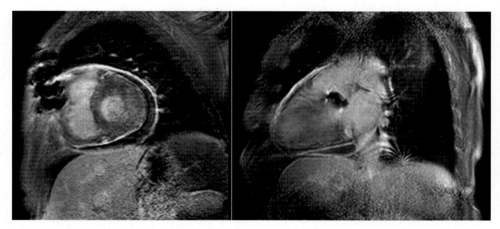

Figure 4-13. CMR hyperenhancement (high signal due to gadolinium contrast and inversion recovery sequence) in parietal and visceral pericardium is seen over extensive surfaces in this patient. There is a small pericardial effusion around the left side of the heart and posteriorly as well, with low signal, that offers higher contrast to the hyperenhancing pericardial layers as the contrast of the two is obvious. There are susceptibility artifacts arising from the sternal wires, confusing the assessment of the anterior pericardium. (Courtesy of Jan-Peter Smedema MD, Capetown, South Africa.)

The Role of Fluid or Tissue Analysis

Unless the patient is very sick, the case is very complicated, or a treatable infectious cause is suspected, the yield of pericardial fluid analysis and of pericardial biopsy in cases of isolated uncomplicated pericarditis, with or without effusion, is too low to routinely justify their routine use.

The Role of Laboratory Investigations

The minimum diagnostic testing for acute pericarditis includes history and physical examination, ECG, chest radiograph, complete blood count, renal function tests, electrolyte determinations, erythrocyte sedimentation rate, and creatine kinase and troponin concentrations. Clinical evaluation (history taking and physical examination) is critical to guide specific investigation of an underlying cause and to determine whether there are symptoms and signs of an associated pericardial effusion with hemodynamic significance.

Troponin levels are elevated in one third (32%) of cases of acute pericarditis. Troponin elevation is not an adverse prognosticator.[6] Creatine kinase elevations are consistent with pericarditis-myocarditis, or postinfarction pericarditis. If clinical suspicion of underlying disease is prominent, the appropriate testing is SLE serology, thyroid function, and rheumatoid arthritis. Echocardiography is not required for a first uncomplicated episode. Admission to the hospital is reasonable for those in need of pain control, those in whom there is need to exclude an underlying cause, and those in whom there is or may be tamponade.

COMPLICATIONS OF ACUTE PERICARDITIS

Potential complications of acute pericarditis include the following:

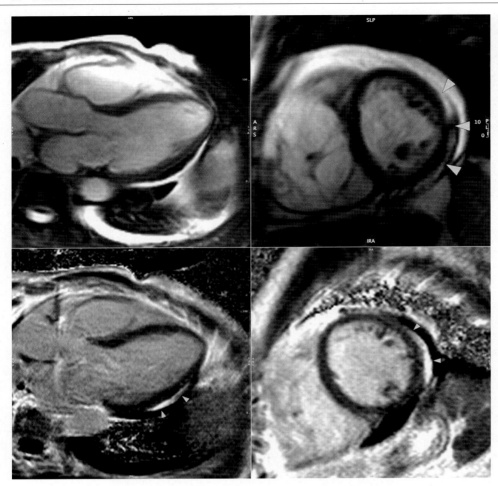

Figure 4-14. Regional pericarditis. TOP, CMR SSFP sequences. BOTTOM, Late gadolinium enhancement. LEFT IMAGES, Four-chamber views. RIGHT IMAGES, Short-axis views. The SSFP images reveal a small pericardial effusion, a left pleural effusion, and thickening of the epicardial surface of the heart over the left ventricle. The same area of thickening demonstrates late gadolinium enhancement. (Courtesy of Matthias Friedrich, MD, Calgary.)

- Recurrences (involve 10% to 25% of all cases)
- Pericardial effusions do develop in some cases; most do not progress.
- Tamponade occurs but is not usual.

Other potential complications include the following:

- Effuso-constriction
- Constriction
- Atrial arrhythmias
- Heart failure may develop if the myocarditis component of combined myocarditis-pericarditis is prominent.

TREATMENT OF ACUTE PERICARDITIS

Bed rest is appropriate to avoid aggravation of pericarditis pain and lessens analgesic needs. Analgesia and anti-inflammatories (aspirin or NSAIDs) should be taken as needed. Concurrent anticoagulation use during pericarditis increases the chance of effusion and of tamponade; therefore, anticoagulation must be used cautiously during acute pericarditis (e.g., consider changing warfarin to heparin during the acute phase). Steroids are effective to relieve pain but if given for more than a week may increase the chance of relapse when they are tapered.[15] Clinical follow-up is needed. Prophylactic methylprednisolone does not reduce the incidence of postpericardiotomy syndrome in children.[16]

Colchicine for Relapsing Pericarditis

Repeated relapses may occur in 10% to 25% of all cases. Colchicine has been shown to be generally well tolerated and effective in reducing episodes of relapse and in getting patients off chronic prednisone treatment. In a study in which 51 patients were treated for ≤10 years for recurrent pericarditis, the combination of prednisone (20 to 60 mg/day) and colchicine (1 mg/day) enabled patients to undergo tapering and discontinuation of the steroid within 6 months. No recurrences were noted within 18 to 34 months—contrasting with a total of 26 relapses before colchicine.[17] It is unclear and not widely accepted whether colchicine should be used for treatment of uncomplicated first episodes of pericarditis or for its prevention after pericardiotomy.[18] Colchicine is probably best reserved for use after the third or fourth episode or when steroid use is becoming chronic.

In the more recent and larger COPE Trial (COlchicine for acute PEricarditis),[19] 120 patients with a *first* episode of acute idiopathic, postviral, or postpericardiotomy pericarditis were randomized to either ASA alone or ASA plus colchicine 1.0 to 2.0 mg for the first day and then 0.5 to 1.0 mg/day for 3 months. The primary endpoint of recurrence was reduced by two thirds from 32% to 11% ($P = 0.004$; number needed to treat = 5) and the secondary endpoint of symptom persistence at 72 hours was also reduced by two thirds from 37% to 12% ($P = 0.003$). Corticosteroid use was an independent risk for recurrences (OR 4.30; 95% confidence 1.21 to 15.25; $P = 0.024$). Over the 18 months of follow-up, no episodes of tamponade or constriction developed, underscoring the variety of these complications of recurrent pericarditis.[20]

Pericardiectomy for Relapsing Pericarditis

Pericardiectomy may be used to treat chronic relapsing pericarditis that has failed medical management. However, as well as concerns about surgical morbidity and mortality, there clearly are failures to this procedure; complete removal of pericardium is difficult, the inflammatory disorder may persist on the epicardium, and the inflammatory disorder may persist on the pleura. Although some surgical reports have been optimistic,[21] in the series by Fowler and Harbin, followed for 5 to 10 years, only 2 of 9 patients experienced clear improvement with pericardiotomy.[20,22]

CASE 1

History

A 30-year-old man had experienced more than 10 episodes of pericarditis that followed an initial viral illness. The episodes were symptomatic, and many were associated with small- to moderate-sized effusions. Although initially there was good therapeutic response to steroids, each time that steroids were weaned, the pericarditis recurred. There were also steroid-related side effects. An attempt to wean the patient off the steroids with colchicine was unsuccessful, and colchicine-related side effects were bothersome. Recurrent episodes remained debilitating.

▸ No underlying systemic illness or infection was identified.

▸ He underwent surgical pericardiectomy as recurrences continued unabated. After surgery, he was weaned from steroids and has had no recurrences.

Comments

▸ Idiopathic pericarditis with characteristic recurrences during steroid withdrawal

▸ Pericardial effusions did develop in association with the pericarditic episodes, an inconstant occurrence in pericarditis.

▸ No tamponade (or constriction) developed during or after more than a dozen episodes of pericarditis, although effusions were recurrent and the pericardium was developing subclinical thickening.

▸ Surgical pericardiectomy fortunately alleviated the disorder. Pericardiectomy is not without risk or chance of failure, as residual pericardial tissue, including visceral pericardium, may be subject to recurrent pericarditis and could potentially evolve to constriction.

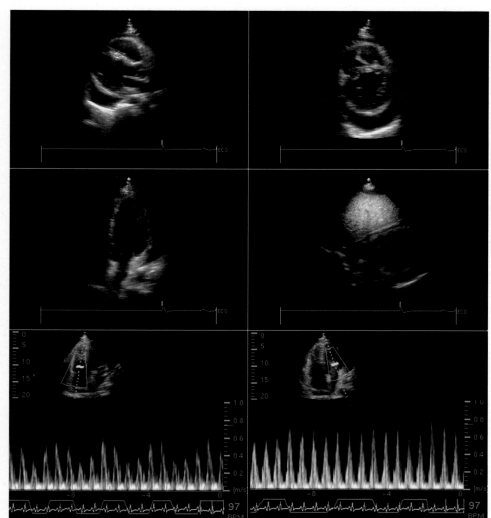

Figure 4-15. Transthoracic echocardiography performed during a clinical recurrence of pericarditis shows a small- to moderate-sized pericardial effusion, principally located to the posterior and left lateral aspect of the heart, without right-sided chamber collapse (TOP IMAGES AND MIDDLE LEFT). The subcostal view suggests thickening of the visceral and parietal pericardium (MIDDLE RIGHT). BOTTOM LEFT, Tricuspid inflow. BOTTOM RIGHT, Mitral inflow. There is phasic variation of the tricuspid valve inflow (mildly increased) associated with the respiratory cycle and normal (lesser) phasic variation of the mitral inflow. The absence of exaggerated mitral inflow variation augers against the compressive states of either tamponade or effuso-constriction.

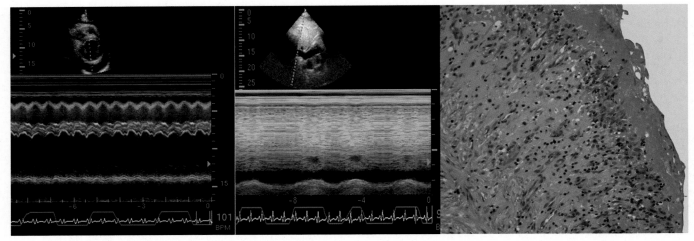

Figure 4-16. Transthoracic echocardiography performed during a clinical recurrence of pericarditis. LEFT, M-mode study at the mid ventricle shows no signs of ventricular interdependence (no increase in right ventricular volume with inspiration with simultaneous fall in left ventricular volume) that would support tamponade or of effuso-constrictive physiology acquired from the many episodes of pericarditis. (Note: inspiration begins with the upward deflection of the red respirometry tracing.) MIDDLE, M-mode study of the inferior vena cava. Normal inferior vena cava diameter (i.e., pressure) and normal decrease in diameter (i.e., fall in pressure) with inspiration, consistent with normal central venous pressures, which was also the clinical impression. RIGHT, Hematoxylin and eosin stain after pericardiectomy shows pericardial thickening with signs of chronic inflammation, granulation tissue, and fibrin, consistent with chronic pericarditis with scarring.

References

1. Sagristà-Sauleda J, Barrabés JA, Permanyer-Miralda G, Soler-Soler J: Purulent pericarditis: review of a 20-year experience in a general hospital. J Am Coll Cardiol 1993;22:1661-1665.

2. Senderovitz T, Viskum K: Corticosteroids and tuberculosis. Respir Med 1994;88:561-565.

3. Sagristà-Sauleda J, Permanyer-Miralda G, Soler-Soler J: Tuberculous pericarditis: ten-year experience with a prospective protocol for diagnosis and treatment. J Am Coll Cardiol 1988;11:724-728.

4. Strang JI, Kakaza HH, Gibson DG, et al: Controlled clinical trial of complete open surgical drainage and of prednisolone in treatment of tuberculous pericardial effusion in Transkei. Lancet 1988;2:759-764.

5. Long R, Younes M, Patton N, Hershfield E: Tuberculous pericarditis: long-term outcome in patients who received medical therapy alone. Am Heart J 1989;117:1133-1139.

6. Imazio M, Demichelis B, Cecchi E, et al: Cardiac troponin I in acute pericarditis. J Am Coll Cardiol 2003;42:2144-2148.

7. Aggeli C, Pitsavos C, Brili S, et al: Relevance of adenosine deaminase and lysozyme measurements in the diagnosis of tuberculous pericarditis. Cardiology 2000;94:81-85.

8. Komsuoglu B, Goldeli O, Kulan K, Komsuoglu SS: The diagnostic and prognostic value of adenosine deaminase in tuberculous pericarditis. Eur Heart J 1995;16:1126-1130.

9. Burgess LJ, Reuter H, Carstens ME, et al: The use of adenosine deaminase and interferon-gamma as diagnostic tools for tuberculous pericarditis. Chest 2002;122:900-905.

10. Lee JH, Lee CW, Lee SG, et al: Comparison of polymerase chain reaction with adenosine deaminase activity in pericardial fluid for the diagnosis of tuberculous pericarditis. Am J Med 2002;113:519-521.

11. Mayosi BM, Burgess LJ, Doubell AF: Tuberculous pericarditis. Circulation 2005;112:3608-3616.

12. Smith KJ, Theal M, Mulji A: Pericarditis presenting and treated as an acute anteroseptal myocardial infarction. Can J Cardiol 2001;17:815-817.

13. Spodick DH: Acute pericarditis: current concepts and practice. JAMA 2003;289:1150-1153.

14. Markiewicz W, Brik A, Brook G, et al: Pericardial rub in pericardial effusion: lack of correlation with amount of fluid. Chest 1980;77:643-646.

15. Godeau P, Derrida JP, Bletry O, Herreman G: Recurrent acute pericarditis and corticoid dependence. Apropos of 10 cases. Semaine des Hopitaux 1975;51:2393-2400.

16. Mott AR, Fraser CD Jr, Kusnoor AV, et al: The effect of short-term prophylactic methylprednisolone on the incidence and severity of postpericardiotomy syndrome in children undergoing cardiac surgery with cardiopulmonary bypass. J Am Coll Cardiol 2001;37:1700-1706.

17. Adler Y: Colchicine treatment for recurrent pericarditis: a decade of experience. Circulation 1998;97:2183-2185.

18. Finkelstein Y, Shemesh J, Mahlab K, et al: Colchicine for the prevention of postpericardiotomy syndrome. Herz 2002;27:791-794.

19. Imazio M, Bobbio M, Cecchi E, et al: Colchicine in addition to conventional therapy for acute pericarditis: Results of the COlchicine for acute PEricarditis (COPE) trial. Circulation 2005;112:2012-2016.

20. Shabetai R: Recurrent pericarditis: Recent advances and remaining questions. Circulation 2005;112:1921-1923.

21. Tuna IC, Danielson GK: Surgical management of pericardial diseases. Cardiol Clin 1990;8:683-696.

22. Fowler NO, Harbin AD III: Recurrent acute pericarditis: Follow-up study of 31 patients. J Am Coll Cardiol 1986;7:300-305.

Pericardial Effusions

KEY POINTS

▸ The "sizing" of pericardial effusions is arbitrary and may be misleading. Ascertaining the physiologic consequence of the effusion is more important than is assigning size.

▸ The interaction of the fluid volume with the pericardial pressure: volume relation, rather than the size of the effusion alone, determines the physiologic consequence of the effusion.

▸ A clinical (including follow-up) and imaging evaluation to establish the cause of the effusion and the physiologic consequence of the effusion is needed in all cases.

▸ Echocardiography and CMR (SSFP sequences) are the most reliable tests to recognize pericardial fluid.

▸ Echocardiography is useful to assess for evidence of tamponade. The anatomic relation of the pericardium to the descending aorta is important to distinguish (by echocardiography) a pericardial from a pleural effusion.

▸ CT scanning is useful in many cases to evaluate related disease in the chest.

▸ Pericardioscopy increases the diagnostic yield from pericardial drainage, which, if it is performed in the absence of tamponade, is low.

Normally, there is a very small amount of pericardial fluid (25 to 35 mL) present within the pericardial space, an amount that is too small to be detected routinely. It serves several purposes, including being a lubricant and normalizing physical forces within the pericardial space. Pericardial effusion, an abnormal and usually pathologic collection of fluid within the pericardial space, occurs when the forces of fluid formation exceed those of removal. In addition to inflammation, infection and tumors may increase fluid formation. Hydrostatic forces may attenuate fluid removal—elevated right atrial pressure increases the likelihood of effusion by impairing the venous drainage through the azygos and hemiazygos veins. Many types of medical disease and surgical procedures may result in pericardial effusion. Pericardial effusions are seen commonly in one of six heart failure cases, one of five valve disease cases, one of six myocardial infarction cases, and seven of eight recent open heart surgery cases. Pericardial effusions are detected in the course of evaluation for related and unrelated complaints and diseases and also in the course of abdominal and chest imaging.

By computed tomography (CT) scanning and cardiac magnetic resonance (CMR) imaging, there is generally no difficulty in distinguishing pericardial from pleural effusions as such an extensive degree of anatomic assessment is obtained by these modalities. However, neither test is a particularly robust test to exclude tamponade physiology. Conversely, echocardiography, because of its limited imaging of the chest, does entail some challenge to distinguish pericardial from pleural effusions; establishment of the relation of the effusion to the descending aorta is critical. The pericardial space resides anterior to the descending aorta, and the pleural space resides posterolateral to the descending aorta; this relationship is most easily imaged on the parasternal long-axis and apical 3-chamber views and can be established in the large majority of individuals (Figs. 5-1 and 5-2).[1] Echocardiography is the best imaging test to determine the presence of compressive tamponade physiology.

Sizing of pericardial effusions is arbitrary, is imprecise (because it does not describe the effusion in volumetric units, only in quantitative dimensional measurements and qualitative terms), and has poor association with hemodynamic consequences, and as well, many effusions are not uniformly distributed. All too frequently, description of an effusion as small generates misunderstanding that tamponade is unlikely and conversely that a large effusion is likely to cause tamponade (Fig. 5-3). Several conventions to size effusions exist. The size of an effusion is more revealing of the chronicity of the disease process and the ease of drainage than it is of the physiologic consequence or responsible underlying disease. A common convention of sizing effusions is as follows:

- Small: <1 cm posteriorly with little fluid anteriorly (Fig. 5-4)
- Moderate: >1 cm posteriorly with fluid anteriorly (Fig. 5-5)
- Large: circumferential with >>1 cm posteriorly or =2 cm in its anterior and posterior distribution (Fig. 5-6)

Pericarditis and pericardial effusion are not synonymous. Most cases of acute pericarditis do not accumulate an effusion, although some do, and only a few will develop tamponade. Similarly, only a few patients with tamponade exhibit the clinical and electrocardiographic findings of pericarditis (see Fig. 5-3).

The diagnostic evaluation and management of pericardial effusions are guided by the clinical context of the case. The diagnostic evaluation of patients with pericardial effusion includes history and physical examination, electrocardiography, chest radiography, basic blood testing, and echocardiography (Table 5-1). CT and CMR are used in a case-specific way. Patients with pericardial effusions should receive follow-up.

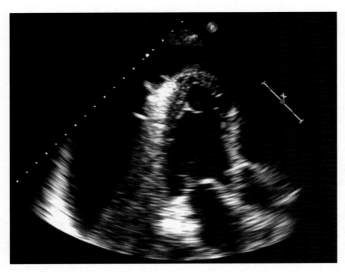

Figure 5-1. Transthoracic echocardiography, apical 3-chamber view. There are fibrinous strands within an effusion, which appears to surround the heart but is actually a left pleural malignant effusion. Without establishment of the relation of the fluid to the descending aorta, pleural effusions are easily mistaken for pericardial effusions.

HISTORY AND PHYSICAL EXAMINATION

The history is directed toward the identification of complaints suggestive of acute inflammatory pericarditis or of tamponade and the review of underlying medical or constitutional disorders and infectious exposures that may define the cause. Large effusions may produce ancillary complaints of cough or dysphagia due to mediastinal distortion or vagal nerve compression. Dyspnea may occur due to the volume of pericardial fluid accruing at the expense of lung volume.

The physical examination focuses on assessment of findings of pericarditis and of pericardial compression of the heart (tamponade and effuso-constrictive pericarditis). It consists of taking vitals (heart rate, blood pressure and pulsus paradoxus, respiratory rate), noting the venous pressure and pattern, presence or absence of edema, and auscultation findings (rub: acute pericarditis; knock: constrictive or effuso-constrictive pericarditis). A large effusion may compress the left lower lobe, resulting in atelectasis and its findings of left basal rales, bronchial sounds, or egophony (Ewart sign). Seemingly paradoxically, a pericardial friction rub may be present in cases of effusion. Several potential explanations exist, including that some pericardial reflections still remain in apposition and may generate the rub or simply that apposition of inflamed surfaces is not necessary to cause a "rub" sound.

Table 5-1. Recommended Minimal Assessment of Pericardial Effusion

History and physical examination
Electrocardiography
Chest radiography
Serum biochemistry, renal indices
Blood counts
Thyroid testing
Immunologic testing if there is clinical suspicion
PPD skin testing if there is clinical suspicion of tuberculosis

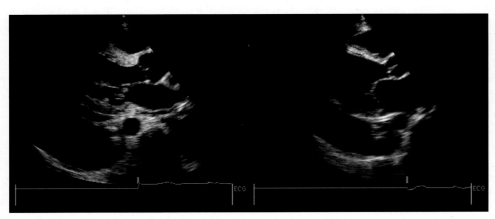

Figure 5-2. Transthoracic echocardiography, parasternal long-axis views. LEFT, There is a fluid-filled cavity posterior to the heart and *posterior* to the descending aorta—a left pleural effusion. RIGHT, There are two fluid-filled cavities posterior to the heart—a pericardial effusion *anterior* to the descending aorta and a fluid-filled cavity *posterior* to the descending aorta—a left pleural effusion. The relation of fluid to the descending thoracic aorta is critical.

LABORATORY TESTING

Serologic Tests

Hypothyroidism should be excluded in all cases. Serologic tests are indicated if there is clinical suspicion of an underlying cause, such as systemic lupus erythematosus or rheumatoid arthritis. Blood cultures are indicated if there is suspicion of infection.

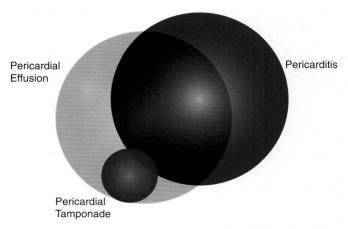

Figure 5-3. The physiologic effect of a pericardial effusion matters more than its size and is not predictable on the basis of its size alone. Only a subset of cases of effusions is associated with tamponade.

Biomarkers of myocardial necrosis should be sought to exclude myocardial infarction in cases of potential recent infarction.

Pericardial Fluid Analysis

Pericardial fluid analysis that is performed in the absence of the clinical syndrome of tamponade has an only 5% etiology detection rate; conversely, pericardial fluid analysis undertaken in the context of tamponade has a 35% to 40% etiology detection rate. If fluid is sampled, it should be analyzed broadly, according to possible etiology. Some assays are not available at all centers. Useful fluid cultures and other laboratory tests are summarized in Table 5-2.

Establishing exudate versus transudate (borrowed Light's criteria for pleural fluid analysis) is seldom helpful in establishing a specific etiology of pericardial effusion. Transudates are seen in congestive heart failure, cirrhosis, and pregnancy. Exudates are seen in inflammatory and infectious states and after trauma. Sanguineous effusions are seen in a range of disorders including infections, inflammation, malignant disease, and trauma.

Skin Testing

Skin testing (PPD) is used to ascertain prior tuberculous exposure; although helpful, it may be confounded by false-negatives. Furthermore, a positive PPD test result is not specific for active tuberculous pericardial disease.

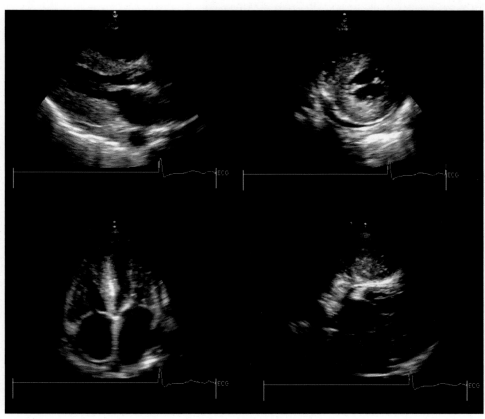

Figure 5-4. Transthoracic echocardiography views of a small pericardial effusion, less than 1 cm in thickness. The fluid is principally posterior and more evident on some views than on others as it is not evenly distributed (amyloidosis case).

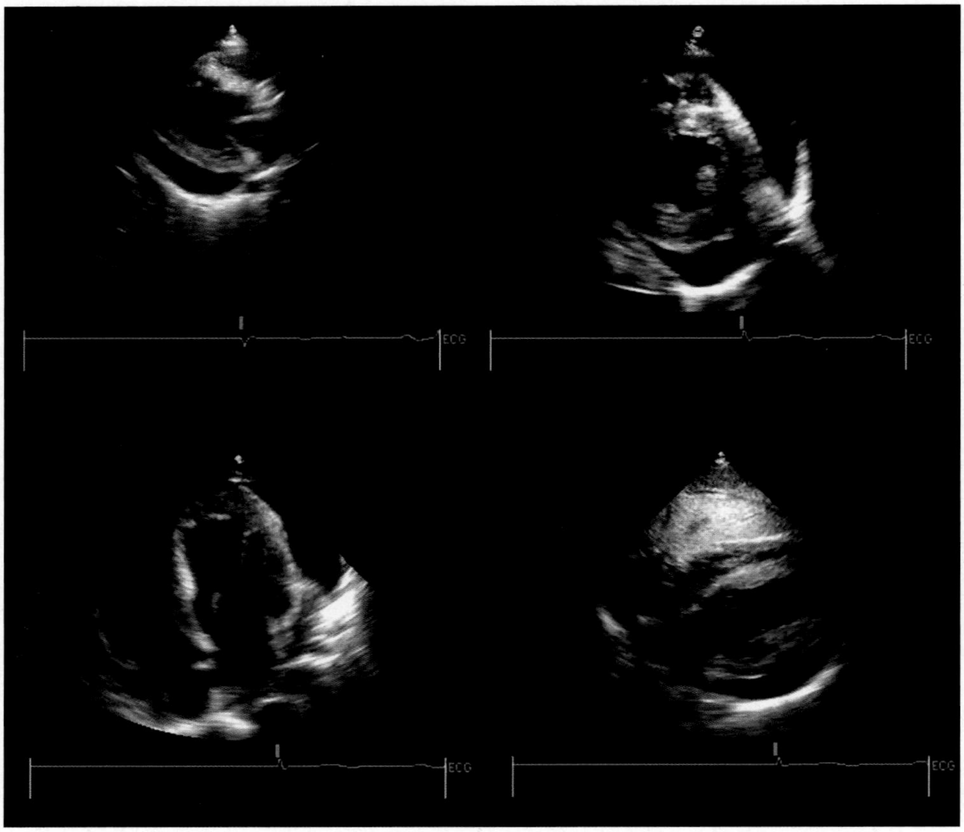

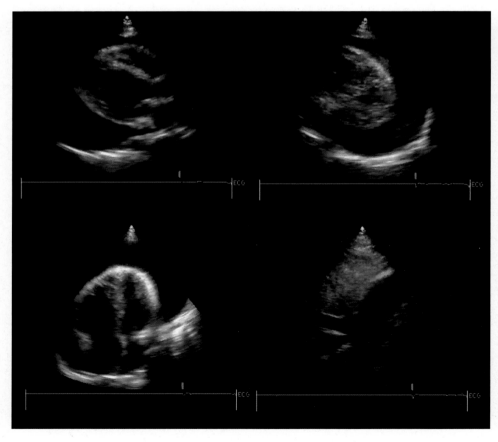

Figure 5-5. Transthoracic echocardiography views of a moderate-sized pericardial effusion, 1 to 2 cm in thickness. The fluid is principally posterior and more evident on some views than on others as it is not evenly distributed.

Figure 5-6. Transthoracic echocardiography views of a large pericardial effusion, more than 2 cm in thickness in several locations. Although the fluid is principally posterior and lateral, there is fluid anteriorly, and the distribution is becoming more uniform.

Table 5-2. Laboratory Tests Useful in the Diagnosis of Pericardial Effusions

Stain and culture

  Bacterial stain and culture

  Tuberculosis stain and culture

  Fungal stain and culture

Cytology

Other tests

  LE cell positive (systemic lupus erythematosus)

  Cholesterol (elevated in myxedema, rheumatoid arthritis, tuberculosis, idiopathic effusions)

  Chylous (thoracic duct damage or obstruction)

  Adenosine deaminase, lysozyme, and interferon-γ (elevated in tuberculous disease)

  Glucose (low in rheumatoid arthritis and in infection)

  Amylase (elevated in pancreatitis)

  Polymerase chain reaction (positive in tuberculous disease)

IMAGING STUDIES

Chest Radiography

Chest radiography should be performed in all cases to assess for associated pleural or parenchymal lung disease, abnormal hilar contours, and abnormal aortic contours. Although "flask-like" enlargement is usual if the effusion is large, multichamber enlargement can produce a similar silhouette, other than the finding of a more tapered superior aspect in the context of pericardial effusion, as the pericardium extends upward along the proximal great vessels, smoothly tapering the silhouette superiorly (Figs. 5-7 and 5-8). Chest radiography is not reliable to detect small pericardial effusions—at least 250 mL of fluid needs to be present to discern a change in the size of the cardiopericardial silhouette. This amount of fluid can be hemodynamically significant. The chest radiograph is also not reliable to exclude the presence of tamponade physiology.

Electrocardiography

Low voltages are uncommonly seen in smaller effusions but are commonly seen in large effusions with tamponade. Electrical alternans is not typical of effusion alone but rather of effusion with tamponade[2] and reflects the presence of a larger effusion and the heart, in distress, dynamically contracting and swinging within it.

Computed Tomography

CT scanning is able to detect all but the smallest effusions. Many pericardial effusions are "incidental findings" of abdominal CT scans. Contrast enhancement is useful to delineate cardiac chambers and hence the pericardial space. Streak artifacts from right-sided heart contrast are common. Electrocardiography (ECG) gating is somewhat useful to improve image clarity.

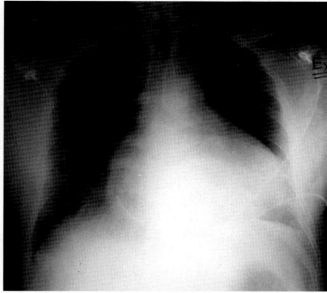

Figure 5-7. Enlarged flask-like cardiopericardial silhouette due to a large pericardial effusion. There is no pulmonary venous engorgement, pleural effusion, or apparent pulmonary parenchymal disease. The appearance of the aorta is normal.

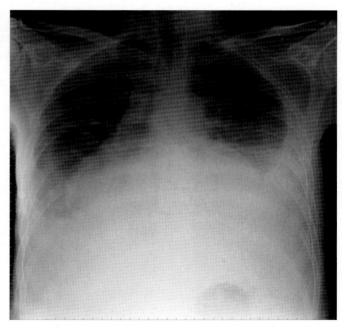

Figure 5-8. Enlarged flask-like cardiopericardial silhouette due to a large pericardial effusion; but because of the presence of adjacent bilateral pleural effusions, establishing the cardiac silhouette size is impossible.

The notable yield from CT scanning is superb delineation of other intrathoracic and intra-abdominal structures (lymph nodes, the aorta, masses). CT scanning also delineates the relation of the fluid to the chest wall and therefore is a useful means by which to guide pericardial fluid drainage (Fig. 5-9).

CT scanning is not well suited to assess the dynamic physiologic consequences of effusions and effuso-constriction (e.g.,

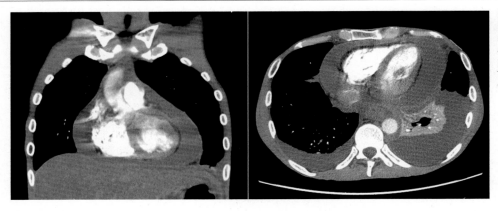

Figure 5-9. CT scans showing a large pericardial effusion around the heart and up the great vessels. A left pleural effusion and left lower lobe atelectasis are also present. The presence or absence of tamponade physiology cannot be reliably established by CT.

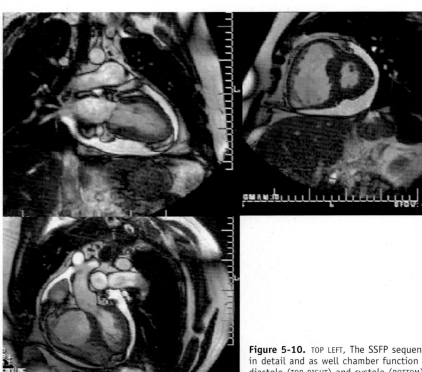

Figure 5-10. TOP LEFT, The SSFP sequence CMR image readily depicts pericardial fluid distribution in detail and as well chamber function and great vessel anatomy. The short-axis images in diastole (TOP RIGHT) and systole (BOTTOM) enable determination of right ventricular diastolic collapse, which is absent in this case. There is right ventricular hypertrophy and hypokinesis. (Courtesy of Steve Schiff, MD, FACC, Fountain Valley, California.)

chamber collapse, ventricular interdependence), although this may be possible with ECG gating. Pericardial effusions often seen to appear larger by CT scanning than they will by echocardiography.

The attenuation characteristics (Hounsfield units) of intrapericardial fluid and soft tissue material do not tend to differ sufficiently to reliably distinguish transudate versus exudate or blood from clot or other tissues.

Cardiac Magnetic Resonance

CMR is able to image pericardial detail and can be useful when echocardiography is inconclusive in detecting pericardial fluid. Steady-state free precession (SSFP) sequences readily detect fluid (high signal) (Figs. 5-10 to 5-12). Epicardial and pericardial fat layers (which appear bright) enable tissue plane identification and assessment of pericardial thickness, particularly on T1-weighted black blood imaging spin echo sequences.

The significance of delayed enhancement of the pericardium with gadolinium contrast inversion recovery gradient echo sequences is unknown. Similar to CT scanning, CMR provides little information on the physiologic and dynamic consequences of an effusion, although SSFP cine sequences will show chamber collapse; but differing from CT scanning, CMR is not a suitable platform to guide drainage and is not a suitable platform to image hemodynamically compromised or unstable patients.

Contraindications to CMR scanning are numerous and include pacers, ICDs, vascular and ocular clips, and hemodynamic instability and inability to breath-hold.

5

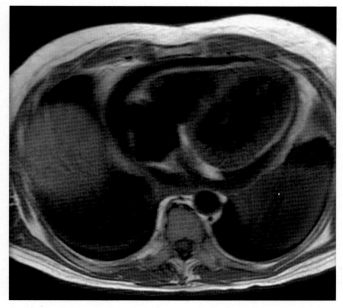

Figure 5-11. T1-weighted black blood axial CMR image. The presence and distribution of the pericardial fluid can be readily appreciated. The presence of epicardial fat establishes a clear interface; the delineation of the interface with the parietal pericardium is less distinct because of less contrast.

Echocardiography

Echocardiography is the diagnostic test of choice for the detection and evaluation of pericardial effusions. Goals of echocardiography are as follows:

- To establish the presence of pericardial fluid
- To distinguish pericardial from pleural effusions
- To identify important underlying causes of effusions, such as infarction, aortic dissection, or masses
- To exclude other causes of the referring complaint
- To recognize the compressive physiology of tamponade
- To evaluate optimal drainage method, when needed
- To guide drainage, when needed

The usual echocardiographic appearance of an effusion is an echolucent space. Other occasional appearances include fluid with specular echoes (if the fluid is purulent or sanguineous); fine specular, often laminated, gelatinous-appearing material echoes (if there is clot); and fibrin strands and fronds (if the fluid is exudative and the protein has precipitated).

Parasternal long-axis, parasternal short-axis, apical 4-chamber, and subcostal views are all important echocardiographic views (Figs. 5-13 to 5-17). The parasternal long-axis view distinguishes pericardial from pleural effusion (as do the apical 2-chamber and 3-chamber views) and is a useful view to determine right ventricular outflow tract collapse. The parasternal short-axis views are among the best to determine the distribution of fluid

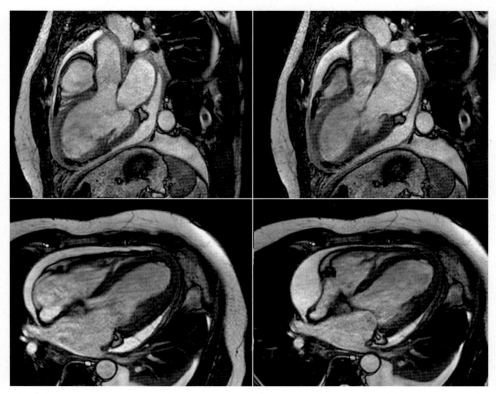

Figure 5-12. SSFP CMR imaging. There is excellent delineation of the location of pericardial fluid, and fluid to parietal layer demarcation, and fluid to epicardium demarcation. Susceptibility artifact actually facilitates delineation of the interfaces.

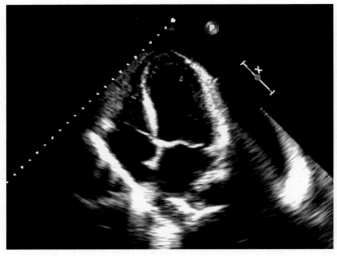

Figure 5-13. Transthoracic echocardiography, apical 4-chamber view. There is a large lucent area (effusion) surrounding the left side of the heart. Although the relation of an effusion to the descending aorta can often be seen on this view, it is obscured by reverberation artifact in this case. Although it is tempting to assume that the effusion is pericardial, as the descending aorta cannot be seen, it would be only an assumption. In fact, this was a pleural effusion.

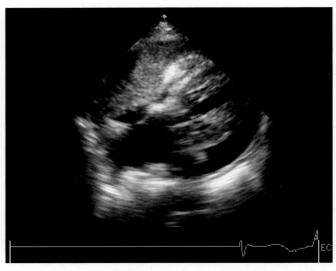

Figure 5-14. Transthoracic echocardiography, subcostal view. Within the pericardial space, there is a large amount of soft tissue with a fine specular pattern. On the far left side of the heart, there is a small amount of pericardial fluid. The appearance of the soft tissue within the pericardial space is similar to that of the liver. Intrapericardial clot.

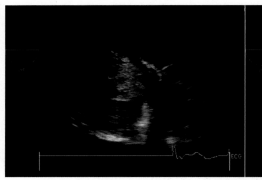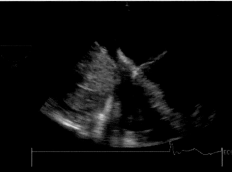

Figure 5-15. Transesophageal echocardiography, lower esophageal 4-chamber views. LEFT, Low gain. RIGHT, Optimal gain. There is a large soft tissue mass lateral to the almost entirely compressed right atrium. The low-gain image depicts the mass, but poorly. The optimal (higher) gain image reveals the fine specular echo "texture" of intrapericardial clot.

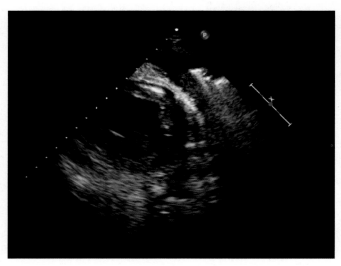

Figure 5-16. Transthoracic echocardiography, parasternal short-axis view at the mid ventricular level. The blood pool and myocardium are apparent. Over the myocardium are both a thick echo-bright layer and a thick echolucent layer. These layers appear to be pericardial as they lie where the pericardium would, but it is actually the pleural cavity filled with malignant mesothelioma, exemplifying how echocardiography, without the ability to depict chest anatomic detail, engenders assumptions.

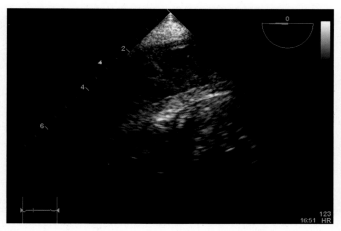

Figure 5-17. Transesophageal echocardiography, transgastric short-axis view of a patient with effusion due to purulent (bacterial) pericarditis. There is a collection of lucent material with complex specular echoes between the liver and a rind of thickened pericardium.

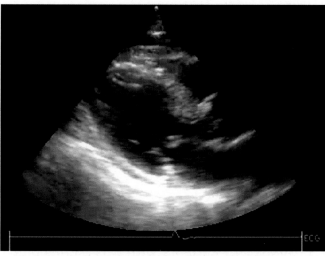

Figure 5-18. The two anterior lucent layers that appear to be fluid are just fat. The more anterior layer is fat on the outside of the pericardium, and the more internal layer is epicardial fat. The pericardium is visible as a very thin layer between them. The lack of circumferential distribution and the specular echoes within make the layers far more likely to be fat than fluid. If needed, CMR would readily delineate epicardial and outside fat planes.

and drainage options and are useful to evaluate for right ventricular, right ventricular outflow tract, and right atrial collapse. The apical 4-chamber view demonstrates right-sided heart collapse well, if it is present, and is the most useful view to record left ventricular inflow variations. Subcostal views are important to determine inferior vena cava distention and right atrial and right ventricular collapse. All views are important to determine the most appropriate means to drain fluid, if pursued.

Fat is normally seen anterior to the right side of the heart. Intrapericardial epicardial fat and pericardial fat on the parietal pericardium may be seen, usually as layers with coarse specular echolucency over the right ventricular outflow tract on the parasternal long-axis view (Fig. 5-18). The differential diagnosis of such includes fat within the pericardial space, fluid, clot, and others. Fluid, if free within the pericardial space, normally resides in the most dependent part of the pericardial space, which, when the patient is lying supine, is posteriorly. Small effusions are generally located posterior to the ventricles and right atrium. Moderate effusions are principally posterior to the ventricles but have more fluid anteriorly than do small effusions. Large effusions are generally circumferential around the ventricles and right atrium and extend to a lesser extent behind the left atrium. When an effusion is under pressure, its extension around the left atrium and into the pericardial sleeves becomes more prominent.

Echocardiography can be limited by poor views in some cases, by incomplete views in others, and by extremely limited evaluation of the thorax in detail.

Differential diagnosis of pericardial fluid beside the heart is listed in Table 5-3.[3]

Pericardioscopy for Acute Pericarditis

To augment the diagnostic yield of pericardial drainage, pericardioscopy can be performed with rigid or flexible systems to visually guide biopsy and to increase diagnostic yield. The availability of pericardioscopy is limited, however.

Table 5-3. Differential Diagnosis of Fluid Beside the Heart

Pericardial fluid

Pericardial thrombus

Pericardial mass

Pericardial cyst

Pericardial pus

Pericardial fibrocalcific peel

Epicardial fat

Pleural effusion

Pleural disease overlying the pericardium

Dilated ascending aorta

Dilated coronary sinus

Left atrial appendage

Esophageal dilation (achalasia, scleroderma esophagus)[4]

Extracardiac mass

From Kuvin JT, Basu AK, Khabbaz KR, et al: Benign lipid envelope of the heart simulating a pericardial hematoma. J Am Soc Echocardiogr 2001;14:234-236. Copyright 2001, with permission from Elsevier.

In a series of 141 consecutive patients with pericardial effusions who underwent pericardioscopy with a rigid mediastinoscope through a subxiphoid window, a diagnosis was achieved in half (49%). There was a 6% in-hospital mortality (none due to mediastinoscopy), and the increase in sensitivity was superior to surgical drainage alone for detection of malignant disease (21%), radiation induced–pericarditis (100%), and purulent effusions (83%).[5]

PERICARDIAL EFFUSION MANAGEMENT ISSUES

There is no specific treatment of pericardial effusion unless it is pyogenic, tuberculous, fungal, or from another infection or treatable systemic illness (e.g., systemic lupus erythematosus) or with associated clinical pericarditis. The physician must observe clinically and echocardiographically for resolution, or evolution, or late complications and investigate for an underlying cause, particularly if the effusion is recurrent or chronic. There is no proven role for routine diagnostic pericardiocentesis unless there is strong clinical suspicion of malignant disease or pyogenic, tuberculous, or fungal infection. There is no role for therapeutic pericardiocentesis unless there is cardiac compression.

Prognosis of Patients with Large Effusions

One observational series of patients with chronic idiopathic large effusions observed that 30% will at some point develop tamponade, potentially suddenly. Pericardiocentesis alleviates tamponade once it has developed but does not convincingly avoid recurrence.[6]

Human Immunodeficiency Virus–Related Pericardial Diseases

Pericardial effusions are seen in one of five patients with HIV infection, of whom the large majority are asymptomatic. Previously, it was observed that the presence of an effusion was associated with a much shorter survival (36% versus 93% at 6 months) for such patients.[7] Many more patients with HIV infection have effusions than have pericarditis or tamponade. On pathologic examination, most effusions have a lymphocytic basis; a minority have an infectious basis (tuberculosis and *Mycobacterium avium-intracellulare* complex, other HIV-related organisms) or a malignant basis (Kaposi sarcoma, lymphomas). Drainage is reasonable if the effusion is symptomatic or a specific cause is sought. HIV-related effusions are a common disorder at inner-city hospitals.[8]

References

1. Haaz WS, Mintz GS, Kotler MN: Two-dimensional echocardiographic recognition of the descending thoracic aorta: value in differentiating pericardial from pleural effusions. Am J Cardiol 1980;46:739-743.
2. Bruch C, Schmermund A, Dagres N, et al: Changes in QRS voltage in cardiac tamponade and pericardial effusion: reversibility after pericardiocentesis and after anti-inflammatory drug treatment. J Am Coll Cardiol 2001;38:219-226.
3. Kuvin JT, Basu AK, Khabbaz KR, et al: Benign lipid envelope of the heart simulating a pericardial hematoma. J Am Soc Echocardiogr 2001;14:234-236.
4. Choe W, Mehlman D: Mediastinal abnormalities in systemic sclerosis. N Engl J Med 2000;343:1771.
5. Nugue O, Millaire A, Porte H, et al: Pericardioscopy in the etiologic diagnosis of pericardial effusion in 141 consecutive patients. Circulation 1996; 94:1635-1641.
6. Sagristà-Sauleda J, Angel J, Permanyer-Miralda G, Soler-Soler J: Long-term follow-up of idiopathic chronic pericardial effusion. N Engl J Med 1999;341:2054-2059.
7. Heidenreich PA, Eisenberg MJ, Kee LL, et al: Pericardial effusion in AIDS: incidence and survival. Circulation 1995;92:3229-3234.
8. Chen Y, Brennessel D, Walters J, et al: Human immunodeficiency virus–associated pericardial effusion: report of 40 cases and review of the literature. Am Heart J 1999;137:516-521.

Pericardial Tamponade

KEY POINTS

- The diagnosis of pericardial tamponade, a clinical syndrome, is made by a combination of observations at the bedside and objective testing—usually echocardiography.

- Neither bedside assessment nor laboratory testing (echocardiography, catheterization, or other) is sufficiently able to resolve the question of tamponade in *all* cases for the use of any approach alone to be encouraged.

- A minority of cases of tamponade remain ambiguous despite repeated assessment and comprehensive testing and can be considered for empirical drainage for attempted therapeutic and diagnostic reasons.

The clinician's goals are (1) to establish and objectify the diagnosis of pericardial tamponade when it is present, (2) to determine the cause of the pericardial tamponade in all cases when it is feasible, and (3) to stabilize the patient and intervene therapeutically for cases of tamponade.

Some causes of tamponade require or are eligible for specific treatment (e.g., tuberculous disease); some causes are themselves life-threatening surgical emergencies (e.g., aortic dissection, postinfarction rupture), and some are medical emergencies (e.g., uremia). The diagnostic yield of pericardial fluid for malignant involvement and infections is highest when drainage is performed for therapeutic relief of tamponade. All patients with tamponade should be admitted to the hospital for stabilization, evaluation, and treatment (see Chapter 7).

Tamponade cases have myriad presentations that depend on the severity and the acuity of the tamponade syndrome (Fig. 6-1): the function, dysfunction, or lesions of the underlying heart; the particular chambers that are collapsed; the mode of respiration and ventilation; the profile of comorbidities; and the overall status of the patient.

PATHOPHYSIOLOGY OF PERICARDIAL TAMPONADE

The normal intrapericardial pressure is approximately −4 to 1 mm Hg. The normal (nonbreathing) intrapleural pressure is about −4 mm Hg and is accentuated in proportion to spontaneous inspiratory effort.

The walls of cardiac chambers are distended by the net force exerted between the pressure in the cavity and the opposing pressure in the pericardial space; this is the transmural distending pressure, which for the right atrium is normally 4 or 5 mm Hg. Transmural filling pressure is the true chamber filling pressure.[1]

The physical properties of the pericardium are normally conferred only by the parietal layer, which has a modest amount of elastin within its connective tissue matrices, imparting a small amount of potential stretch: the pericardial reserve volume. This reserve volume is matched to the maximal advantageous preload reserve of the ventricles (Starling phenomenon). The majority of the matrix of the parietal pericardium is collagen and is stiff and unyielding—effectively limiting acute distention of the ventricles and preserving myocardial sarcomere function, although at the expense of higher diastolic pressures within the pericardial space and the heart cavities. There are very significant differences of pericardial compliance between patients. In a hemodynamic study of tamponade cases, it was noted that the same volume of pericardial fluid was removed from the tamponade group as from the effusion-without-tamponade group, yet the former had an initial intrapericardial pressure of 20 ± 7 mm Hg, and the latter had an intrapericardial pressure of only 5 ± 4 mm Hg.[2] Similarly, in a study of postoperative tamponade cases, early tamponade cases occurred with less fluid (600 mL) than did late tamponade cases (900 mL), consistent with greater compliance allowing more fluid to accumulate before compression of the heart occurred (Fig. 6-2).[3]

Accumulation of freely distributing pericardial fluid past the point of exhaustion of the elastic reserve and remodeling ability of the pericardium leads to elevation of the intrapericardial pressure (significant: >7 mm Hg or >10 mm Hg)[2,4] and elevation (>10 mm Hg) and equilibration (<5 mm Hg pressure difference) of intracardiac diastolic pressures. Loss of cavitary chamber transmural distending pressure results in inward displacement of the chamber walls and eventually chamber wall compression and

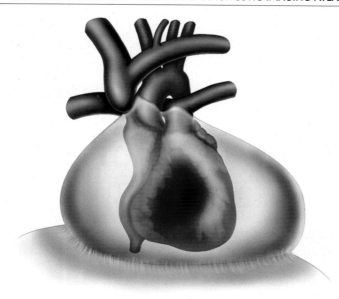

Figure 6-1. Tamponade. Tense pericardial fluid accumulation collapses and compresses the superior and inferior venae cavae and the right atrium (in systole) and the right ventricle (in diastole). The heart is underfilled because of the lessened transmural distending pressure, and therefore the chambers are small. The extrapericardial veins are distended (plethoric).

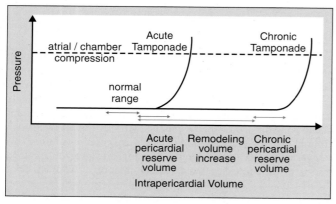

Figure 6-2. The nature of the pericardial pressure : volume (stress : strain) relation is a flat line followed by a steep, nearly exponential rise. The nature of the curve is provided by the histologic composition of the parietal pericardium. A finite amount of stretch or elastic property is conferred by the small amount of elastic tissue, permitting pericardial reserve volume. Once elastic properties have been exceeded and the noncompliant unyielding collagenous pericardial matrix is under stress, the pressure rises rapidly to preserve the intrapericardial volume. Acute (e.g., hemorrhagic) tamponade will occur at a much smaller volume than chronic tamponade, as the heart has no time to remodel the pericardial collagen matrix, and the finite acute pericardial reserve volume is exceeded. Chronic effusions can be accommodated by remodeling of the connective tissue (elastin and collagen) matrices of the pericardium, but the limited elastin again allows only a finite reserve volume.

collapse, limiting diastolic filling of the heart and resulting in a small stroke volume and therefore, in turn, a smaller pulse pressure. As intracardiac pressures vary through the cardiac and respiratory cycles, chamber collapse is specific to an interval of the cardiac cycle and varied by the respiratory cycle. The cardiac chambers effectively compete for volume against the intrapericardial accumulation of volume and pressure. Clear-cut cases of tamponade have an intrapericardial pressure of about 20 mm Hg before pericardiocentesis.[2]

Table 6-1. Hemodynamics of Experimental Tamponade[7]

Intrapericardial pressure (mm Hg)	0	10	20	30
Transmural distending pressure (mm Hg)	3	−2	−4	−6
Right atrial pressure (mm Hg)	3	8	11	14
Percent change (%):				
Stroke volume	0	−55	−62	−74
Heart rate	0	13	19	23
Arterial pressure	0	−3	−5	−15

The cavae, both of which have intrapericardial portions, are also subject to compression by pericardial fluid,[5] as may be the pulmonary veins. Angiographic studies demonstrate that in tamponade, the superior vena cava in particular experiences compression in phase with the respiratory cycle similar to right atrial collapse.[5]

During spontaneous inspiration, venous return to the right side of the heart increases, increasing right-sided heart volume and right-sided heart intracavitary pressure, increasing the transmural distending pressure transiently until expiration. During spontaneous inspiration, venous return to the left side of the heart falls somewhat as the pulmonary venous capacitance increases as lung volume increases. The differential effects of right- and left-sided heart filling, occurring within the confines imparted by the accumulated intrapericardial volume, lead to ventricular interdependence or interaction—the right-sided heart filling occurs to the detriment of left-sided heart filling. In tamponade, the pattern of left-sided heart (atrial) filling changes and becomes systolic predominant.[6]

Pulsus paradoxus is a common but not universal finding seen within the respiratory cycle. It reflects variation in left-sided heart inflow gradients and the interaction of right- and left-sided heart filling within the confinement of the heart chambers by the surrounding pericardial effusion as the venous return varies to the right and left sides of the heart according to the phase of the respiratory cycle (Fig. 6-3).

Hypotension is usual, but blood pressure, despite being easily recorded and often emphasized, is a poor surrogate of cardiac output and tissue perfusion. Furthermore, the usual blood pressure of the patient is seldom known, and therefore the extent of fall of blood pressure—*relative hypotension* (a good marker of hemodynamic distress)—is usually also unknown. Some patients experience a hyperadrenergic respons to the distress of tamponade that raises their blood pressure, making blood pressure a confounded marker of hemodynamic distress from tamponade.

Elevation of heart rate and vasoconstriction are compensatory mechanisms reactive to the low stroke volume. Once these are exhausted, blood pressure will fall. However, hypotension is not a good marker for tamponade severity because its fall is a late or terminal event, it does not correlate well with cardiac output (Fig. 6-4), and as well hyperadrenergic and hypertensive responses to tamponade occur (Fig. 6-5). A small stroke volume and therefore small pulse pressure are nearly constant findings.

As can be seen in Table 6-1, experimentally increasing intrapericardial pressure from baseline (0 mm Hg) to 10, 20, and 30 mm Hg results in increases of right atrial pressure from 3 mm Hg to 8, 11, and 14 mm Hg; that is, the increase in intrapericardial pressure exceeds (twofold) what is apparent from the

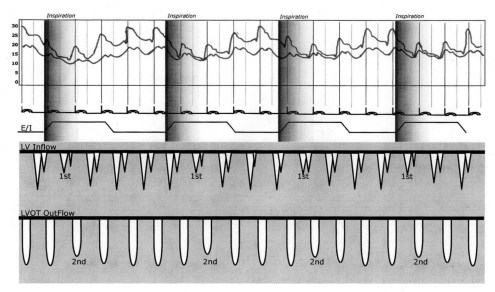

Figure 6-3. Tamponade. Respiratory variation of pulmonary capillary wedge pressure (PCWP) and intrapericardial pressure (IPP) as a basis of pulsus paradoxus. The upper panel denotes the PCWP tracing and the IPP tracing. The ECG is below, as is the respirometry tracing—upward deflection denotes inspiration, which is also indicated by shading. At functional residual capacity (end-expiration), the PCWP and the IPP are both prominently elevated. With inspiration, both fall, although the fall in PCWP is greater, presumably because of the additive effect of increased pulmonary venous capacitance. As a result of the fall in the PCWP:IPP gradient, the diastolic inflow to the left ventricle (LV) falls prominently with the first cardiac cycle of inspiration, underloading the left ventricle. (Ventricular interdependence may further the underloading of the left ventricle.) The next cardiac cycle ejection is therefore underloaded (second cardiac cycle of inspiration), relaying the underloading to the aorta one cardiac cycle later. LVOT, left ventricular outflow tract.

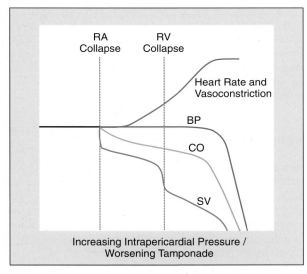

Figure 6-4. As right atrial (RA) pressure rises, blood pressure (BP) is kept constant until very late, by rising heart rate and vasoconstriction, to compensate for smaller stroke volume (SV). Once blood pressure has begun to fall, small changes in RA pressure and transmural distending pressure and cardiac output (CO) are not related linearly to tamponade severity. Blood pressure is a poor sign of tamponade because it changes only late in the course of the disease process. RV, right ventricular.

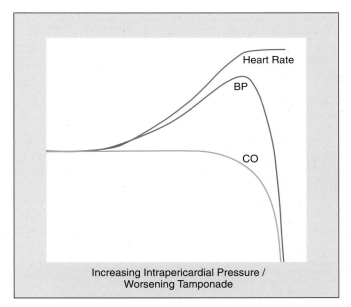

Figure 6-5. In hypertensive or hyperadrenergic tamponade, the distress of tamponade elicits a hypertensive response, which can be highly misleading as to the state of tamponade. In hyperadrenergic tamponade, there is excess vasoconstrictor response and tachycardia that mask tamponade findings until critically late and mislead with respect to the diagnosis and the severity. BP, blood pressure; RA, right atrial.

recorded venous pressure. Furthermore, the impression that the right atrial filling pressure is adequate as it rises to supranormal is misleading as the increase in intrapericardial pressure from baseline (0 mm Hg) to 10, 20, and 30 mm Hg exceeds the right atrial pressure and results in a change in transmural distending pressure from positive at baseline (3 mm Hg) to negative: −2, −4, and −6 mm Hg, respectively. The stroke volume is rapidly compromised (−55%, −62%, −74%) as transmural distending pressure falls to negative. The increase in heart rate (+13%, +19%, +23%), as intrapericardial pressure rises, is less revealing than the fall in stroke volume, which is threefold greater. Arterial pressure shows the least revealing changes: −3%, −5%, −15%.[8]

Unlike in pericardial constriction, in pericardial tamponade there is compression of the heart and therefore limitation of diastolic filling throughout diastole; whereas in constriction, the early diastolic recoil of the pericardium results in supranormal early diastolic filling. Hence, in tamponade, the y descents are blunted (by compression occurring in early diastole—as well as through the rest of the cardiac cycle); whereas in constriction, the y descent is augmented by the recoil of the pericardium in early diastole.

Most cases of chronic tamponade involve at least 500 mL of fluid, often 1000 to 1500 mL of fluid and occasionally up to 2000 mL. Most cases of acute (e.g., perforation, hemorrhagic) tamponade occur with 175 to 250 mL of fluid. Although the size of pericardial effusion roughly corresponds to the extent of tamponade physiology, the correlation is clinically so imperfect that the more important notion is to establish the physiologic consequence of the effusion through physical diagnosis and imaging testing, rather than to make assumptions simply on the basis of the size of the effusion. Acute hemorrhagic effusions are commonly due to trauma and interventional cardiology and electrophysiology misadventure; they are generally small and yet may be life-threatening because their acuity exceeds the remodeling time needed for the pericardium to accommodate the increase in intrapericardial volume.

Prior pericardial disease, such as prior post open heart surgery pericarditis, may result in stiffer than normal pericardium and tamponade with smaller volumes of pericardial fluid.

DIFFERENTIAL DIAGNOSIS OF RIGHT-SIDED HEART FAILURE

Many cases of tamponade present with predominant right-sided heart failure symptoms or findings. The differential diagnosis of

Table 6-2. Differential Diagnosis of Right-Sided Heart Failure

Causes of Acute Right-Sided Heart Failure	Causes of Chronic Right-Sided Heart Failure
Tamponade	Chronic tamponade
Pulmonary embolism	Constrictive pericarditis
Right ventricular infarction	Effuso-constrictive pericarditis
Tension pneumothorax	Restrictive cardiomyopathy
	Dilated cardiomyopathy
	Cor pulmonale (all causes)
	Congenital heart lesions
	Tricuspid regurgitation and stenosis

right-sided heart failure can be divided into acute right-sided failure and chronic right-sided failure (Table 6-2).

HISTORY

Patients have complaints that vary according to the severity of the tamponade, the particular comorbidities, and the overall status of the patient. Complaints include fatigue, exertional fatigue (reduced, limited cardiac output), presyncope, syncope when standing or walking (preload reduction when standing, fixed cardiac output), shortness of breath (from mild elevation of the pulmonary venous pressures and from the volume of pericardial blood within the chest competing with lung volume), cough, dysphagia (mass effect of the increased weight of the heart on the esophagus), and edema if it is chronic. A review of systems may help establish the underlying disease state responsible for the tamponade syndrome.

PHYSICAL EXAMINATION

Venous Pressures

Venous pressures are normal early in tamponade but rise in proportion to the severity of tamponade and may be above the angle of the jaw and not well appreciated in late-stage tamponade. Concurrent hypovolemia, which is encountered regularly in trauma patients, competes against venous distention and therefore masks this basic tamponade finding and, importantly, also masks compensation. Atypical localized pericardial effusions, such as those against the left-sided heart chambers, may not produce significantly elevated central venous pressures. Only about 60% to 75% of tamponade cases are actually recognized to have elevation of jugular venous pressures when they are assessed at the bedside.[9,10]

Venous Contours

There is loss ("blunting" or "obliteration") of the y descent because there is impairment of ventricular filling (and atrial emptying) throughout all of diastole by compression from the pressurized pericardial effusion. Although the x descent is dominant, it is usually not steepened. A prominent x descent alone without a steep y descent usually indicates tamponade or effuso-constriction, even in the presence of atrial fibrillation.

Kussmaul Sign

Typically, Kussmaul sign is not present in pericardial tamponade.

Pulsus Paradoxus

Pulsus paradoxus is defined as variation (fall) of systolic blood pressure of more than 10 mm Hg *with normal respiration*. An even more traditional definition includes also that the pulse pressure falls as the systolic pressure falls more than does the diastolic pressure. The "paradox" of pulsus paradoxus, a historic and anachronistic term, is not that the blood pressure falls with inspiration, which to a degree is normal, but rather that the peripheral pulse may be reduced or absent, despite a cardiac contraction being evident by auscultation. Pulsus paradoxus may be palpated (if the variation in blood pressure is prominent) or recorded by sphygmomanometry and auscultation or direct pressure recording.[1,2]

The basis of pulsus paradoxus appears to be multifactorial. It includes (1) ventricular interdependence, such that the left-sided heart filling and stroke volume are compromised by the increase in right-sided heart filling in inspiration; (2) that pulmonary venous pressure falls in inspiration as lung capacitance increases with increase in lung volume; and (3) the inspiratory superimposition of negative intrapleural pressure onto the heart and aorta. In observational studies of patients with tamponade, it has been demonstrated that the intrapericardial pressure varies less (variation: 7 ± 1 mm Hg) than does the pulmonary capillary wedge pressure (variation: 17 ± 2 mm Hg)—creating constantly varying pulmonary capillary wedge : intrapericardial pressure gradients that are least with the first cardiac cycle of inspiration, reducing the pulmonary capillary : intrapericardial pressure gradient and left-sided heart filling[11] and ejection.

Pulsus paradoxus is most likely to be present in tamponade if the heart is structurally normal, the respirations are spontaneous, and the pericardial fluid is circumferential, not loculated. Only about 35% of tamponade cases are recognized to have pulsus paradoxus when they are assessed at the bedside.[10]

Pulsus paradoxus is a classic but neither invariable nor specific finding of tamponade. Pulsus paradoxus may also be seen in other disease states: respiratory distress from pulmonary disease of any type, hypovolemic shock, right ventricular systolic failure (e.g., right ventricular infarction, acute massive pulmonary embolism), and constrictive pericarditis.

Although it is detected in a large number of cases of tamponade, pulsus paradoxus is not a sufficiently sensitive sign for the diagnosis of tamponade, given the range of underlying cardiac abnormalities and also comorbidities that may be present. Pulsus paradoxus may be absent or attenuated in situations in which there is normalization of the left-sided heart volume loading through the respiratory cycle, such as with an atrial septal defect, severe aortic insufficiency, or left ventricular failure, thereby obviating the ventricular interdependence effect (Fig. 6-6). Localized pericardial tamponade (localized effusions that compress the left-sided heart chambers) commonly do not produce pulsus paradoxus. Positive-pressure mechanical ventilation also commonly obscures a pulsus paradoxus (Fig. 6-7).

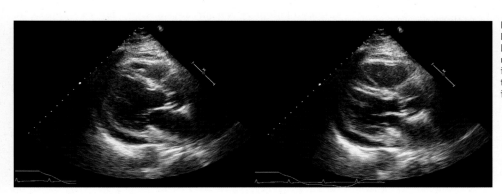

Figure 6-6. Parasternal long-axis view. Note the respirometry tracing along the bottom. With inspiration (denoted by an upward deflection of the tracing), the interventricular septum briskly shifts from the right to the left side (ventricular interdependence).

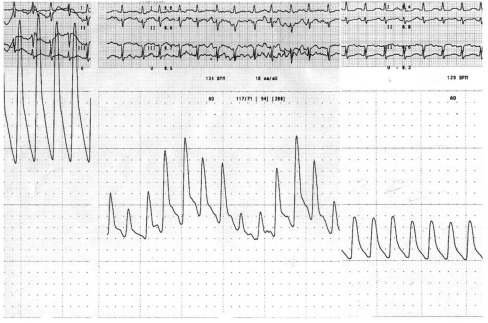

Figure 6-7. Aortic pressure tracings. LEFT, Hypertensive state during catheterization. MIDDLE, After attempted percutaneous coronary intervention resulting in acute tamponade. There has been a significant fall in the blood pressure, but more significantly there is now a pulsus paradoxus. The systolic pressure falls by more than 10 mm Hg through the respiratory cycle, and the fall in the systolic pressure is greater than the fall in diastolic pressure (i.e., the pulse pressure falls with inspiration). RIGHT, After intubation, sedation, and mechanical ventilation (and before drainage), the pulsus paradoxus is completely lost. There is tachycardia, though.

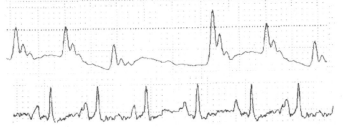

Figure 6-8. With the fourth cardiac cycle, during inspiration, there is a marked fall in the spectral flow profile velocity within the left ventricular outflow tract, associated with a severe, nearly total fall in the pulse pressure, hence the absence of a pulse, despite a cardiac contraction, due to ventricular interdependence in pericardial tamponade (total pulsus paradoxus). If progressive, it is apparent how terminal tamponade results in pulseless electrical activity.

Total Pulsus Paradoxus

Strikingly, in advanced tamponade, the pulse (pressure) disappears during inspiration. This is referred to as total paradox (Fig. 6-8). It requires verification for occurrence of regular cardiac cycles.

Pericardial Rub

A significant number of patients with effusions and tamponade do have a pericardial rub.[1]

Heart Sounds

Heart sounds are often distant in the context of larger effusions or chronic tamponade and normal in the context of smaller effusions or acute tamponade.

ELECTROCARDIOGRAPHY

In tamponade, electrocardiography (ECG) is usually abnormal, although nonspecifically so. *Low voltages* (<5 mm in the standard limb leads or <10 mm in the precordial leads) are seen in about half (61%) of chronic tamponade cases[3] because of increased distance between the heart and the surface recording. The finding of reduced voltages is likely to be less common in the context of acute tamponade resulting from small effusions because less distance is interposed between the chest wall and the cardiac chambers.

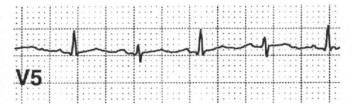

Figure 6-9. Electrical alternans. The mean QRS voltage and axis are varying in alternate cycles, as the heart swings to-and-fro within a larger pericardial effusion, hypercontractile from the distress of tamponade.

Electrical alternans, a phasic variation of the R-wave amplitude, usually best seen in precordial leads and with a beat-to-beat cycle length (every second beat has smaller voltages), is consistent with large chronic effusions that achieved significant tamponade and widely swinging motion of an underlying normal heart responding with vigorous contraction that varies the orientation of the mean electrical vector of the heart. Electrical alternans is a specific but insensitive (seen in only 20% of cases) sign of tamponade. The sign is strongest when the variation in amplitude includes the QRS *and the P wave amplitude* and will be present only if the effusion is large and the heart normal and able to respond to tamponade stress with dynamic contraction that results in swinging. Electrical alternans is often seen with advanced chronic malignant effusions; it is not seen with acute tamponade that occurs without substantial swinging motion of the underlying heart chambers (Fig. 6-9).

CHEST RADIOGRAPHY

The chest radiograph is useful to recognize that the heart size and shape are consistent with the presence of excess pericardial fluid. Such findings are usual for chronic tamponade cases that accrue larger and more obvious effusions and less common in acute tamponade produced by smaller effusions. At least 200 to 250 mL of pericardial fluid needs to accumulate before the chest radiograph reliably shows a difference that exceeds the variation due to the cardiac and respiratory cycles. Chest radiography is useful to identify associated pleural effusions and lung disease. The distinction of pericardial tamponade from pericardial effusion without tamponade by the chest radiograph is difficult because the size of the heart (the size of the pericardial effusion) is not accurately predictive of the likelihood of compressive (tamponade) effect.

ECHOCARDIOGRAPHY

Echocardiography is the test of choice to objectify pericardial tamponade and should always be obtained to confirm the diagnosis and to plan drainage safely, unless the patient's status is unsustainable. Transthoracic echocardiography (TTE) is usually adequate; transesophageal echocardiography (TEE) is increasingly rarely needed.[4-6] Goals of echocardiography in all tamponade cases include the following:

- Determination of the presence of pericardial fluid
- Determination of the exact distribution of pericardial fluid

- Determination of the presence of echocardiographic signs of tamponade
- Determination of the cause of tamponade, if possible
- Determination of the safest and most logical method of pericardial drainage, if needed

Although echocardiography is the single most useful test to recognize tamponade and to plan drainage procedures, echocardiographic signs of tamponade are not definitively predictive in all cases. Clinical assessment to establish a "pretest" probability of tamponade is essential, as is consideration of proceeding to hemodynamic study in cases that remain unclear or with clinical:echocardiographic discordance. Echocardiographic signs, alone or in combination, are not predictive of all cases of tamponade (Tables 6-3 and 6-4).

Echocardiographic Signs of Tamponade

There are both 2-dimensional and Doppler signs of pericardial tamponade. Two-dimensional echocardiography is used to acquire views that definitively establish that the accumulated fluid

is pericardial, not pleural, and to gather signs of chamber compression or collapse (right atrial collapse, right ventricular diastolic collapse), raised central venous pressure (IVC plethora), and ventricular interdependence (marked respiratory variation of chamber size—inspiratory septal shift) (Fig. 6-10). As the right-sided heart diastolic pressure increases in inspiration (and the left-sided heart pressure decreases in inspiration), the interventricular septum and often the interatrial septum are displaced to the left during inspiration as the systemic venous return increases and the pulmonary venous return falls.

Doppler signs of pericardial tamponade include marked variation of ventricular inflow velocities in parallel to 2-dimensional changes: right-sided heart (right ventricular) inflow velocities increase substantially (>40%) in inspiration, and left-sided heart (left ventricular) inflow velocities decrease substantially (>25%) in inspiration.

The likelihood of chamber collapse is influenced by its transmural distending pressure and the thickness of its wall—both of which resist the inward forces of pericardial fluid under pressure. Therefore, the right atrium is the most likely to collapse; the right ventricle, second most likely; the left atrium, less so; and the left ventricle, the least likely to collapse. Exceptions to this

Table 6-3. Right-Sided Chamber Collapse and Venous Inflow[10]

	Sensitivity (%)	Specificity (%)	PPV (%)	NPV (%)
Any collapse	90	65	58	92
RA collapse	68	66	52	80
RV collapse	60	90	77	81
RA and RV collapse	45	92	74	76
Abnormal inflow	71	95	82	88
Abnormal inflow and collapse of one chamber	67	91	80	84
Abnormal inflow and collapse of two chambers	37	98	90	75

NPV, negative predictive value; PPV, positive predictive value; RA, right atrial; RV, right ventricular.

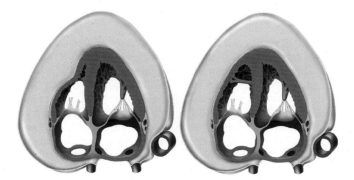

Figure 6-10. In tamponade (LEFT, note right ventricular diastolic collapse), within the confines imparted by the compressive pericardial effusion, with inspiration (RIGHT), the right side of the heart fills, but at the expense of the left side of the heart (ventricular interdependence). Note the shift of the interatrial and interventricular septa to the left side. The fall in left ventricular filling with inspiration is a component of the pulsus paradoxus in pericardial tamponade.

Table 6-4. Echocardiographic Two-Dimensional Signs[12-14]

		Sensitivity (%)	Specificity (%)	PPV (%)	NPV (%)
RA collapse	Reported range	55-100	68-100	90+	90
	High PTP			89	86
	Medium PTP			49	98
	Low PTP			8	>99
RV collapse	Reported range	48-93	50-100	90	90
	High PTP			88	78
	Medium PTP			45	97
	Low PTP			7	>99
IVC plethora	Reported range	97-100	40-75		
	High PTP			62	93
	Medium PTP			15	99
	Low PTP			2	>99

IVC, inferior vena cava; NPV, negative predictive value; PPV, positive predictive value; PTP, pretest probability; RA, right atrial; RV, right ventricular.

include disorders in which the distribution of pressure is not generalized, such as a loculated left-sided effusion (under pressure), which may compress only the adjacent left-sided chamber and not the right-sided chambers, and when chamber wall thickness is abnormal, such as pulmonary hypertension resulting in right ventricular hypertrophy, rendering the right ventricle less likely to collapse than the left atrium.

Two-Dimensional Echocardiographic Signs: Chamber "Collapse"

Chamber "collapse" (inversion, inflexion) signifies that the pericardial pressure exceeds the intracavitary pressures (that the chamber wall transmural distending pressure is now negative), resulting in chamber collapse and underfilling. Although the tendency is to dichotomize chamber collapse as either present or absent, it behaves as a linear variable with respect to the diagnosis of tamponade: the more it is present, the greater the specificity. Chamber collapse is most apparent when the contour of the chamber experiences inflexion (concavity or indentation), which does not normally occur when a chamber contracts. Although chamber collapse is a sought after sign, chamber collapse is imperfectly predictive of clinical or hemodynamic evidence of tamponade. M-mode study is useful in timing the chamber collapse of tachycardic hearts, but the combined effects of collapse and translation of the heart are not easy to distinguish on all views.

Right ventricular diastolic collapse is a useful but imperfect sign of tamponade physiology. The developed right ventricular systolic pressure is almost always sufficient to resist compression and collapse by the raised intrapericardial pressure, which only dips in tamponade in systole. Right ventricular diastolic pressure is lowest in early diastole, and if intrapericardial pressure exceeds the intracavitary pressure, collapse occurs. The predictive value of this sign is dependent on the pretest probability of the patient's having tamponade based on clinical assessment.[15] Right ventricular diastolic collapse is more sensitive in depicting elevated intrapericardial pressure than is pulsus paradoxus and is seen when cardiac output has fallen 20%, but before arterial blood pressure has fallen.[8-10] False-negatives occur from right heart–predominant diseases that result in right ventricular hypertrophy and a stiffer, less easily deformed right ventricular wall. Furthermore, chronic right ventricular hypertrophy is likely to be associated with higher right ventricular diastolic pressures, maintaining transmural distending pressure later in the course of tamponade.

In some cases, persistent collapse (due to very elevated intrapericardial pressure) of the right ventricle is unrecognized (Fig. 6-11). Some false-negatives defy clear explanation. Some false-negatives may be effuso-constrictive. False-positives occur as well. It has been elegantly shown in an experimental model that right ventricular diastolic collapse may be produced by the presence of large bilateral pleural effusions, presumably due to the hydrostatic weight imposed onto the right ventricular wall, and an elevation of the intrapericardial pressure.[16] In this study, it was shown that right ventricular diastolic collapse occurs at similar elevations of intrapericardial pressure, whether it is due to infused pleural effusion (9.5 mm Hg) or infused pericardial effusion (8.2 mm Hg).[16] A combined echocardiographic and hemodynamic observational study of patients with tamponade undergoing drainage in which the initial intrapericardial pressure was 25 ± 1 mm Hg revealed that right ventricular diastolic collapse disappeared at an average intrapericardial pressure of 4 ± 13 mm Hg. At the point of disappearance of right ventricular diastolic collapse, the stroke volume nearly doubled to 61 ± 10 mL from 37 ± 12 mL (Fig. 6-12).[2]

Right atrial collapse is a common finding in suspected tamponade cases as the right atrial wall is thin, compliant, and mobile and often exhibits striking concavity. Collapse of the right atrium occurs in systole in tamponade as the right atrial pressure is lowest with the x descent (which is dominant to the y descent in tamponade), and it is at this time that the intracavitary pressure is most likely to fall below the raised intrapericardial pressure. As well, the right atrial volume is least at the end of diastole. The right atrial pressure will rise only through ventricular systole as venous return fills and pressurizes the atrium. The greater the intrapericardial pressure, the more negative the transmural distending pressure, and the more filling of the right atrium must occur before the intracavitary pressure exceeds the intrapericardial pressure; that is, the higher the intrapericardial pressure, the longer the duration of right atrial collapse. Right atrial collapse continues well into systole in significant tamponade; hence, significant right atrial collapse in tamponade is predominantly a ventricular systolic event (in contradistinction to right ventricular collapse in tamponade, which is diastolic). Late diastolic right atrial collapse is extremely sensitive but not specific; right atrial collapse alone has excellent sensitivity (100%) but significantly lacks positive predictive value—only 50%. Exemplifying that the echocardiographic sign of right atrial collapse is a linear variable describing tamponade severity, and that the longer the collapse, the higher the intrapericardial pressure, a "cutoff" of one third of

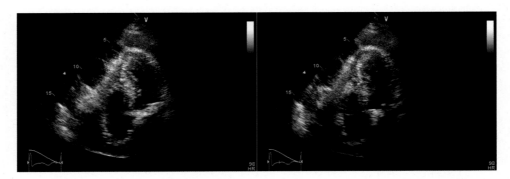

Figure 6-11. An 80-year-old man 5 days after re-do surgery for aortic valve replacement, mitral valve replacement, and aortocoronary bypass. LEFT, Diastole. RIGHT, Systole. There is a large pericardial effusion with extensive fibrinous stranding over the right side of the heart. The right atrium is not collapsed in either systole or diastole. The right ventricle, though, is collapsed in its apical half through the cardiac cycle. Chamber collapse occurring dynamically through the cardiac cycle is a more obvious finding than persisting collapse, as in this case. The clue is the absence of any cavity distal to the moderate band at any time during the cardiac cycle. The case was surgically proven.

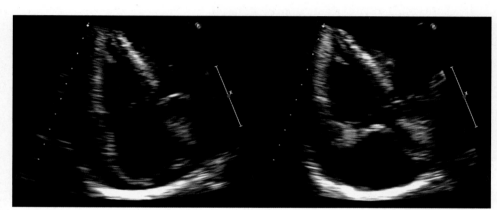

Figure 6-12. Apical 4-chamber views showing a large pericardial effusion. LEFT, Right atrial (ventricular systolic) collapse (concavity) is present as the right atrial transmural distending pressure is negative. MIDDLE, Right ventricular early diastolic collapse is present as the right ventricular transmural distending pressure is negative. RIGHT, End-diastolic (post–P wave/A wave) pressure rise; the right atrial and right ventricular pressures are greater, and their transmural distending pressures are positive.

Figure 6-13. Two-dimensional echocardiographic views of right atrial collapse. The right atrial free wall exhibits concavity or indentation—an entirely abnormal configuration—as the transmural distending pressure becomes negative because the intrapericardial pressure exceeds intracavitary pressure. The size of the right atrial cavity is correspondingly decreased. Normally, the right atrium expands in ventricular systole as the tricuspid valve is closed and venous return progressively fills the atrium.

the cardiac cycle (duration of right atrial collapse/cardiac cycle, 0.34) is used because it has good sensitivity (94%), specificity (100%), and positive predictive value (100%) as longer durations of right atrial collapse are increasingly hemodynamically relevant. Although, in general, right atrial collapse is a sensitive sign, the predictive value of the sign is heavily influenced by the clinically derived pretest (Bayesian) probability of tamponade.[15] The absence of sinus rhythm does not appear to confound the sign of right atrial inversion.[17] Right atrial collapse may be viewed as an "earlier" sign of tamponade, whereas right ventricular collapse is a "later" sign that occurs once cardiac output has fallen but before blood pressure has fallen (Figs. 6-13 and 6-14).

Experimental studies demonstrate that the combination of right atrial and right ventricular diastolic collapse results in significantly greater fall in cardiac output and rise in heart rate than does tamponade of the right ventricle alone, establishing that even if right atrial collapse is not alone a highly predictive sign, it is a significant or even dominant pathophysiologic component.[8]

The most important echocardiographic views are the parasternal long-axis view for right ventricular outflow tract (RVOT) collapse (Fig. 6-15); the parasternal short-axis view for right atrial, right ventricular, and RVOT collapse (Figs. 6-16 and 6-17) and for fluid distribution in potential drainage; the apical 4-chamber view for right atrial and right ventricular collapse (Fig. 6-18); and the subcostal view for right atrial and right ventricular collapse, IVC plethora, and fluid distribution in potential drainage.

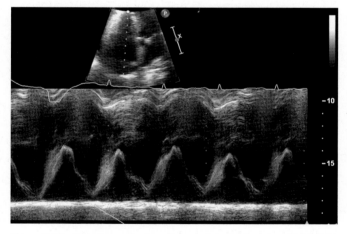

Figure 6-14. M-mode sample from the apical 4-chamber view. Right atrial collapse is seen through systole and half of diastole (more than one third of the cardiac cycle). Problems of M-mode sampling from this perspective include that the atrioventricular plane normally moves apically in systole, and tracking of the heart, if it is swinging, may be difficult. The determination of the fraction of the cardiac cycle during which the right atrial free wall is collapsed is usually made visually, without measurement.

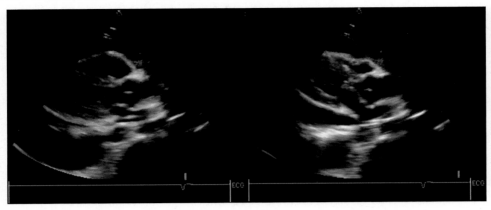

Figure 6-15. Parasternal long-axis views in systole (LEFT) and diastole (RIGHT). Note the diastolic collapse (concavity) of the RVOT due to pericardial tamponade and loss of diastolic transmural distending pressure. As well, the left-sided heart chamber dimensions are reduced because of loss of transmural distending ("filling") pressure. Normally, the right ventricle and outflow tract are expanded during diastole as they fill.

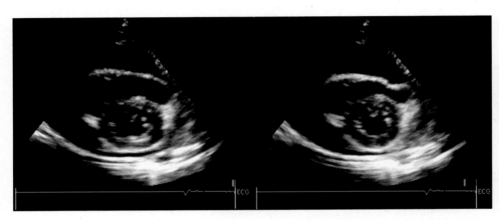

Figure 6-16. Parasternal short-axis views in end-diastole (LEFT) and mid-diastole (RIGHT). Note the mid-diastolic collapse (concavity) of the RVOT due to tamponade. With atrial contraction and the A-wave pressure rise in the right ventricle, at end-diastole, the RV transmural distending pressure is sufficient to distend the right ventricular free wall.

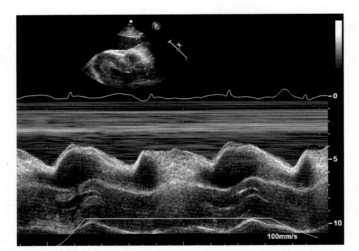

Figure 6-17. M-mode sample from the parasternal long-axis view. Right ventricular diastolic collapse is present due to pericardial tamponade. Normally, the right ventricle and outflow tract are expanded during diastole as they fill. In inspiration (note respirometry tracing), due to augmentation of venous return, there is some reduction of right ventricular collapse.

Chamber collapse may be absent in tamponade due to (1) pulmonary hypertension and right ventricular hypertrophy, (2) tricuspid regurgitation, or (3) pacing.

Doppler Signs

Doppler signs of tamponade include marked respiratory variation of right and left ventricular early-inflow velocities. The early (E wave) variation is twice as great as the variation of the atrial contraction (A wave) and is what is to be assessed. The normal (and post-pericardiocentesis) variation of left ventricular inflow is less than 10%, and the normal right ventricular inflow variation is less than 25%.[11]

Doppler signs of tamponade include marked respiratory variation of right (>40%; average, 85% ± 53%) and left (>25%; average, 43% ± 9%) ventricular early (E wave) inflow velocities.[11] The accentuation of the left-sided heart inflows is far more specific for pericardial disease as any pulmonary disease will accentuate variation in right-sided heart filling.

Variation of E-wave inflow velocities is markedly influenced (dampened) by positive-pressure ventilation. Inflow variations are prominent as well in other disease states, such as with any form of respiratory distress, pericardial constriction, or pericardial effuso-constriction. Adequate sampling of inflow velocities is difficult in a significant proportion of cases because of the small size of the heart cavities and the swinging motion in many cases (Fig. 6-19).

Inferior Vena Cava Dimensions and Motion

The infrahepatic shape and dimensions of the inferior vena cava (IVC) depend substantially on body position, presumably because of the variable weight of the liver transmitted to the underlying IVC.[18] Normally, in the left lateral decubitus position, the IVC diameter is less than 1 cm, the area is less than 2 cm², and the IVC diameter and area fall with inspiration[9,18] and fall briskly with a "sniff" maneuver. The greater the IVC diameter, the higher the

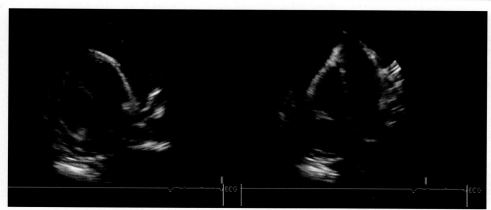

Figure 6-18. Apical 4-chamber views. Note the systolic collapse (concavity) of the right atrium almost to the tricuspid annulus level due to pericardial tamponade. Normally, the right atrium expands in ventricular systole as the tricuspid valve is closed and venous return fills the atrium.

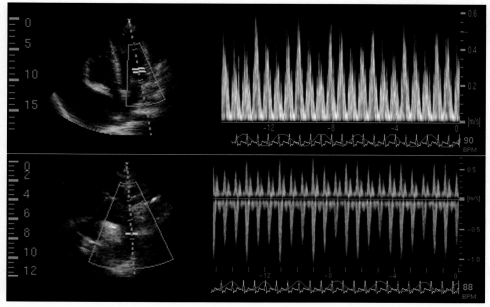

Figure 6-19. TOP, Left ventricular inflow recording. With inspiration, denoted by the upward deflection of the respirometry tracing, the early (E wave) inflow velocity falls prominently (>25%). These tracings are typical as they engender some uncertainty as to distinction of the E wave and the A wave because of summation of the two. BOTTOM, Proximal descending aortic flow velocity recorded from the suprasternal position shows a corresponding pattern. With inspiration, there is a prominent fall in velocity, commensurate with the pulsus paradoxus phenomenon. The variation in blood pressure due to the pulsus paradoxus was similar in proportion to the variation in velocity.

IVC distending pressure, and the less the "collapsibility."[18] Also, as IVC pressure rises, the diameter reduction that occurs with inspiration (or a sniff maneuver) decreases. "Plethora" of the IVC is said to occur as the deep inspiration IVC diameter decrease is 50% or less (Fig. 6-20). An IVC diameter greater than 10 mm achieves an 84% sensitivity, a 96% specificity, and a positive predictive value of 95% for a right atrial pressure greater than 8 mm Hg. An IVC cross-sectional area greater than 2 cm^2 offers a 73% sensitivity, a 100% specificity, and a positive predictive value of 100% for a right atrial pressure greater than 8 mm Hg.[9,18] The predictive value of this sign is dependent on the pretest probability of the patient's having tamponade on the basis of clinical assessment.[15]

Although logical as a means to objectify the beside physical diagnosis visual (subjective) impression, it is noteworthy that IVC assessment is more sensitive for the presence of tamponade than clinical assessment of venous distention (97% versus 61%).[9]

Patients with plethora and tamponade have higher heart rate (111 ± 21 versus 98 ± 20 bpm), greater pulsus paradoxus (24 ± 15 versus 12 ± 4 mm Hg), jugular venous distention (14 ± 5 versus 8 ± 3 mm H$_2$O), greater right atrial pressure (17 ± 6 versus 12 ± 6 mm Hg), and lower blood pressure (109 ± 22 versus 132 ± 27 mm Hg; all $P < .05$) (Fig. 6-21).[9]

CATHETERIZATION FINDINGS

Right- and left-sided cardiac catheterization is not necessary for the diagnosis of most tamponade cases (given the widespread availability of echocardiography), but it is useful if volume status is unclear,[4] if the echocardiographic findings are inconclusive, or if other cardiac disorders are considered. In pericardial tamponade (with uniform distribution of pericardial fluid around the heart), typical findings at catheterization include the following (Fig. 6-22):

- Elevation and "equilibration" (<5 mm Hg difference) of the average diastolic pressures (if the heart is otherwise normal) that often range between 15 and 25 mm Hg
- The right atrial and right ventricular pressure tracings reveal a blunted or an absent *y* descent; hence, there is no "square-root" (or "dip-and-plateau") sign and no Kussmaul sign.

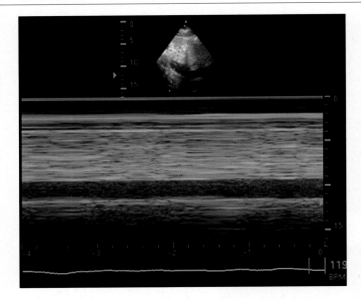

Figure 6-20. M-mode views of IVC diameter. In this case of tamponade, the IVC diameter is increased (>1 cm) and without inspiratory fall, typical of severely raised central venous pressure.

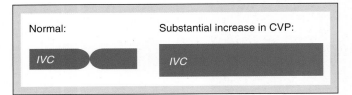

Figure 6-21. Normal recumbent IVC diameter is less than 1 cm, and there is prominent inspiratory collapse of the IVC as IVC volume and pressure fall as venous return to the thorax augments (normally to more than a meter a second) as inspiration reduces intrapleural and intrathoracic pressure. Hence, normally, a sniff maneuver will elicit a prompt fall in the IVC diameter. With raised central venous pressure (CVP), as with tamponade, the IVC diameter is greater, and the IVC diameter does not fall with spontaneous respiration (inspiration) or with a sniff maneuver.

- An elevated systemic vascular resistance
- Reduced cardiac output
- The arterial pressure waveform usually shows a pulsus paradoxus.
- Arterial blood pressure: Arterial hypotension is typical of advanced cases, but many patients with "normal" blood pressure are in fact hypotensive relative to their usual pressure. Some patients experience a striking hyperadrenergic response and are in fact hypertensive due to, and in spite of, the tamponade. The heart rate is usually also prominently elevated.
- The definition of tamponade is elevation (>10 mm Hg) and equilibration (<5 mm Hg) of intrapericardial and right atrial pressure, with a transmural distending pressure of less than 2 mm Hg. Classic tamponade is said to be present when the intrapericardial pressure is elevated above 7 mm Hg[4] or above 10 mm Hg[17] and the right atrial pressure is adequate, that is, 4 mm Hg or more after drainage (establishing the lack of intravascular volume depletion). Low-pressure tamponade is said to be present when the intrapericardial pressure is below 7 mm Hg and above 2 mm Hg before drainage and the right atrial pressure is less than 4 mm Hg after drainage (consistent with lesser intravascular volume).

Typically, if drainage is undertaken while there is hemodynamic monitoring, normalization or near-normalization of arterial waveforms, blood pressure, cardiac output, and filling pressures occurs with drainage of as little as 50 mL, unless there is underlying effuso-constrictive pericarditis or other cardiac structural abnormalities. If intrapericardial pressure is monitored, it falls to zero with drainage. Another important issue concerning catheterization is that many patients with critical tamponade cannot lie flat.

PERICARDIAL EFFUSION VARIANTS

Several variants of pericardial tamponade exist. They are important to recall because they have atypicality with respect to physical findings, imaging findings, and therapy.

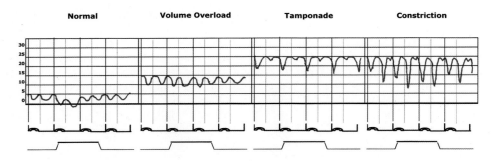

Figure 6-22. Right atrial pressure tracing in different states. Normal right atrial pressure is 0 to 5 mm Hg, with equal A and V waves and equal and gently sloping x and y descents. There is a fall in pressure associated with inspiration. With hypervolemia, the right atrial pressure rises, and the A and C waves and x and y descents rise simply in proportion. With tamponade, the right atrial pressure is elevated, and the y descent is diminished or obliterated; the x descent predominates. There is loss of inspiratory fall in pressure. With constriction, the right atrial pressure is elevated, and the x and y descents are exaggerated and steepened. The x and y descents may be equal or the y descent may predominate. With inspiration, there is less or no fall in mean right atrial pressure, but the x and y descents usually accentuate.

Postoperative Tamponade

After cardiac surgery or in anyone with prior adhesions from pericarditis, effusions may accumulate with atypical distributions and thus cause atypical tamponade syndromes. Prior valve surgery is twice as commonly responsible as is aortocoronary bypass surgery.[3] Early postoperative tamponade (<7 days) is associated with excessive (65%) or therapeutic (8%) use of anticoagulation. Late postoperative tamponade (after 7 days) is associated with use of anticoagulation (65%) and postpericardiotomy syndrome (34%).[3] Potential atypical aspects of postoperative cases include an underlying abnormal heart, possible prior pulmonary hypertension that renders right-sided heart compression less likely, stiffness of the myocardium due to imperfect "pump protection," atypical distribution of fluid, possible pericardial adhesions, volume overload, intravascular depletion from diuretics, concurrent pleural effusions, acquired or prior pulmonary disease increasing respiratory effort, and possible mechanical ventilation.

Early and late postoperative tamponade are notable for the concurrence of atrial fibrillation in half of cases.[3] Postoperative tamponade cases have a substantial number of noncircumferential effusions, although the reported range of loculated effusion is widely ranging. Among a series of 18 postoperative tamponade cases, only 3 of 18 cases had circumferential effusions, whereas 15 of 18 cases had loculated effusions. Chamber collapse less predictably occurs with right-sided chambers and may involve left-sided chambers; right atrial collapse was seen in only 3 of 15 loculated tamponade cases, right ventricular diastolic collapse was seen in only 1 of 15 loculated cases, left atrial collapse was seen in 3 of 15 loculated cases, but left ventricular collapse was seen in all cases of loculated effusions. Among a larger series of 209 late postoperative effusions, 70% were described as circumferential, 17% as posterior loculated, 7% as anterior loculated, and 7% as loculated in other positions.[3]

An experimental study demonstrated that localized tamponade does not result in typical hemodynamic findings; for example, experimental collapse of the left ventricle results in a fall in cardiac output and hypotension but not an increase in atrial pressure—a potential caveat about seeking usual signs (jugular venous distention) of tamponade in potentially atypical cases.[8] Similarly, tamponade of the right ventricle alone results in a rise in right atrial pressure alone, not of the left atrium (Figs. 6-23 and 6-24).[8]

Hypertensive-Hyperadrenergic Tamponade

An important subset of tamponade cases, generally with prior hypertension, experience a hypertensive response to tamponade, with arterial pressures in some cases above 200 mm Hg.[19] The believed mechanism is an excessive sympathetic-adrenergic response to distress. Such cases poorly tolerate vasodilation (such as sedation) and exemplify the poor and sometimes misleading association of arterial blood pressure with cardiac output and tissue perfusion. The discordance of blood pressure and cardiac output is illustrated in an experimental hemodynamic study, which demonstrated that in anesthetized mongrels with isolated right ventricular tamponade, arterial blood pressure increased while cardiac output fell.[8]

Low-Pressure Tamponade

Low-pressure tamponade is a variably defined entity but held to describe about 20% of tamponade cases that fulfill catheterization criteria of tamponade and that have only modestly elevated intrapericardial pressure *but also have modest degrees of concurrent intravascular depletion, compounding the effect of raised intrapericardial pressure.* Patients with low-pressure tamponade have fewer symptoms (mainly only dyspnea on exertion) and lesser severity of tamponade hemodynamic findings compared with classic tamponade (clinical diagnosis of tamponade, 24% versus 71%; jugular venous distention, 22% versus 55%; pulsus paradoxus, 7% versus 50%) but have significant increase in cardiac output after drainage (before, 3 ± 1.3, versus after, 3.2 ± 1.1 L/min/m^2).[4] Interestingly, echocardiographic findings of tamponade do not differ significantly between low-pressure tamponade and classic tamponade: effusion thickness (30 ± 12 versus 34 ± 14 mm; NS), no collapse (27% versus 21%), right atrial collapse (74% versus 76%; NS), right ventricular collapse (33% versus 51%; NS), exaggerated inflow velocity variations (54% versus 59%; NS).[4] The effect of volume loading such patients to correct the volume component of the tamponade syndrome has not been well studied.

MANAGEMENT

The definitive management of pericardial tamponade is pericardial fluid drainage by the most appropriate method—percutaneous or surgical.

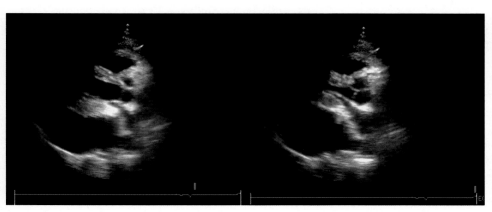

Figure 6-23. Systolic (LEFT) and diastolic (RIGHT) frames of a patient with postoperative left ventricular diastolic collapse due to a localized effusion. There is no fluid over the RVOT, hence no compression there.

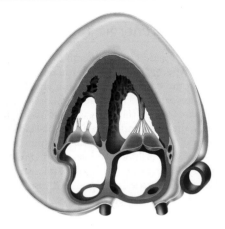

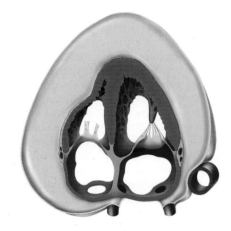

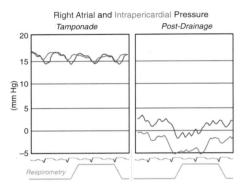

Right Atrial and Intrapericardial Pressure

Tamponade   *Post-Drainage*

(mm Hg)

Respirometry

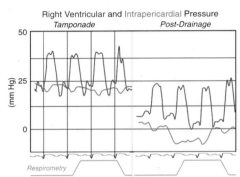

Right Ventricular and Intrapericardial Pressure

Tamponade   *Post-Drainage*

(mm Hg)

Respirometry

Figure 6-24. LEFT, Right atrial systolic collapse diagram and hemodynamics. RIGHT, Right ventricular diastolic collapse diagram and hemodynamics. Collapse of the right atrium is a concavity curvature of the free wall. In tamponade, the right atrial and intrapericardial pressures are elevated and similar. Right atrial pressure falls most with the dominant *x* descent in (ventricular) systole and is most likely at this time to fall beneath the intrapericardial pressure, resulting in systolic atrial collapse due to loss of transmural distending pressure. With drainage, there is normalization of the right atrial and intrapericardial pressure and of the transmural distending pressure through the cardiac and respiratory cycles, alleviating collapse. Collapse of the right ventricle is also a concavity curvature, which may occur anywhere along the free wall or RVOT. In tamponade, the right ventricular diastolic pressure and intrapericardial pressure are elevated and similar. The right ventricular diastolic pressure falls beneath the intrapericardial pressure in early diastole, resulting in loss of transmural distending pressure and collapse. With drainage, there is normalization of the right ventricular and intrapericardial pressure and of the transmural distending pressure, alleviating collapse.

Medical stabilization with volume loading or inotropes is controversial, although seemingly useful, while drainage is being arranged and effected. Medical stabilization has little chance to definitively stabilize the patient unless severe intravascular volume depletion was the major pathophysiologic culprit, greatly compounding the consequences of elevated intrapericardial pressure.

Although volume depletion exacerbates the effect of pericardial tamponade, volume expansion in euvolemic cases does not clearly improve hemodynamics. Excessive volume expansion infusion has the potential to exacerbate ventricular interdependence by further expanding the right-sided heart volume, at further expense to the filling of the left side of the heart. Therefore, unguided volume infusion is controversial and potentially futile, if not harmful, in tamponade cases.

Institution of mechanical ventilation, with its requirement of profound sedation, is relatively contraindicated in cases of pericardial tamponade. Both profound sedation and positive-pressure ventilation reduce preload to the right side of the heart and may precipitously drop the blood pressure.

SUMMARY

- Tamponade will occur when the compliance properties of the pericardium and their rate of accommodation are exhausted by the amount and rate of fluid accumulation.
- Acute tamponade occurs with rapid pericardial fluid accumulation (e.g., iatrogenic) of smaller effusions that rapidly exceeds existing compliance; chronic tamponade occurs with slower accumulation of larger effusions that finally exhaust both compliance reserve and remodeling abilities.

- The recognition of tamponade may be rendered difficult by the presence of underlying heart disease, comorbidities, localized effusions, and mechanical ventilation.

- Physical diagnosis is very helpful in most cases but does have limitations, especially in mechanically ventilated patients.

- When the transmural distending pressure (intracavitary pressure minus pericardial pressure) becomes negative (as the intrapericardial pressure exceeds the intracavitary pressure), the chamber is increasingly susceptible to collapse.

- Echocardiography is the single most useful test but must be interpreted in a context of clinical evaluation–derived probability. Echocardiographic 2-dimensional signs of tamponade include chamber collapse and IVC dilation or plethora. Echocardiographic Doppler signs include wide variation of left ventricular early (E wave) inflow velocities (>25%). Some echocardiographic studies will be nondiagnostic. Cardiac catheterization is usually not necessary but will be helpful in some cases of echocardiographic uncertainty, and some cases of tamponade occur in the catheterization laboratory; hence, familiarity with catheterization findings is important.

- The cause of tamponade should always be determined because it may be as life-threatening as the tamponade state itself or even more so.

- Medical stabilization is most successful if there is concurrent volume depletion that can be remedied by volume infusion; but routine volume infusion is controversial, as is routine use of adrenergic agents.

- Therapeutic drainage should be obtained to alleviate tamponade.

CASE 1

History

▸ 25-year-old man with recently diagnosed diffuse B-cell non-Hodgkin lymphoma, before treatment
▸ 3 weeks of progressive shortness of breath and cough

Physical Examination

▸ Elevated JVP (to the angle of the jaw)
▸ BP 110/80; pulsus paradoxus 25 mm Hg
▸ HR 140 bpm
▸ No pericardial rub or knock

Outcome

▸ Pericardiocentesis and drainage of 900 mL of serous fluid
▸ Cytologic test result was negative.

Comments

▸ Typical chronic tamponade case with a large effusion and nearly all clinical and echocardiographic signs present. Remodeling of the pericardium over time allows an increase in compliance and ability to accommodate a large volume of fluid before compression of the heart finally occurs.
▸ The effusion was presumed to be malignant from the lymphoma (there was documented intrathoracic disease—mediastinal adenopthy).
▸ The negative cytologic test result does not exclude that the effusion was malignant, as the sensitivity of pericardial cytology for malignant involvement is imperfect.
▸ Striking swinging motion of the heart and electrical alternans associated with the swinging motion

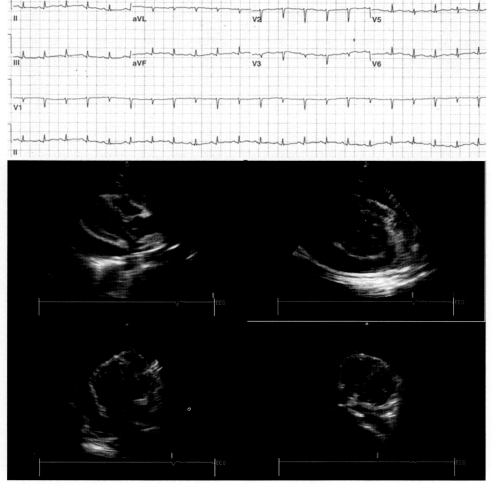

Figure 6-25. TOP, ECG shows right axis deviation, low voltages (<5 mm in the standard limb leads, <10 mm in the precordial leads), and electrical alternans. MIDDLE AND BOTTOM, TTE views reveal a large pericardial effusion and a small heart. The parasternal long-axis view demonstrates right ventricular diastolic collapse. The apical 4-chamber view demonstrates right atrial collapse. There is marked swinging of the heart (LOWER IMAGES), which generates the electrical alternans.

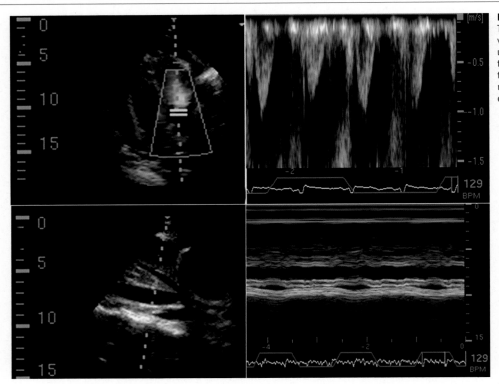

Figure 6-26. TOP IMAGES, Mitral inflow. There is a significant fall in early inflow velocity with inspiration (denoted by the upward deflection of the respirometry tracing). BOTTOM IMAGES, M-mode study of the IVC. The IVC is dilated and without respiratory variation, consistent with elevated central venous pressure.

CASE 2

History

▸ 45-year-old man with uncomplicated coronary artery bypass grafting 10 days previously
▸ Commenced warfarin day 5 for suspected pulmonary embolus, after initial anticoagulation with heparin IV
▸ Presented with increasing shortness of breath; INR: 3.7

Physical Examination

▸ Normal venous pressure
▸ Normotensive
▸ No pulsus paradoxus
▸ No pericardial rub or knock

Outcome

▸ Uneventful course after a pericardial window drainage procedure and removal of 450 mL of old blood, which was under pressure
▸ The appearance and motion of the heart normalized with drainage of the fluid, and the dyspnea resolved.

Comments

▸ Tamponade after aortocoronary bypass from a localized, loculated pericardial effusion
▸ As with this case, atypical findings abound in postoperative cases, and diastolic collapse of the left side of the heart, rather than of the right-sided heart chambers, is common.
▸ Early anticoagulation increases the risk of postoperative tamponade.

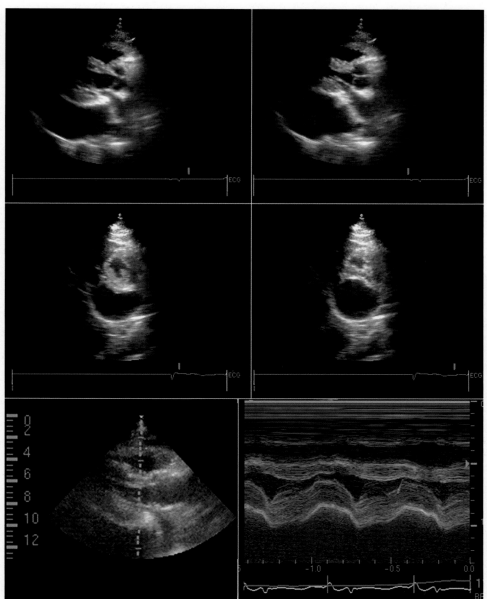

Figure 6-27. TTE. TOP LEFT, Parasternal long-axis view in systole. TOP RIGHT, Parasternal long-axis view in diastole. MIDDLE LEFT, Parasternal short-axis view in systole. MIDDLE RIGHT, Parasternal short-axis view in diastole. There is a posterior (only) pericardial effusion. The posterior wall of the left ventricle displaces outward in systole but collapses inward in diastole. BOTTOM IMAGES, M-mode study through the basal left ventricle. The diastolic collapse of the left ventricular posterior wall is depicted against the ECG. (Note: the P wave is the positive ECG deflection, and the QRS is the smaller complex.)

CASE 3

History

▸ 55-year-old woman undergoing PCI for an acute coronary syndrome
▸ During the coronary dilations, she developed chest pain and hypotension, and a pulsus paradoxus was observed on the arterial tracing.

Outcome

▸ Prompt resuscitation by pericardiocentesis
▸ No reaccumulation

Comments

▸ Acute tamponade
▸ Tamponade from a small amount of rapidly accumulating fluid
▸ Alleviation of tamponade by drainage of only 50 mL of fluid (only 250 mL in total was drained), revealing the small amount of additional intrapericardial volume needed to exhaust normal pericardial compliance and result in tamponade

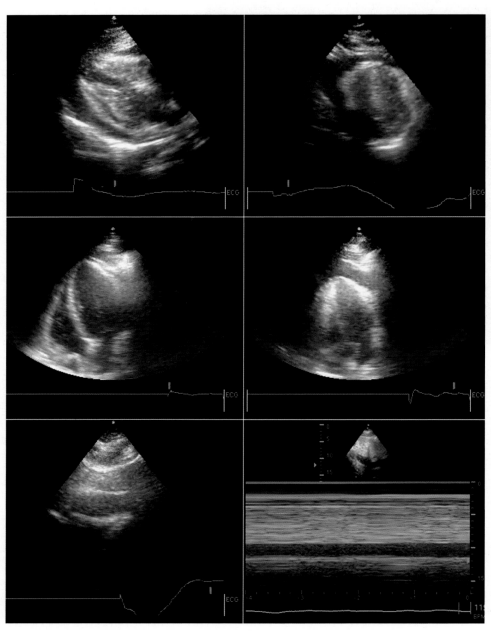

Figure 6-28. TTE. Due to loss of transmural distending pressure, the cardiac chamber cavities are very small—the left ventricular cavity is diminutive. There is a medium-sized pericardial effusion. The right ventricle collapses in diastole, and the right atrium collapses in systole. The IVC is dilated and does not exhibit respiratory variation.

CASE 4

History

A 77-year-old man 12 days after repeated aortocoronary bypass grafting was noted to be increasingly hypotensive. His jugular veins had been distended the day before and his legs edematous; in the belief that he was volume overloaded, he underwent diuresis of 1.2 liters within a 12-hour period. It was also considered whether he had developed pulmonary emboli, given the longer postoperative course, the neck veins, and a clear chest radiograph. Anticoagulation had already been started because of atrial fibrillation. His blood pressure fell from 150/85 mm Hg to 90/65 mm Hg. There was a 20 mm Hg pulsus paradoxus. His heart rate increased from 65 to 85 bpm, but he was taking beta-blockers for his recent myocardial infarction.

Outcome

▸ Volume infusion corrected the hypotension.
▸ Oliguria did not develop.

▸ Because he was receiving an anticoagulant (warfarin) and tolerating the tamponade, he was observed rather than being directly drained.
▸ Within 2 days, his neck veins had normalized (without diuresis), and the pericardial effusion had largely subsided.

Comments

▸ Intolerance to intravascular volume depletion is typical of tamponade.
▸ Restoration of volume corrected the blood pressure.
▸ Localized, asymmetric pericardial fluid distribution in a postoperative patient (twice operated on) is common.
▸ Concurrent beta-blocker use is common in postoperative patients, attenuating heart rate response and compensation (and a sign of tamponade), and anticoagulation use is also common, adding a factor into considerations of drainage.
▸ Left-sided chest views through pleural effusions assist with imaging of the heart.

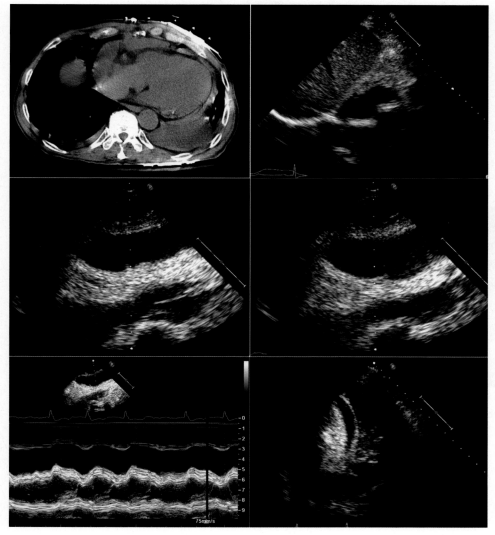

Figure 6-29. TOP LEFT, Non–contrast-enhanced CT scan axial image. There is a left pleural effusion but also a pericardial effusion that appears principally loculated to the right side of the heart lateral to the right atrium and ventricle. TOP RIGHT, Subcostal echocardiographic image of the fluid collection lateral to the right atrium-ventricle, which has a shape similar to the fluid collection as seen on the CT scan. MIDDLE IMAGES, Zoom views of the fluid pocket, the atrial wall, and the right atrium. The linear structure on the right of the very narrowed RA cavity is the closed tricuspid valve, denoting systole. The RA and the RV are larger in systole than they are seen to be in the right middle image in diastole (tricuspid valve opened), where they are compressed by the pericardial fluid collection. BOTTOM LEFT, M-mode study depicting the pandiastolic collapse of the right ventricle. BOTTOM RIGHT, Imaging through the left side of the chest and the pleural effusion contained therein; a small pericardial effusion can be seen lateral to the left ventricle.

CASE 5

History

A 19-year-old man, who had been stabbed in the heart 4 weeks previously and undergone successful repair of a myocardial puncture, was noted to have an enlarging cardiopericardial silhouette. He had been anticoagulated during this time. He had also developed mild hypotension (95/60 mm Hg; usual, 130/70 mm Hg), and his heart rate was 110 bpm. The venous pressures were elevated to the angle of the jaw. No pulsus paradoxus was present.

Outcome

▸ The patient underwent surgical resection of the parietal pericardium, which was very thickened.

▸ Fluid under pressure was removed.
▸ Thickening of the serosal layer was noted.

Comments

▸ Nonuniform pericardial fluid distribution in a postoperative patient
▸ Atypical tamponade signs (right ventricular collapse throughout the cardiac cycle and no right atrial collapse) are common in postoperative patients.

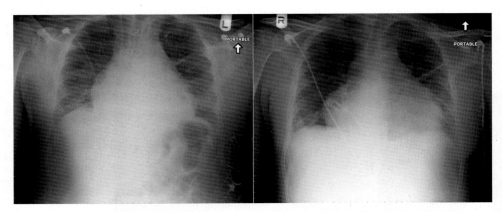

Figure 6-30. Chest radiographs taken after initial surgical repair (LEFT) and 4 weeks later (RIGHT). The cardiopericardial silhouette has enlarged and assumed a frankly globular shape, consistent with development of a pericardial effusion.

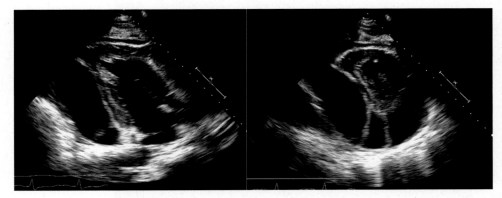

Figure 6-31. TTE parasternal long-axis (LEFT) and short-axis (RIGHT) views. There is a large pericardial effusion with nonuniform distribution—the anterior surface of the heart is adherent to the parietal pericardium, and the fluid, which contains some fibrin strands, is posterior. The posterior walls of the left and right ventricles are collapsing in diastole.

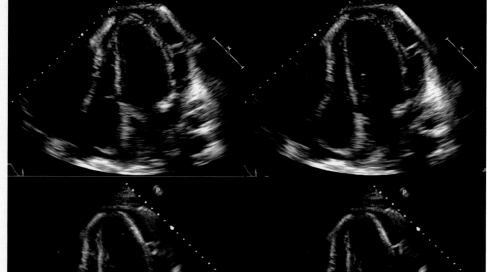

Figure 6-32. TTE apical 4-chamber views during different phases of the cardiac cycle. TOP LEFT, Systole (note the closed tricuspid valve). The basal and mid right ventricular free wall is compressed. TOP RIGHT, Diastole (note open tricuspid valve). The right ventricular free wall is even more compressed. BOTTOM, Deeper field images in diastole (LEFT) and systole (RIGHT). The right ventricle is collapsed and compressed throughout the cardiac cycle. It therefore does not exhibit the usual conspicuous collapse motion in each diastole, and its finding of collapse, despite being more severe than usual, is less obvious. Interestingly, the right atrium does not exhibit collapse.

References

1. Spodick DH: Acute cardiac tamponade. N Engl J Med 2003;349:684-690.
2. Singh S, Wann LS, Schuchard GH, et al: Right ventricular and right atrial collapse in patients with cardiac tamponade: a combined echocardiographic and hemodynamic study. Circulation 1984;70:966-971.
3. Tsang TSM, Barnes ME, Hayes SN, et al: Clinical and echocardiographic characteristics of significant pericardial effusions following cardiothoracic surgery and outcomes of echo-guided pericardiocentesis for management: Mayo Clinic experience, 1979-1998. Chest 1999;116:322-331.
4. Sagristà-Sauleda J, Angel J, Sambola A, et al: Low-pressure cardiac tamponade: clinical and hemodynamic profile. Circulation 2006;114:945-952.
5. Miller SW, Feldman L, Palacios I, et al: Compression of the superior vena cava and right atrium in cardiac tamponade. Am J Cardiol 1982;50:1287-1292.
6. Louie EK, Hariman RJ, Wang Y, et al: Effect of acute pericardial tamponade on the relative contributions of systolic and diastolic pulmonary venous return: a transesophageal pulsed Doppler study. Am Heart J 1995;129:124-131.
7. Fowler NO, Gabel M, Buncher CR: Cardiac tamponade: a comparison of right vs. left heart compression. J Am Coll Cardiol 1988;12:187-193.
8. Fowler NO, Gabel M: The hemodynamic effects of cardiac tamponade: mainly the result of atrial, not ventricular, compression. Circulation 1985;71:154-157.
9. Himelman RB, Kircher B, Rockey DC, Schiller NB: Inferior vena cava plethora with blunted respiratory response: a sensitive echocardiographic sign of cardiac tamponade. J Am Coll Cardiol 1988;12:1470-1477.
10. Mercé J, Sagristà-Sauleda J, Permanyer-Miralda G, et al: Correlation between clinical and Doppler echocardiographic findings in patients with moderate and large pericardial effusion: implications for the diagnosis of cardiac tamponade. Am Heart J 1999;138:759-764.
11. Appleton CP, Hatle LK, Popp RL: Cardiac tamponade and pericardial effusion: respiratory variation in transvalvular flow velocities studied by Doppler echocardiography. J Am Coll Cardiol 1988;11:1020-1030.
12. Gillam LD, Guyer DE, Gibson TC, et al: Hydrodynamic compression of the right atrium: a new echocardiographic sign of cardiac tamponade. Circulation 1983;68:294-301.
13. Himelman RB, Kircher B, Rockey DC, Schiller NB: Inferior vena cava plethora with blunted respiratory response: a sensitive echocardiographic sign of cardiac tamponade. J Am Coll Cardiol 1988;12:1470-1477.
14. Leimgruber PP, Klopfenstein HS, Wamm LS, et al: The hemodynamic derangement associated with right ventricular diastolic collapse in cardiac tamponade: an experimental echocardiographic study. Circulation 1983;68:612-620.
15. Eisenberg MJ, Schiller NB: Bayes' theorem and the echocardiographic diagnosis of cardiac tamponade. Am J Cardiol 1991;68:1242-1244.
16. Vaska K, Wann LS, Sagar K, Klopfenstein HS: Pleural effusion as a cause of right ventricular diastolic collapse. Circulation 1992;86:609-617.
17. Gillam LD, Guyer DE, Gibson TC, et al: Hydrodynamic compression of the right atrium: a new echocardiographic sign of cardiac tamponade. Circulation 1983;68:294-301.
18. Nakao S, Come PC, McKay RG, Ransil BJ: Effects of positional changes on inferior vena caval size and dynamics and correlations with right-sided cardiac pressure. Am J Cardiol 1987;59:125-132.
19. Ramsaran EK, Benotti JR, Spodick DH: Exacerbated tamponade: deterioration of cardiac function by lowering excessive arterial pressure in hypertensive cardiac tamponade. Cardiology 1995;86:77-79.

Pericardial Fluid Drainage

KEY POINTS

▸ Pericardial drainage can be performed by a variety of techniques; clinicians should be familiar with more than pericardiocentesis.

▸ The stronger indication for pericardiocentesis is as a therapeutic intervention rather than as a diagnostic technique. Pericardiocentesis performed to relieve tamponade has a much greater diagnostic yield than

does pericardiocentesis performed as a diagnostic procedure.

▸ Whenever possible, pericardiocentesis should be performed with imaging guidance.

▸ Although it is not widely available, pericardioscopy appears to increase the diagnostic yield of pericardial drainage.

Drainage of pericardial fluid is performed either to attempt to achieve a diagnosis (of bacterial infection, tuberculous or fungal infection, or malignant disease) or to alleviate compression by the fluid of the cardiac chambers (tamponade). The underlying disease processes responsible for the need of pericardial fluid drainage are numerous (Tables 7-1 and 7-2). The diagnostic yield of pericardial fluid analysis is far less in the absence of tamponade than in the presence of tamponade.

Diagnostic procedures consist of fluid analysis, biopsy, and pericardioscopy. Drainage procedures include pericardiocentesis (tap) with a needle, pericardiocentesis (catheter drainage), percutaneous balloon pericardiostomy, surgical pericardial window, and surgical pericardiectomy.

DRAINAGE PROCEDURES

Pericardiocentesis is the removal of pericardial fluid for therapeutic (decompression) or diagnostic sampling purposes. Only 50 to 100 mL of fluid needs to be removed to alleviate tamponade; therefore, pericardiocentesis itself may be therapeutic (Fig. 7-1), if only temporarily so.[1,2]

Catheter drainage (the insertion of a drainage catheter) is commonly performed at the time of pericardiocentesis to attempt to completely drain the pericardial space of fluid and thereby to lessen the likelihood of symptomatic recurrence and need for repeated procedures. Pericardial catheter drainage has become the most common primary treatment strategy (75%) (Fig. 7-2).[1]

Chest tube drainage techniques can also be used. A chest tube can be inserted into the pericardial space by several surgical approaches (through subxiphoid incision, thoracotomy, or ster-

notomy). A chest tube is usually left briefly after a pericardial window procedure is performed to ensure that the window is working.

A *pericardial window,* also known as a fenestration or decompression procedure (from the French *fenêtre,* window), can be performed through several surgical approaches (subcostal, sternotomy, thoracotomy, thorascopic). A subxiphoid approach can be managed without general anesthesia in some cases. A section of the pericardium, usually about the size of a matchbox, is removed, allowing drainage of pericardial fluid into the left pleural cavity, obviating fluid accumulation in the pericardial space and thereby the development of tamponade, as well as providing a tissue specimen for stain, culture, and histology.

Among drainage procedures, pericardial windows provide the longest lasting benefit. However, there is still a low but definite failure rate over time (Fig. 7-3). Presumably the margins of the excised parietal pericardium adhere to the visceral pericardium, re-establishing integrity of the pericardial space and excluding it from the pleural space, allowing fluid, and pressure, to reaccumulate within the pericardial space.

In cases of critically severe compression of the heart by tamponade or clot, surgical drainage procedures that use general anesthesia run the risk of precipitating extreme hypotension when anesthesia is induced because of sympatholysis, which diminishes afterload and preload. Typically, vasopressor support is temporarily needed in such cases. As is seen regularly in pericardial drainage cases, predrainage vasopressor need is typically followed by vasopressor-induced hypertension when the tamponade is relieved.

Pericardiostomy is a percutaneous balloon dilation of the pericardium that is performed to fistulize the pericardial cavity into the pleural cavity, percutaneously achieving a result similar

Table 7-1. Etiology of Pericardial Effusions Undergoing Drainage

Malignancy (lung cancer >> others)	32%
Tuberculosis	18%
Other infections	14%
Collagen disease	18%
Hypothyroidism	18%
Aortic dissection	4%

Modified from Zayas R, Anguita M, Torres F, et al: Incidence of specific etiology and role of methods for specific etiologic diagnosis of primary acute pericarditis. Am J Cardiol 1995;75:378-382.

Table 7-2. Causes of Effusions Undergoing Drainage

Malignancy	25%
Postoperative	28%
Cardiac perforations from procedures	14%
Infection	7%
Connective tissue disease	4%
Idiopathic	8%
CAD related	2%
Other	12%

CAD, coronary artery disease.
From Tsang TS, Enriquez-Sarano M, Freeman WK, et al: Consecutive 1127 therapeutic echocardiographically guided pericardiocenteses: clinical profile, practice patterns, and outcomes spanning 21 years. Mayo Clin Proc 2002;77:429-461.

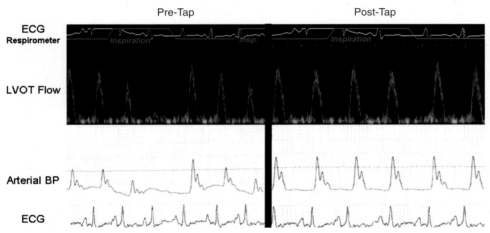

Pre-Tap   Post-Tap

ECG
Respirometer

LVOT Flow

Arterial BP

ECG

Figure 7-1. A 53-year-old woman with known rheumatoid arthritis presented with severe fatigue, venous distention, blood pressure of 70/50 mm Hg, and total pulsus paradoxus (absence of pulse with inspiration). Echocardiography showed a large effusion and tamponade. The pre-tap panel on the left shows a nearly total fall in left ventricular outflow tract (LVOT) flow with inspiration and total pulsus paradoxus. After removal of 70 mL, there is normalization of flow and blood pressure. Two liters were drained. She was alive 5 years later. The pericardial fluid was positive for LE cells, and her disease has evolved into frank systemic lupus erythematosus.

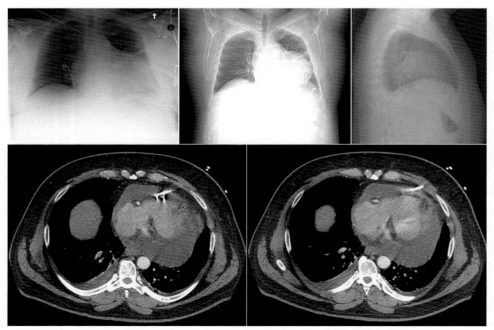

Figure 7-2. A 58-year-old man who had been observed for a chronic idiopathic large pericardial effusion that progressed to tamponade. Pigtail catheter drainage was performed through an apical approach. TOP LEFT, Anteroposterior chest radiograph after drain insertion. The cardiopericardial silhouette remains large. TOP MIDDLE AND TOP RIGHT, CT scan scout images also reveal the globular enlargement of the heart and the drainage catheter. BOTTOM, Contrast-enhanced CT scan image shows the pigtail drain in the interior pericardial effusion but with extensive residual pericardial infusion due to loculation.

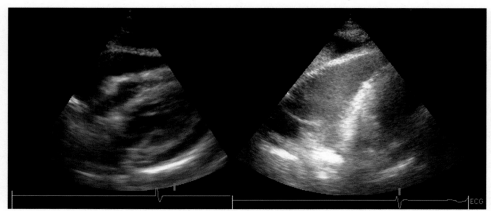

Figure 7-3. LEFT, Initial presentation of cardiac tamponade (subcostal view). There is a circumferential effusion. The right atrium is collapsed, and the right ventricle is small. Lung carcinoma was responsible. A window was performed, and the patient was treated with chemotherapy. RIGHT, The patient presented again a year later in tamponade, which was percutaneously drained. He survived only 8 more weeks.

to a surgical pericardial window procedure. The procedural success rate is approximately 88% when it is performed by experienced operators in patients with large effusions due to malignant disease. Complications include fevers and pneumothoraces (Table 7-3).[3]

Diagnostic Yield

Drainage performed as a therapeutic procedure often provides both therapy and a diagnosis, whereas drainage performed in the absence of tamponade with the intention of achieving a diagnosis achieves only a low diagnostic yield. Pericardiocentesis with effusion but without tamponade achieves an approximately 6% diagnostic yield, and pericardiocentesis of effusion with tamponade achieves an approximately 29% diagnostic yield.[4] Similarly, pericardial biopsy of effusion without tamponade achieves an approximately 5% diagnostic yield, and pericardial biopsy of effusion with tamponade achieves an approximately 54% diagnostic yield.[4] In a series of 100 consecutive cases of effusion with tamponade that were drained, the overall diagnosis rate was 22%, with 90% of the diagnoses made in the subset with tamponade. Although the diagnostic yield of diagnostic-intention pericardiocentesis is low, identification of treatable infections of the pericardium is relevant.

IMAGING GUIDANCE

To achieve the highest success rate and to minimize complications, percutaneous drainage procedures should be guided, preferably by an imaging modality (Figs. 7-4 to 7-7). Critical instability necessitates drainage or attempted drainage without imaging guidance. However, whenever possible, guidance should be used. Electrocardiographic, fluoroscopic, computed tomographic (CT), and echocardiographic guidance may be used; the availability and local experience generally determine the choice.

Electrocardiographic Guidance

Pre-imaging guidance is feasible through electrocardiographic recording of current through a metal finder needle to which an alligator clip is attached that allows recording of electrocardio-

Table 7-3. Hemodynamic Values Before and After Drainage

Parameter	Pre-Tap	Post-Tap	P
CO (L/min)	4.0 ± 1.4	7.9 ± 2.0	<.001
HR	112 ± 19	103 ± 14	<.05
SV	37 ± 14	78 ± 18	<.01
RAP	18 ± 9	9 ± 6	<.01
PCWP	23 ± 8	16 ± 8	<.01
IPP	21 ± 7	2 ± 4	<.01
MAP	98 ± 6	128 ± 8	<.05

CO, cardiac output; HR, heart rate; IPP, intrapericardial pressure; MAP, mean arterial pressure; PCWP, pulmonary capillary wedge pressure; RAP, right atrial pressure; SV, stroke volume.
From Singh S, Wann LS, Schuchard GH, et al: Right ventricular and right atrial collapse in patients with cardiac tamponade: a combined echocardiographic and hemodynamic study. Circulation 1984;70:966-971, table 1.

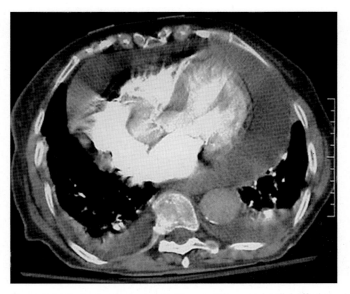

Figure 7-4. Contrast-enhanced axial CT scan. A large pericardial effusion is seen around all four cardiac chambers, particularly over the left-sided heart chambers. There are prominent streak artifacts over the right heart especially and (cardiac) motion artifact, as the image is not ECG gated.

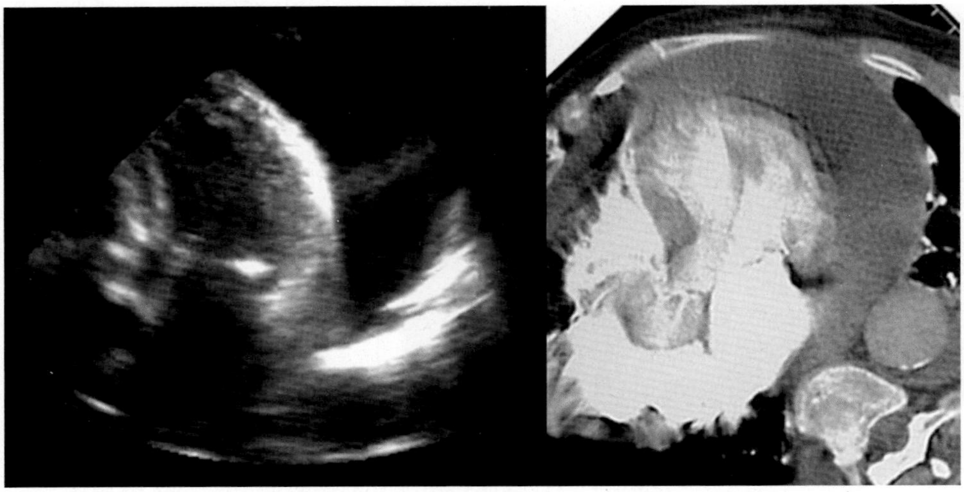

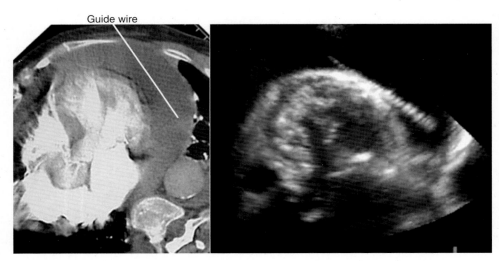

Figure 7-5. LEFT, Apical transthoracic echocardiographic view oriented into the effusion. RIGHT, The contrast-enhanced CT scan axial image is rotated to match the transthoracic echocardiographic image.

Figure 7-6. A wire is present in the pericardial space, oriented toward the greatest depth of fluid.

Guide wire

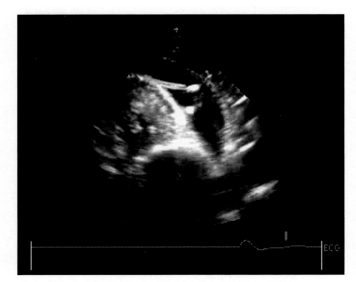

Figure 7-7. A pigtail catheter is in the pericardial space, with partial reduction of the pericardial effusion size.

graphic (ECG) complexes. Should the finder needle encounter straw-colored fluid, the drainage procedure can proceed with the needle kept at that position. Should the needle encounter bloody fluid, the fluid is less likely to be from a cardiac chamber if there is no ST elevation recorded from the needle. If ST elevation is noted, the needle tip is against or in the epicardium (current of injury). When the needle tip is withdrawn slightly and the ST elevation subsides, the tip should be in the pericardial space. ECG guidance often achieves some degree of trauma to the heart chambers and possibly the overlying coronary arteries.

Fluoroscopic Guidance

The interventional cardiac catheterization laboratory provides an excellent environment within which to perform almost any invasive procedure, including pericardiocentesis. The ability to rotate the x-ray tower to achieve an optimal tangential image of the cardiopericardial silhouette usually displays the lucent stripe of the epicardial fat layer over the darker myocardium and under the pericardial fluid layer (see Fig. 3-16). Furthermore, the catheterization laboratory readily provides for transducing and recording of pressures from any cavity entered, which may useful to guide the procedure and to evaluate the extent of hemodynamic benefit of drainage, especially in suspected effuso-constrictive cases.

Computed Tomographic Guidance

The combination of CT scanning and interventional radiology also provides an excellent means and venue with which to perform pericardial drainage. Among the many virtues of CT scanning of the heart is the depiction of the heart within complete anatomic reference of the rest of the chest. Echocardiography, although very useful, offers imaging without the same extent of delineation of the heart to chest and chest wall anatomy.

Echocardiographic Guidance

Echocardiography is the most common means by which pericardial drainage is guided. It is a portable modality, is available at bedside, is suitable for unstable patients, and has considerable versatility, even if it has substantially limited depiction of anatomic field of imaging and is limited by tomographic planes of imaging that render delineation of curved structures, such as wires, very difficult.

With echocardiography, as with CT scanning, it is possible to determine the safest access site (the one with the largest fluid dimension behind it) and the easiest access site (the one with the shortest distance into the effusion) and the orientation of the approach into the effusion (such that the needle tip is oriented preferably not at the heart chambers but away from the heart chambers, into the effusion). By use of either modality, the distance into the effusion can be accurately determined, which assists substantially with the procedure (Figs. 7-8 to 7-10).

Ultrasound imaging can be performed during the procedure; a sterile sleeve over the transducer allows the operator to scan simultaneously to image the needle, wire, catheter, or injected agitated saline. Alternatively, a second operator can scan. Although this requires skill, it is readily mastered.

In development and not well validated is a device that enables imaging with color Doppler study of the needle tip in real time. There are also probe-mounted needle holders that are feasible, but again with limited validation.

PERICARDIOCENTESIS

Pericardiocentesis is performed to withdraw fluid from the pericardial cavity for therapeutic or diagnostic reasons. Pericardiocentesis is often the first step toward insertion of a drainage catheter into the pericardial space to drain it completely.

The most common causes of effusions that require drainage are malignant disease, post–open heart surgery, perforation from interventional procedures, infection, connective tissue disease, idiopathic, and coronary artery disease related as well as others. Malignant involvement and postoperative causes account for more than 50% of cases at most hospitals.

The introducer needle tip and its bevel are sharp and may lacerate structures; therefore, the needle should be introduced from a location, at an angle, with knowledge of the depth not to be exceeded. Wires and catheters are less traumatic as they are not sharp. The introducer needle must be inserted for a minimum of time, undertaking verification maneuvers (imaging or agitated sterile saline injection), withdrawal of the needle, or insertion of the wire. If fluid return is straw colored, the needle tip is most likely in the pericardial space and is clearly not in the heart chambers. There are some uncommon occasions when straw-colored fluid return is from a pleural effusion (transthoracic approach) or from ascites (xiphocostal approach). If the fluid return is bloody, the possibilities are that the needle tip is in a bloody pericardial effusion, within a cardiac chamber, or, if it is subcostally inserted and oriented too low, in the spleen (Table 7-4). Both bloody pericardial fluid and right-sided heart intracardiac chamber blood may return under pressure. The appearance of pericardial fluid is quite variable.

The risks of pericardiocentesis are influenced by operator experience. Major complications arise in about 1% of cases except at centers with high volume and proficiency.[5] Major risks include death, cardiac arrest, cardiac cavitary laceration requiring surgery,

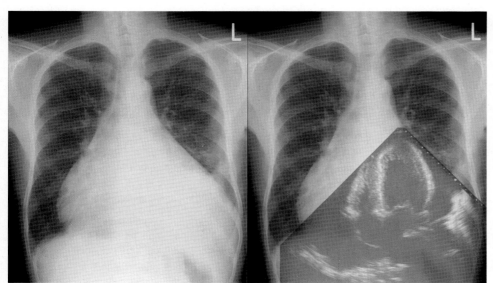

Figure 7-8. LEFT, Posteroanterior chest radiograph of a patient with tamponade due to dialysis. RIGHT, Chest radiograph with the patient's echocardiography image superimposed. Although the projections are not directly comparable, the point can be made that there is a large amount of fluid, extensively to the right of the heart and also to the left side. The only location where pericardial fluid is typically not present in tamponade due to large effusions is posterior to the mid left atrium.

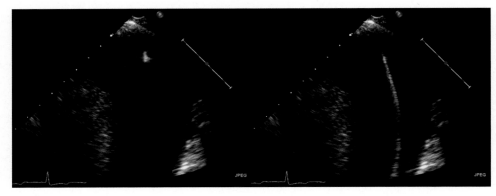

Figure 7-9. Zoom apical views of a pericardial effusion, left ventricle wall on the left side. LEFT, The needle tip has been advanced only 0.5 cm into the effusion but is clearly seen within the effusion. Because the wire is metallic, its artifact is more prominent than its image. RIGHT, The wire can be seen within the pericardial space. As the wire is following a planar course for a substantial distance, and as the imaging plane has been aligned to match it, a considerable length of the wire is seen.

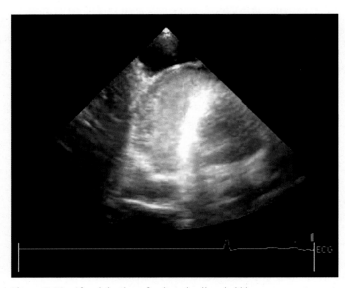

Figure 7-10. After injection of agitated saline, bubbles are present within the pericardial space (coarser echoes). There is also a fresh thrombus over the right ventricle (finer specular echoes), whose motion was that of gelatin. Repeated needle passes had traumatized the heart, resulting in a significant intrapericardial hematoma.

Table 7-4. Appearance of Pericardial Effusion in Postoperative Tamponade Cases

Bloody	47%
Serosanguineous	28%
Serous	20%
Chylous	2%
Purulent	0.4%
Stranding	20%
Partially coagulated	3.7%

From Tsang TS, Barnes ME, Hayes SN, et al: Clinical and echocardiographic characteristics of significant pericardial effusions following cardiothoracic surgery and outcomes of echo-guided pericardiocentesis for management: Mayo Clinic experience, 1979-1998. Chest 1999;116:322-331.

Table 7-5. Common Sites of Pericardiocentesis

Subxiphoid	17%
Chest wall	71%
Right parasternal	2%
Left parasternal	5%
Midclavicular line	12%
Anterior axillary line	52%
Not identified	12%

From Kopecky SL, Callahan JA, Tajik AJ, Seward JB: Percutaneous pericardial catheter drainage: report of 42 consecutive cases. Am J Cardiol 1986;58:633-635.

coronary artery laceration requiring surgery, injury to intercostal arteries requiring surgery (Fig. 7-11), pneumothoraces requiring chest tubes, ventricular arrhythmias, and sepsis. Minor risks include bleeding, pneumothoraces not requiring chest tubes, vasovagal reflexes, nonsustained ventricular tachycardia, and pleuropericardial fistula. Among 1127 echocardiographically guided pericardiocenteses at the Mayo Clinic, the success rate was 97% and the complication rate was 4.7%, of which 1.2% were major and 3.5% were minor.[1] Another Mayo Clinic series identified the most common sites of pericardiocentesis (Table 7-5).[6] Common difficulties encountered in pericardiocentesis are shown in Table 7-6. Figures 7-12 and 7-13 illustrate the common access sites and the procedure itself.

PERICARDIAL FLUID ANALYSIS

Fluid analysis is undertaken to directly document infections and malignant involvement and to indirectly support other disorders.

Stains and cultures objectify and specify bacterial, fungal, and tuberculous infections and establish antimicrobial sensitivities. Rare infections may necessitate use of uncommon stains and cultures. Cytology is performed to detect malignant cells. Biochemical testing is performed to establish the following:

- Reduced glucose concentration is consistent with rheumatoid arthritis and bacterial infection.
- Elevated cholesterol level is consistent with hypothyroidism, rheumatoid arthritis, and tuberculosis.
- Elevated lipid levels document chylous effusion.
- Elevated adenosine deaminase and interferon-γ levels, if available, suggest tuberculosis.

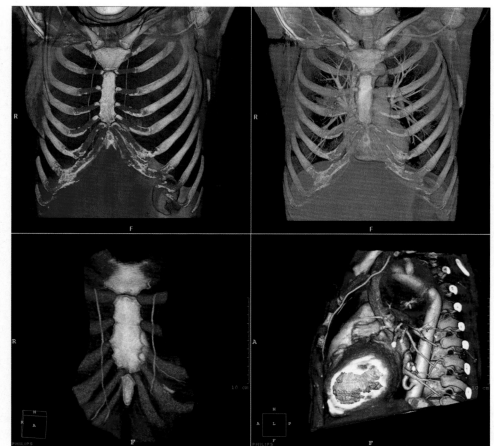

Figure 7-11. These 3D reconstructed cardiac CT images demonstrate the relation of the chest wall, the heart, and the internal thoracic/internal mammary arteries. CT is performed, when possible, with a deep breath; therefore, the diaphragm and heart are lower in the chest than with usual respiration. The internal thoracic/mammary arteries are depicted on the left images (UPPER LEFT IMAGE, view from the outside of the chest; LOWER LEFT IMAGE, view from the inside of the chest.) The internal thoracic/mammary arteries can be seen to lie against the back of the anterior chest ribs/costral cartilages, 1- to 2-finger breadths lateral to the margin of the sternum. Inferiorly, they give rise to some anterior subcostal arteries, as can be seen in the LOWER LEFT IMAGE. The relation of the heart (chambers) to the chest wall (on deep inspiration) is apparent in the RIGHT UPPER IMAGE. The RIGHT LOWER IMAGE depicts the course of the left internal thoracic artery along the inside of the left anterior chest wall. Although not depicted on this arterial phase angiogram, there are actually internal thoracic/mammary veins immediately lateral to the internal thoracic arteries. (Courtesy of Michael Regan, Philips, Canada.)

Table 7-6. Common Difficulties in Performing Pericardial Catheter Drainage

Difficulty	Potential Causes and Responses
Selection of a suboptimal access site	Review echocardiography or CT to optimize selection.
Awkward positioning	Ensure optimal positioning of the patient, the operator, and the equipment with use of a large sterile field.
Excess resistance in passing the catheter over the wire	Skin nick may be inadequate, the course of the wire may be angulated, or the dilator tunnel may be too short or kinked from the needle's course having been varied excessively. This is most commonly encountered with a subxiphoid puncture that was too steep and the course redirected more shallowly. Also, thickened parietal pericardium may engender resistance.
Unsure of needle, wire, or catheter location	Means by which to establish the location of the needle tip, wire, or catheter tip include the following: Imaging of the needle, wire, or catheter Recording of the waveform (although ventricular pressure tracings are generally distinguishable from atrial and intrapericardial pressure tracings, atrial and intrapericardial pressures tracings may not be) Injection of agitated saline and imaging by ultrasonography Injection of contrast dye and imaging by fluoroscopy Electrocardiographic recording to exclude ST elevation
Needle is inserted farther than the distance seen on echocardiography or CT between the skin and the effusion and there is no fluid return	Needle is not following the planned course. Withdraw, reorient, and reinsert. Also, intrapericardial material may not be fluid, or needle lumen may be plugged.
Excessive ongoing drainage	Suggests that the catheter tip is within a heart cavity or a vessel or that there is ongoing leakage into the pericardial space. Consider the cause. Withdraw or replace.
Ambiguous saline or dye injection findings	Saline may be poorly prepared (poorly agitated), or too little volume of agitated saline or dye may have been injected. The catheter (if multiholed) may be half into a heart cavity and half into the pericardial effusion. Withdraw or replace.
Patient distress	Use adequate local anesthesia. Consider light sedation if hemodynamics are not critical and the patient is distressed. Verify that procedural complications have not occurred.
Worsened hypotension after sedation	Avoid unnecessary sedation in cases of critical tamponade that are dependent on vasoconstriction for blood pressure.

If tamponade is absent, the overall diagnostic rate from fluid analysis is 5%; if tamponade is present, the diagnostic rate is approximately 50%.

PERICARDIAL BIOPSY

Pericardial biopsy has a similar or slightly higher diagnostic rate for the detection of malignant involvement and infection; some cases have positive biopsy findings with negative fluid analysis results, or vice versa. For example, among 32 diagnostic and 44 therapeutic cases, there was no difference in the diagnosis rate by fluid analysis (19%) and biopsy (22%).[4] The detection rate of malignant involvement by pericardial biopsy is not 100%, and it is lower yet for the detection of tuberculosis. Many patients with tuberculosis of the pericardium will have typical tuberculi bacilli without acid-fast bacilli on staining and without positive culture; such cases cannot be reliably distinguished from other fungal diseases. Thus, the contribution of standard pericardial

biopsy to fluid analysis at the time of pericardiocentesis is controversial.

PERICARDIOSCOPY

Pericardioscopy is an uncommon technique of limited availability that uses rigid or flexible thoracscopes or mediastinoscopes to visually assess the pericardium. The rationale is that visual guidance of sampling increases diagnostic yield by targeting biopsy to nonuniformly distributed pathologic changes within the pericardium. In a series of 141 consecutive patients with pericardial effusions undergoing pericardioscopy with a rigid mediastinoscope through a subxiphoid window, a diagnosis was achieved in 49% of the cases. There was 6% in-hospital mortality, but none due to mediastinoscopy. The increase in sensitivity was superior to surgical drainage alone for detection of malignant involvement (21%), radiation-induced pericarditis (100%), and purulent effusions (83%) (Fig. 7-14).[7] The ongoing development of laparoscopic and thorascopic techniques and technologies may provide superior diagnostic yield of undifferentiated large pericardial effusions when an important or treatable cause is suspected.

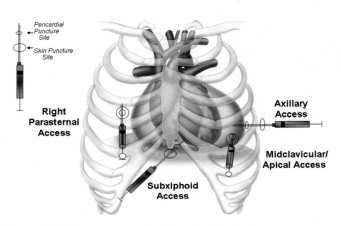

Figure 7-12. Common access sites for pericardiocentesis.

PERICARDIAL CATHETER DRAINAGE

Indwelling catheter drainage appears to decrease the recurrence rate of tamponade and therefore reduce the need for repeated procedures. Pericardial catheters, if carefully and aseptically inserted and maintained, can be left in for days. From a series of 42 consecutive cases of percutaneous catheter drainage, the mean duration of an indwelling catheter was found to be 3.5 days (1 to 19 days), of which only 3% became occluded and 2% became infected.[6] At the Mayo Clinic, use of catheter drainage procedures has been associated with a 50% reduction of early and late recurrences of tamponade and thereby reduction of need for pericardial surgery.[1,2]

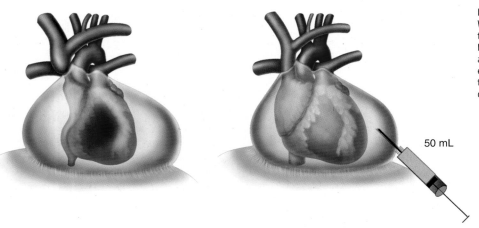

Figure 7-13. Pericardiocentesis. Withdrawal of only 50 to 75 mL eliminates tamponade (compression) in most cases. Note relief of right atrial, right ventricular, and caval compression and of venous engorgement and the increase in size of the left side of the heart after alleviation of cardiac compression by tamponade.

50 mL

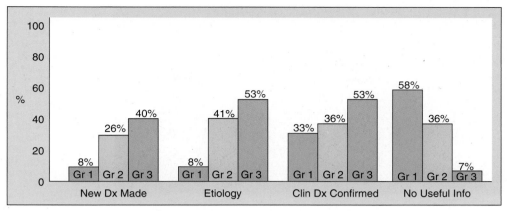

Figure 7-14. Pericardioscopy in 49 consecutive patients with large effusions. Group 1: biopsy under fluoroscopy alone; group 2: biopsy under pericardioscopic guidance (4 to 6 samples); group 3: biopsy under pericardioscopic guidance (18 to 20 samples). (From Seferovic PM, Ristic AD, Maksimovic R, et al: Diagnostic value of pericardial biopsy: improvement with extensive sampling enabled by pericardioscopy. Circulation 2003;107:978-983.)

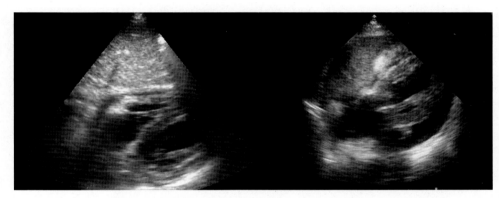

Figure 7-15. LEFT, Subcostal view. This patient was severely hypotensive from tamponade. The effusion was located only on the left side of the heart, by the left atrium. Pericardial adhesions along the diaphragmatic surface, presumed to be from remote aortocoronary bypass operation, made drainage from that approach unwise. RIGHT, This patient was severely hypotensive from tamponade but also from a large blood clot compressing the right side of the heart. The liquid effusion was located only on the left side of the heart. A subcostal percutaneous approach would encounter only clot, before entering the heart chamber, and would be unwise for that reason to be an attempted drainage site and also unsuccessful because the clot cannot be aspirated.

XIPHOCOSTAL ANGLE DRAINAGE (LARREY'S POINT)

Before imaging guidance became available, pericardiocentesis was performed with use of physical diagnosis skills to establish the presence of pericardial tamponade and use of external landmarks to orient needle introduction into the pericardial space. As with many procedures, pericardiocentesis was honed through practice in wars, as traumatic tamponade was abundant because of blunt and penetrating trauma (Figs. 7-15 to 7-17). Two surgeons deserve particular recognition: Dominique-Jean Larrey (1766-1842) and Franz Schuh (1804-1864).

Dominique-Jean Larrey, a military surgeon and Napoleon's personal physician, traveled with Napoleon's army on their military campaigns. He improvised field ambulances and developed the technique of limb amputations—the only treatment at the time for serious penetrating limb injury. He performed more than 300 amputations on the night of the Battle of Borodino alone. Larrey's point is the left xiphosternal angle, the traditional site of blind pericardiocentesis (Fig. 7-18).

Franz Schuh performed the first pericardiocentesis of the modern era. His technique for drainage of traumatic tamponade became popular during the Crimean War.

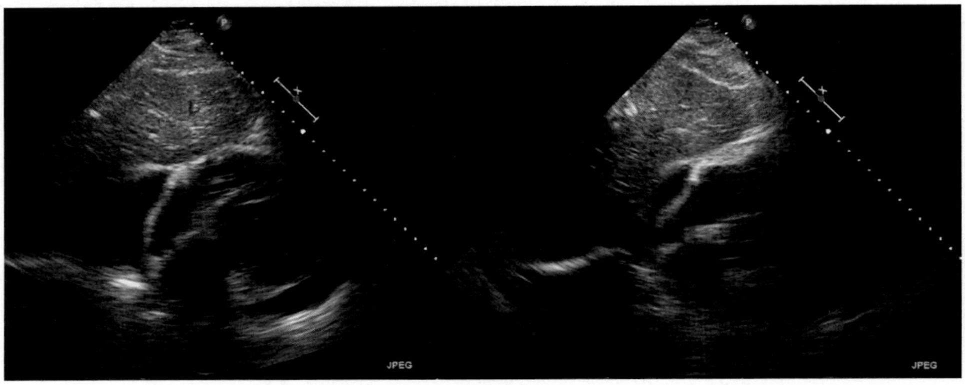

Figure 7-16. This patient developed pericardial tamponade a week after undergoing bypass surgery. These subcostal views demonstrated that the pericardium is adherent along most of the diaphragmatic surface of the heart. The relevance is that most subxiphoid approaches for percutaneous drainage have no pericardial space to enter into; the first fluid return would be anticipated to be from entering the right side of the heart. The other implication is that surgical drainage through the same approach has to be directed far to the left to avoid the same complication—entering the right ventricle.

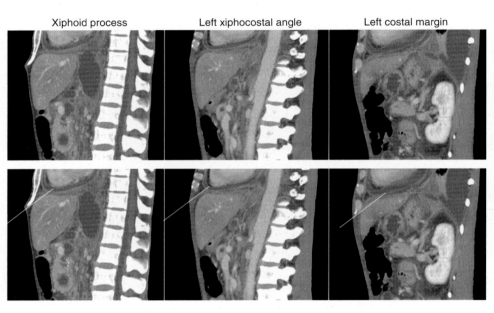

Xiphoid process | Left xiphocostal angle | Left costal margin

Figure 7-17. These sagittal contrast-enhanced CT images depict the course of a wire or needle entering the pericardial space from three different positions. LEFT, The course of a needle entered beneath the xiphoid process—the track, entering low, tends to traverse the top of the liver. MIDDLE, The course from a point of insertion at the xiphocostal angle; the track passes over the liver (this is the surgical approach that avoids liver). RIGHT, The track with insertion along the costal margin, again showing the tendency to traverse the liver. Therefore, the optimal site is the xiphocostal angle, also referred to as Larrey's point.

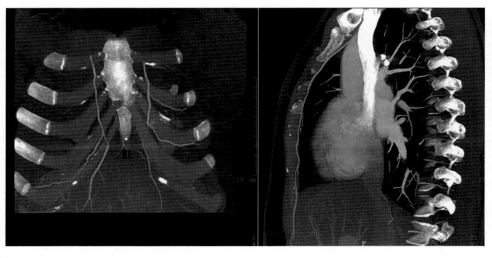

Figure 7-18. CT angiogram images. The internal mammary (thoracic) arteries (and veins) run beside and down the length of the sternum, and the anterior intercostal arteries run behind the inferior margin of the rib. The intercostal interspaces away from the sternum, especially over the ribs, are generally free of arteries, as is the xiphocostal angle, also known as Larrey's point.

CASE 1

History

▸ 43-year-old man with severe fatigue
▸ HIV-positive, under treatment for bronchogenic carcinoma

Physical Examination

▸ BP 80/40 mm Hg (pulsus paradoxus of 25 mm Hg); HR 105 bpm, RR 20/min
▸ Venous distention to the angle of the jaw
▸ Heart sounds distant, no rub
▸ No edema
▸ Clear chest

Management and Outcome

▸ 1 L drained directly, with definite improvement in symptoms, fall in venous pressure, and elimination of pulsus paradoxus and electrical alternans.
▸ There was little drainage after 36 hours, and the drain was pulled on the third day. The patient was discharged on the day after.
▸ The syndrome recurred 6 weeks later, concurrent with belief by the oncologist that the lung carcinoma was failing to respond to chemotherapy. The effusion was drained again. The patient was again discharged.

▸ The tumor continued to grow, and the effusion recurred, as did the tamponade. It was drained percutaneously once more, as a surgical window seemed unwarranted in the context of terminal malignant disease. The patient died as a result of metastases within a few weeks.

Comments

▸ Recurrent pericardial effusion and tamponade due to malignant disease unresponsive to treatment
▸ Large pericardial effusion consistent with chronicity and pericardial remodeling
▸ Typical physical diagnosis and echocardiographic signs of tamponade
▸ Prominent swinging motion and electrical alternans are common in tamponade cases due to malignant disease. The adrenergic response to distress from the tamponade syndrome accentuates the motion and swinging of the heart.
▸ The effusion was so large and evenly distributed that many sites of drainage may have been feasible, but apical access to the lateral pericardial space always seemed the shortest way in to the largest depth of fluid.
▸ Percutaneous treatment was employed repeatedly to obviate a surgical drainage procedure during chemotherapy. A pericardial window would have afforded more reliable drainage.

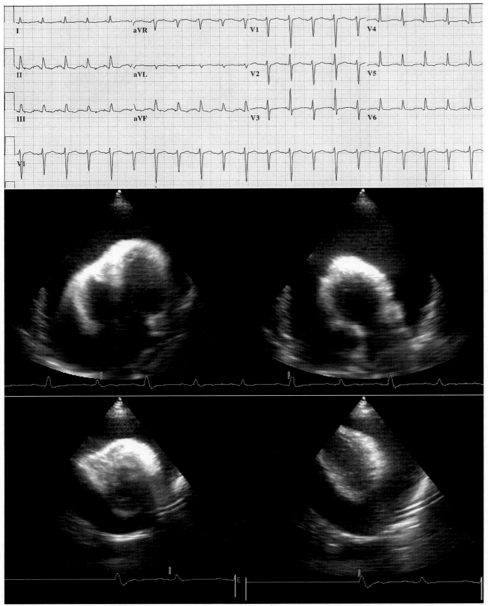

Figure 7-19. TOP, Electrical alternans and sinus tachycardia: signs of cardiac distress from pericardial tamponade. The heart is swinging prominently; its electrical axis variations are responsible for the electrical alternans. BOTTOM IMAGES, Transthoracic echocardiographic apical 4-chamber and short-axis views show a large pericardial effusion, and there is both right atrial and right ventricular collapse. MIDDLE AND LOWER IMAGES, The swinging of the heart on successive cardiac cycles.

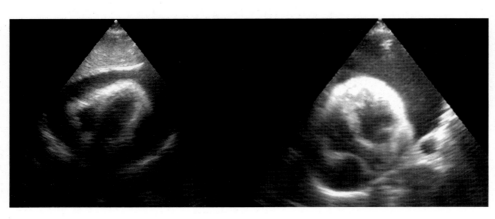

Figure 7-20. Transthoracic echocardiography. LEFT, Subcostal image. RIGHT, Apical 4-chamber view. The shorter distance from the skin puncture site to the pericardial site and the greater dimension of pericardial (fluid) space make the apical approach in this case more amenable to fluid drainage than the subcostal approach.

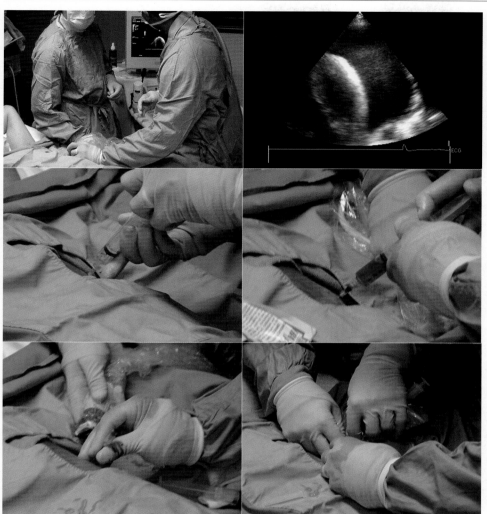

Figure 7-21. Pericardiocentesis. TOP LEFT, Apical echocardiographic images taken with use of a sterile sleeve. TOP RIGHT, Corresponding view, establishing the optimal orientation into pericardial fluid along the left lateral aspect of the heart. MIDDLE LEFT, Introduction of needle and saline in syringe. MIDDLE RIGHT, Fluid return shows tinged blood. BOTTOM LEFT, Spontaneous return of bloody fluid. BOTTOM RIGHT, Two syringes on a three-way stopcock being attached, with attention to maintain a stable needle position.

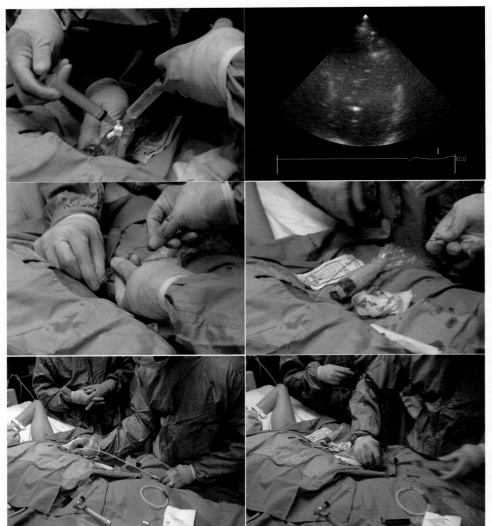

Figure 7-22. TOP, Injection of agitated saline. Injected microbubbles confirm position of the needle tip in the pericardial space. MIDDLE, Wire being inserted. BOTTOM, Catheter being inserted.

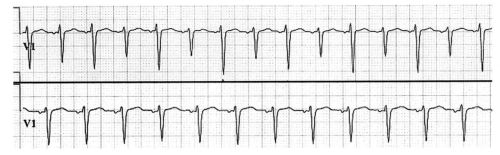

Figure 7-23. TOP, Tracing before pericardiocentesis shows electrical alternans from swinging motion. BOTTOM, Tracing after pericardiocentesis shows no alternans after evacuation of pericardial fluid and stabilization of the heart motion.

CASE 2

History

▸ A 74-year-old man presented to the emergency department with severe dyspnea.
▸ He had initially presented with tamponade, resulting in a diagnosis of bronchogenic carcinoma 15 months before. Initial drainage was percutaneous.

Physical Examination

▸ BP 80/50 mm Hg (pulsus paradoxus of 25 mm Hg), HR 90 bpm, RR 22/min
▸ Venous distention to the angle of the jaw
▸ No rub

Management and Outcome

▸ Complete drainage was performed.
▸ The patient's dyspnea improved only partially, as there were extensive concurrent pulmonary complications of his carcinoma.
▸ He died in hospital 7 weeks later of postobstructive pneumonia and debility.

Comments

▸ Untreatable malignant disease responsible for 3 episodes of tamponade
▸ Failure of a pericardial window is a rare occurrence; ascitic fluid potentially confused the percutaneous drainage, but proper planning of the procedure (knowing the distances exactly) and confirmation with injection of agitated saline (bubbles) assisted.
▸ Poor clinical outcome is common in tamponade due to malignant involvement

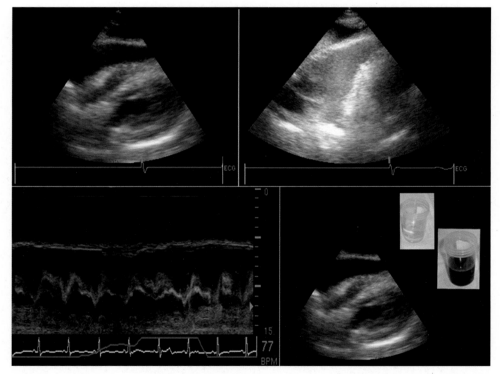

Figure 7-24. TOP LEFT, Transthoracic echocardiographic subcostal image at initial presentation 15 months before shows pericardial effusion, right-sided heart collapse, and ascites. TOP RIGHT, Transthoracic echocardiographic view at re-presentation again shows a pericardial effusion, severe collapse of the right side of the heart, and ascites. BOTTOM LEFT, M-mode study from the subcostal view into the heart. The first dark space is ascites (5 cm). The second black space is pericardial fluid (further 3 cm). The right ventricular free wall and the small right ventricular cavity are beyond. The right ventricular cavity increases in dimension with inspiration. The tap was planned on the basis of distance, but unexpectedly it was obvious when the pericardial cavity was entered because the ascitic fluid was yellow and the pericardial fluid was blood tinged. BOTTOM RIGHT, Fluid withdrawn during tap: yellow ascites fluid and blood tinged pericardial fluid.

CASE 3

History

▸ 74-year-old man 7 days after aortocoronary bypass
▸ Developed dyspnea

Physical Examination

▸ BP 85/50 mm Hg (pulsus paradoxus of 25 mm Hg), HR 95 bpm, RR 22/min
▸ Venous distention to the angle of the jaw
▸ No rub

Management and Outcome

▸ The patient was clinically in tamponade. Echocardiography identified a localized effusion with very little access by subcostal or transthoracic percutaneous approaches.
▸ The case was referred for surgical drainage and creation of a pericardial window. The surgeon was notified that most of the right ventricle was adherent to the parietal pericardium. The window was performed by subxiphoid approach, the heart and pericardium were inspected: the right ventricle was adherent to the pericardium over most of the surface of the heart, but laterally, fluid within the pericardial space could be identified, and the window was created there. Iatrogenic laceration, or puncture of the right ventricle, was avoided by recognizing the localized nature of the effusion and the inability to safely approach it by standard subcostal access techniques.

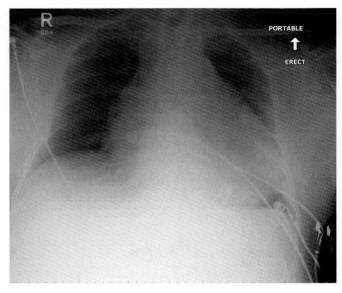

Figure 7-25. Cardiomegaly is evident on the chest radiograph.

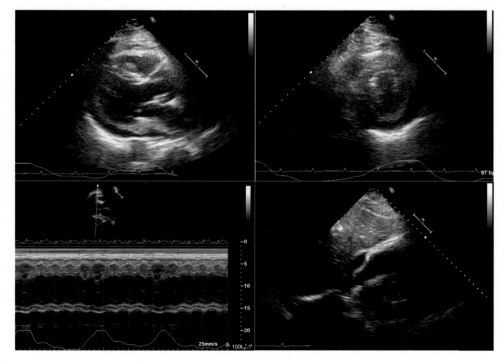

Figure 7-26. Transthoracic echocardiography. TOP LEFT, Parasternal long-axis view. TOP RIGHT, Parasternal short-axis view. Both views show a pericardial effusion located posteriorly only, not anteriorly. BOTTOM LEFT, M-mode study across the basal left ventricle. Left ventricular septal motion indicates ventricular interdependence ("bounce" toward the left ventricle with the first or second cardiac cycle of respiration). BOTTOM RIGHT, Subcostal long-axis view shows pericardial fluid beside part of the right atrium, collapsing it, but some of the right atrium and all of the right ventricle are adherent to the parietal pericardium.

CASE 4

History

▸ A 20-year-old man was admitted to the hospital after being stabbed 7 times in the abdomen. He was hemodynamically stable with these wounds. He underwent exploratory laparotomy.
▸ 5 days later, he was short of breath.

Physical Examination

▸ BP 85/50 mm Hg (pulsus paradoxus of 25 mm Hg), HR 95 bpm, RR 22/min
▸ Venous distention to the angle of the jaw, no y descent
▸ No pericardial rub or murmurs

Management and Outcome

▸ The patient was clinically and echocardiographically in tamponade.
▸ Surgical drainage was chosen because it afforded the means to evacuate thrombus within the pericardial space, to drain blood or fluid within the pericardial space, and to inspect the heart for the source of bleeding and the cause of LV apical systolic dysfunction.
▸ At surgical inspection, it was found that there was puncture of the pericardium and apical RV/LV myocardium with coronary laceration. Presumably, the coronary artery was responsible for the bleeding, which had stopped. Coronary damage resulted in apical myocardial dysfunction, but the patient survived.

Comments

▸ Surgical drainage also affords the means and opportunity to inspect the heart for bleeding sources responsible for tamponade.
▸ Surgery affords the only realistic means to evacuate intrapericardial blood clot.
▸ The lucent track seen on subcostal echocardiographic imaging was very nearly identical to the knife track upward that injured the heart.

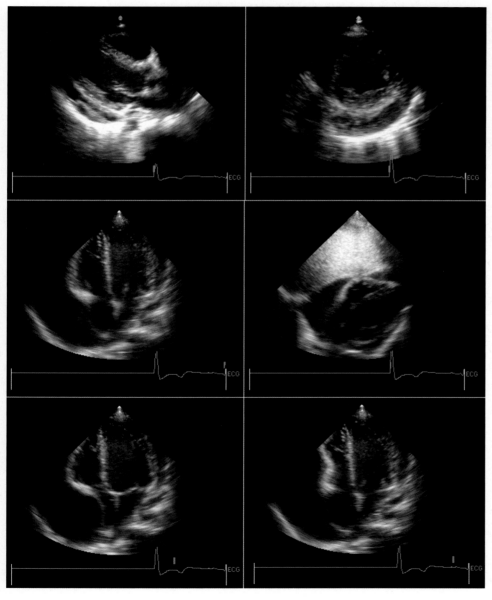

Figure 7-27. Transthoracic echocardiographic views show a large pericardial effusion lateral to the right side of the heart. Under the left ventricle, there appears to be thrombus. The subcostal views depict adherence of the right ventricle to the parietal pericardium and a peculiar, suspicious lucent track from the apex of the sector to that site that may be the knife wound. There are both right ventricular diastolic collapse and right atrial systolic collapse.

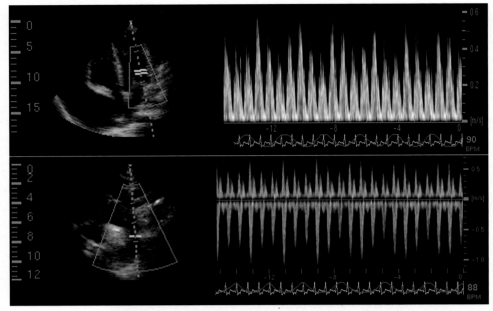

Figure 7-28. TOP ROW, Left ventricular inflow. There is prominent respiratory variation of the early diastolic inflow velocity. BOTTOM ROW, Aortic flow velocity in the descending aorta falls with inspiration—a surrogate of pulsus paradoxus.

CASE 5

History

▸ A 44-year-old woman, a smoker with a known lung mass, presented to the hospital with a stroke and a lowered level of consciousness. Her initial assessment was focused on neurologic issues.

Physical Examination

▸ BP 110/80 mm Hg, pulsus paradoxus of 15 mm Hg (respiratory effort was reduced because of lowered level of consciousness), HR 95 bpm
▸ Neck veins distended but difficult to assess because the patient could not be positioned
▸ Predominant x descent; no pericardial rub

Management and Outcome

▸ 1.4 L of fluid was removed.
▸ Cytologic test result was positive for adenocarcinoma.
▸ The patient underwent chemotherapy but died within 2 months.

Comments

▸ Malignant effusion and tamponade
▸ Circumferential effusion
▸ Imaging of the wire, with use of a sterile sleeve over the ultrasound transducer, confirms the location.
▸ The 1-year survival rate of malignant tamponade is only 15%.

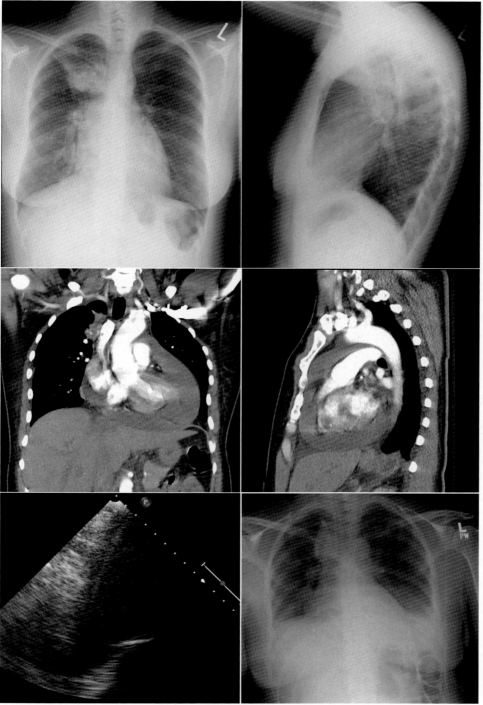

Figure 7-29. TOP, Posteroanterior and lateral chest radiographs. The left upper lobe lung mass is obvious. There are no pleural effusions. The cardiopericardial silhouette is increased slightly, but the lung volumes (against which the heart size is assessed) are increased because of emphysema. MIDDLE, Contrast-enhanced chest CT scan revealing a significantly sized pericardial effusion. There is considerable motion artifact, as the acquisition is not gated. BOTTOM LEFT, Apical transthoracic echocardiographic view showing the pericardial space and a wire introduced into it during the drainage procedure. BOTTOM RIGHT, Pigtail catheter in place.

CASE 6

Case Synopsis

A 47-year-old dialysis patient experienced exertional fatigue and exertional near-syncope, which was clearly exacerbated by hemodialysis and ultrafiltration. His blood pressure fell prominently with hemodialysis and ultrafiltration, which was not the usual case for him. The venous pressures were increased more than was typical before dialysis. A 15 mm Hg pulsus paradoxus was present before dialysis, and a 30 mm Hg pulsus paradoxus was present after dialysis. Chest radiographs before and after drainage are shown in Figure 7-31.

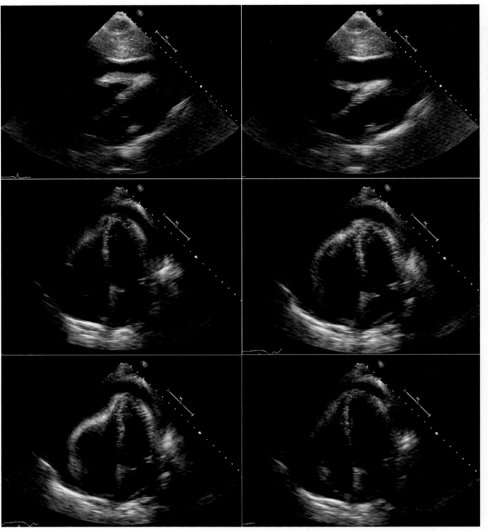

Figure 7-30. TOP, Subcostal views in diastole (LEFT) and systole (RIGHT) show right ventricular diastolic collapse. MIDDLE, Apical 4-chamber view in systole. MIDDLE LEFT, There is right atrial collapse (wall inversion). MIDDLE RIGHT, By late systole, venous return to the right atrium has increased the intracavitary pressure sufficiently to restore transmural distending pressure and to restore normal right atrial free wall curvature. BOTTOM LEFT, In diastole, there is right ventricular diastolic collapse. BOTTOM RIGHT, After atrial contraction, the right ventricle no longer experiences wall collapse as the post–A wave pressure is high enough to confer a transmural distending pressure against the elevated intrapericardial pressure.

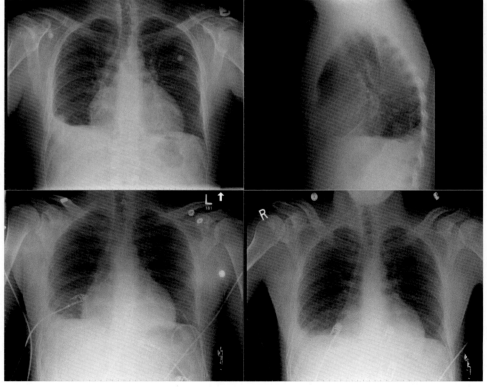

Figure 7-31. TOP, Posteroanterior and lateral chest radiographs before drainage. The cardiopericardial silhouette is enlarged, with a tapered, flask-like shape. The azygos vein is significantly dilated, consistent with elevated central venous pressure. BOTTOM LEFT, Pigtail drain in place through an anterior apical puncture site. BOTTOM RIGHT, After drain withdrawal, the cardiopericardial silhouette is smaller than before drainage, the azygos vein is smaller (consistent with reduction of the central venous pressure), and the lung volumes are larger.

CASE 7

Case Synopsis

A 94-year-old woman developed dyspnea and exertional intolerance. She had been started on warfarin 2 months previously because of atrial fibrillation. She had lost 15 pounds in the preceding year. She had been treated for hypertension for two decades. A chest radiograph had demonstrated cardiomegaly that led to an echocardiogram. Further physical examination revealed distended jugular veins, a pulsus paradoxus of 15 mm Hg, and an elevated BP of 190/75 mm Hg. Chest radiographic and echocardiographic findings are shown in Figures 7-32 and 7-33.

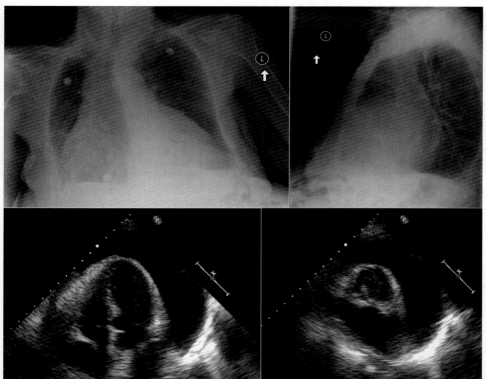

Figure 7-32. TOP, Posteroanterior and lateral chest radiographs demonstrating enormous cardiomegaly, clear lung fields, and no pleural effusions. BOTTOM LEFT, Transthoracic echocardiographic apical 4-chamber view. BOTTOM RIGHT, Transthoracic echocardiographic parasternal short-axis view. Both views show a large circumferential pericardial effusion. The apical 4-chamber view shows right atrial collapse, and the parasternal short-axis view shows a small, collapsed right ventricle.

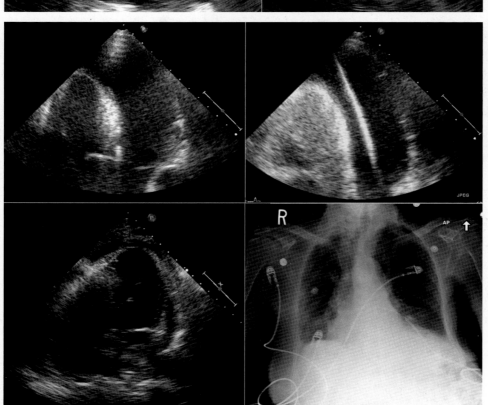

Figure 7-33. TOP, Echocardiographic images during pericardial drainage. TOP LEFT, Apical 4-chamber view revealing a shallow distance into the pericardial fluid and an ideal site and orientation for "apical" puncture into the pericardial space. TOP RIGHT, The guide wire is clearly seen in the pericardial space. BOTTOM LEFT, After removal of 1.2 L of fluid, there is very little remaining pericardial fluid. BOTTOM RIGHT, Chest radiograph confirming position of the pigtail drain and absence of pneumothorax.

CASE 8

Case Synopsis

A 55-year-old woman, a lifelong nonsmoker, presented with dyspnea and exertional presyncope. Venous pressures were elevated. There was tachycardia (105 bpm) and hypotension (95/60 mm Hg), with a 25 mm Hg pulsus paradoxus. There was no pericardial rub. The patient was not only dyspneic but also hypoxic. Ultrasound-guided drainage of the pericardial effusion and bilateral pleural effusions alleviated the symptoms. Imaging investigations revealed a lung mass, and pericardial fluid, which was bloody, yielded adenocarcinoma of the large-cell type. Case findings are shown in Figures 7-34 to 7-38.

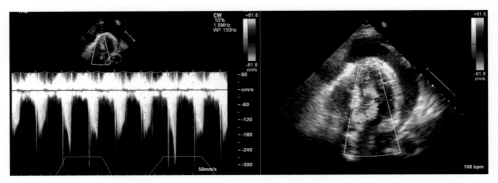

Figure 7-34. LEFT, Spectral Doppler study of the lower LVOT flow with respirometry tracing along the bottom. With inspiration (denoted by the upward deflection of the respirometer), the outflow velocity nearly doubles and assumes a dagger-shaped contour consistent with dynamic obstruction. RIGHT, A systolic frame with color flow mapping showing the site of intracavitary obstruction due to papillary muscle: septal apposition. Because of the tamponade, the left side of the heart was so underfilled that it generated an intraventricular gradient that was dynamically aggravated by inspiration, which further reduced left ventricular filling. These findings were entirely eliminated by the relief of the tamponade and served to illustrate the underloading of the left side of the heart as an integral part of tamponade physiology.

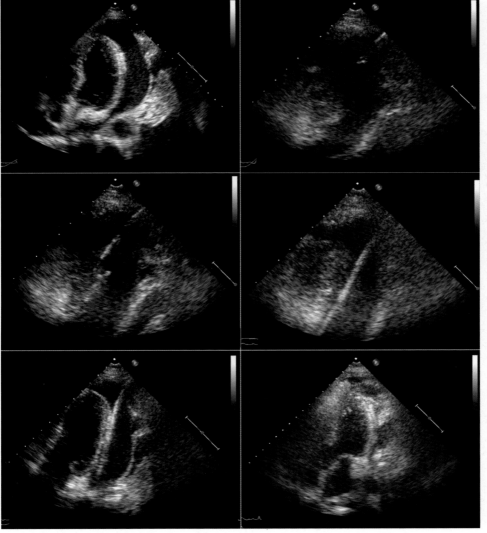

Figure 7-35. TOP LEFT, Apical 4-chamber view displaced slightly laterally to image the pericardial effusion. The effusion is large and extends between the descending aorta and the left AV groove. The left atrium is collapsed, as is the right atrium. TOP RIGHT, The introducer needle is imaged entering the pericardial fluid space. The image is obtained with use of a sterile sheath held in the same interspace immediately beside the introducing needle. MIDDLE LEFT, The J wire has been introduced through the introducing needle that is seen in the pericardial fluid. MIDDLE RIGHT, The wire has been advanced farther into the pericardial space. BOTTOM LEFT, A deeper view of the pericardial effusion showing the wire alongside the heart. BOTTOM RIGHT, After drain insertion and drainage of 850 mL of fluid. There is little remaining pericardial fluid. The left atrium is now larger as the left side of the heart is filling better as a result of the relief of the tamponade.

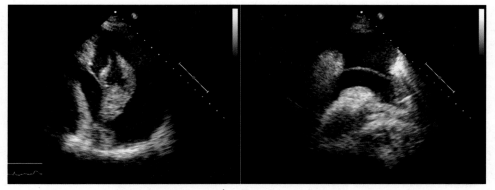

Figure 7-36. These transthoracic echocardiography images obtained from the chest wall reveal both pleural effusion and pericardial effusion separated by the thin parietal pericardium. Atelectatic lung is present within both pleural spaces.

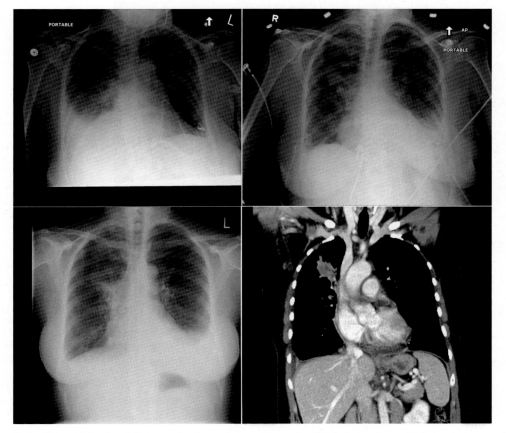

Figure 7-37. TOP LEFT, Pericardial and left pleural drains are in place. TOP RIGHT, The pericardial drain has been withdrawn, and a new drain is also present in the right pleural space. BOTTOM LEFT, After withdrawal of the pleural drains, a small effusion has occurred on the right side and a somewhat larger one on the left side. BOTTOM RIGHT, Contrast-enhanced chest CT revealing the right upper lobe mass also visible on the chest radiographs. This mass was a large-cell bronchogenic carcinoma responsible for the pleural effusions and also the pericardial tamponade.

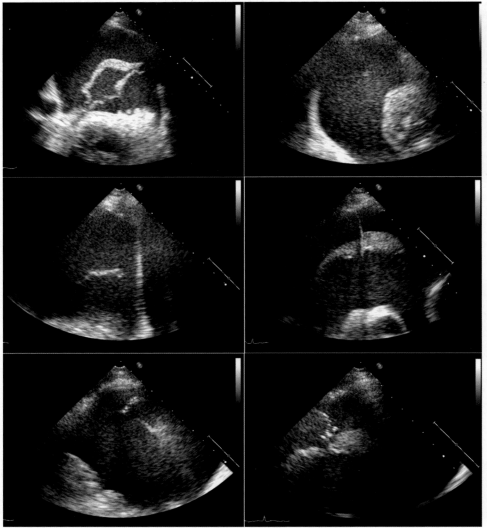

Figure 7-38. LEFT, Left pleural effusion drainage. RIGHT, Right pleural effusion drainage. The upper images reveal large pleural effusion bilaterally with small atelectatic lung within. The atelectasis was the cause of right-to-left shunting and hypoxemia. The middle images confirm wire entry into the pleural space, and the lower images confirm placement of the pigtail catheter into the pleural cavity. A total of 6 liters was drained in this patient.

References

1. Tsang TS, Enriquez-Sarano M, Freeman WK, et al: Consecutive 1127 therapeutic echocardiographically guided pericardiocenteses: clinical profile, practice patterns, and outcomes spanning 21 years. Mayo Clin Proc 2002;77:429-461.

2. Fagan SM, Chan KL: Pericardiocentesis: blind no more! Chest 1999; 116:275-276.

3. Wang HJ: Technical and prognostic outcomes of double-balloon pericardiotomy for large malignancy-related pericardial effusions. Chest 2002;122:893-899.

4. Permanyer-Miralda G, Sagristà-Sauleda J, Soler-Soler J: Primary acute pericardial disease: a prospective series of 231 consecutive patients. Am J Cardiol 1985;56:623-630.

5. Tsang T: Rescue echocardiographically guided pericardiocentesis for cardiac perforation complicating catheter-based procedures: the Mayo Clinic experience. J Am Coll Cardiol 1998;32:1345-1350.

6. Kopecky SL, Callahan JA, Tajik AJ, Seward JB: Percutaneous pericardial catheter drainage: report of 42 consecutive cases. Am J Cardiol 1986;58:633-635.

7. Nugue O, Millaire A, Porte H, et al: Pericardioscopy in the etiologic diagnosis of pericardial effusion in 141 consecutive patients. Circulation 1996;94:1635-1641.

Intrapericardial Thrombus

KEY POINTS

▸ Intrapericardial thrombus may occur for several reasons.

▸ It is important to anticipate and to identify intrapericardial thrombus because it cannot be remedied by aspiration, and if it is hemodynamically compromising, it requires evacuation. Attempting to evacuate

thrombus by aspiration expends time and confers risk of cardiac chamber perforation.

▸ Because clot and frank blood are best distinguished by echocardiography, it is important to have familiarity with echocardiographic findings.

DEFINITION AND ETIOLOGY

Intrapericardial thrombus, or clot, may arise in several situations. If the amount of thrombus is sufficient, it may result in compression of the underlying cardiac chambers or vessels within the pericardial space. The relevance of intrapericardial thrombus is that, first, the compression syndromes it causes are generally with atypical features of tamponade, and second, evacuation of thrombus cannot be achieved through pericardiocentesis needles or drainage catheters, rendering surgical evacuation the preferred method.

Causes of intrapericardial thrombus are listed in Table 8-1. Anticoagulant, antiplatelet, and fibrinolytic medications augment bleeding into the pericardium and intrapericardial thrombus formation.

CLINICAL PRESENTATION

The site of intrapericardial thrombus accumulation depends on the site of bleeding, the potential pericardial space, and the body position at the time. Because many cases are postoperative, accumulation dependently (posterolateral to the right atrium) is the most common site. Accumulation beside the right ventricle is also common.[1] Thrombus may accumulate anywhere within the pericardial space, including over the pulmonary artery or around the intrapericardial aspects of the superior vena cava and the inferior vena cava. Some recesses of the pericardial space are difficult to image, short of computed tomographic (CT) scanning or surgical inspection.

Intrapericardial thrombus is more likely than intrapericardial fluid to accumulate locally and not distribute through the

pericardial space. The reasons for this are unclear and may pertain to localized sites of bleeding or concurrent pericardial adhesions that loculated the accumulating thrombus.

Intrapericardial thrombus may be present in an amount too small to result in hemodynamic compromise or in an amount with sufficient bulk to compress the heart globally or, more commonly, to compress an adjacent chamber or vessel. The syndrome that arises is typically one dominated by low cardiac output. Elevation of venous pressure is usually present when the right atrium or ventricle is compressed, but it may be disproportionately less than the extent of hypotension if a left-sided chamber is compressed. Usually, the "full picture" (elevation and equilibration of diastolic pressures) of tamponade findings is absent. Furthermore, as intrapericardial thrombus is most commonly seen after open heart surgery and interventions, the heart itself often has structural abnormalities that will contribute to the atypicality of the diastolic pressures.

DIAGNOSTIC IMAGING

Echocardiography is the single most useful imaging means by which to identify intrapericardial thrombus. Echocardiography can also determine signs of compression of adjacent cardiac chambers or great vessels. Importantly, both transthoracic echocardiography (TTE) and transesophageal echocardiography (TEE) may be performed at the bedside of urgent and unstable cases (Fig. 8-1).[2-4] Clot can generally be distinguished from fluid by the gelatinous wobbling appearance of fine specular echoes—a texture akin to liver, but finer, and with fine motion consistent with its gelatinous nature. In contrast, fluid is echolucent and typically black in appearance on pre–harmonic imaging and dark gray on harmonic imaging. TTE is increasingly sufficient, but TEE

Table 8-1. Causes of Intrapericardial Thrombus

Post–open heart surgery, particularly if there has been

    Abnormal bleeding or coagulopathy

    Early use of anticoagulants

    Re-do surgery

    Valve surgery

    Aortic surgery

Postinfarction myocardial rupture

Aortic dissection with intrapericardial rupture

Trauma

    Penetrating

    Blunt

    Iatrogenic

        Pacemaker lead insertion or revision

        Implantable defibrillator lead insertion or revision

        Coronary or electrophysiologic interventional procedures

        Central lines insertion

is usually superior although not always necessary. However, challenges are still encountered with echocardiography, including transesophageal, when thrombus accumulation is deep within recesses that are not well within the field of view.

CT scanning is useful to detect intrapericardial fluid, blood, and thrombus, but it generally does not reliably distinguish the blood and blood clot because their attenuation coefficients (Hounsfield units) are not reliably different. CT does not reliably establish that the heart shows physiologic, or real-time, signs of compression. CT scanning entails transportation of the patient and intravenous administration of contrast material.

Surgical inspection is the "gold standard" for identification and correction of the source of bleeding, and evacuation of clot and drainage of fluid.

MANAGEMENT

If hemodynamics are not perturbed, no interventions are needed. Stabilization consists of volume loading optimization and inotropes and vasopressors. Correction of bleeding diatheses and anticoagulation are important.

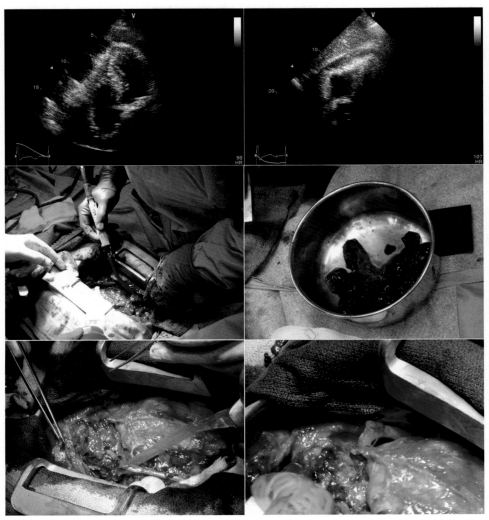

Figure 8-1. This 78-year-old man underwent a re-do aortic and mitral valve replacement as well as a three-vessel coronary artery bypass 5 days previously. Severe and then critically low output developed in the CVICU. TOP LEFT, Bedside TTE revealing a large pericardial effusion with extensive fibrinous stranding over the right ventricular free wall. The right atrium is not collapsed. TOP RIGHT, Subcostal view of the heart reveals adhesion of the right ventricle to the pericardial surface and no pericardial fluid accessible by subcostal approach. MIDDLE, Surgical evacuation of the pericardium. Despite supportive vasopressors, when anesthesia was induced, blood pressure was lost, and 300 to 400 mL of dark red-black fluid gushed out of the pericardial space. There was an equal volume of clotted blood of variable consistency, from gelatinous to tough and rubbery, which was carefully dissected away. BOTTOM LEFT, The ascending aorta has rough and irregular appearance on the outside from multiple previous cardiac surgeries. The suction catheter is underneath the vein graft to the posterior descending coronary artery arising from the right side of aorta. BOTTOM RIGHT, The vein graft is coming off the ascending aorta running out to the obtuse marginal coronary circulation. The anastomosis of the vein graft to the marginal circulation was the bleeding source that had resulted in postoperative cardiac tamponade and pericardial blood clot.

Pericardiocentesis is unwise if clot is probable. If there is only clot and little or no free fluid, pericardiocentesis is usually fruitless ("dry"), as thrombus will not be evacuated through a needle. Furthermore, pericardiocentesis may be dangerous as the tendency is to advance the needle until fluid withdrawal, which may occur only as the needle enters a cardiac cavity (i.e., only after chamber perforation).

The definitive management of intrapericardial thrombus resulting in hemodynamic compromise is surgical evacuation. Importantly, surgery enables inspection for, identification of, and correction of a responsible "bleeder" lesion or site to prevent recurrence (see Fig. 8-1).

CASE 1

History and Physical Examination

▸ 70-year-old man who, while in the ICU 2 days after aortic valve replacement for aortic stenosis, developed progressive hypotension and tachycardia, with elevation of the central venous pressures but not of the pulmonary artery or pulmonary capillary wedge pressure

▸ No pulsus paradoxus; no pericardial rub

Evolution

▸ Prompt return to the operating room for evacuation of a large amount of intrapericardial clot. No culprit source of bleeding was identified.

▸ Other than additional ventilator time, recovery was uneventful.

Comments

▸ Clot posterolateral to the right atrium is the most common site of accumulation.

▸ As is often seen, there is no pulsus paradoxus when the clot compresses the right atrium alone.

▸ Surgical evacuation is the definitive remedy and the best means to exclude a remediable (surgically correctable) lesion.

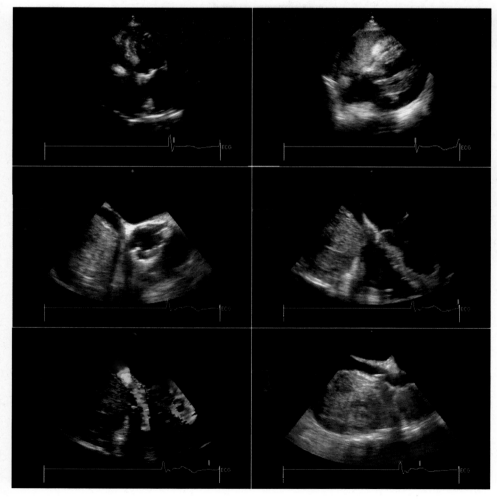

Figure 8-2. TOP LEFT, Apical 4-chamber view. The right ventricle appears small, and the right atrium is difficult to recognize. The left-sided heart cavities on this plane appear unremarkable. TOP RIGHT, Subcostal view. There is a large bulk of clot compressing the right ventricle and seemingly obliterating the right atrial cavity. The fine specular echo pattern of clot is apparent. MIDDLE IMAGES, TEE view oriented toward the right atrium revealing the large round bulk of intrapericardial thrombus severely compressing the right atrium, leaving only a very small slit-like cavity. BOTTOM LEFT, Color Doppler flow mapping demonstrates flow acceleration at the tricuspid valve level caused by the narrowing. BOTTOM RIGHT, TTE vertical view demonstrating the height of and superior extent of the clot, which extends well up the pericardial sleeve around the superior vena cava.

CASE 2

History and Physical Examination

▸ A 59-year-old woman recently diagnosed with bronchogenic carcinoma presented with 2 weeks of increasing shortness of breath.
▸ Elevated neck veins; BP 120/80 mm Hg with no pulsus paradoxus; no pericardial rub

Evolution

▸ Pericardiocentesis removed a few hundred milliliters of serosanguineous fluid. The fluid was initially serous but rendered partially sanguineous from cardiac trauma by the repeated attempts at percutaneous drainage.

▸ An indwelling catheter was left for several days. There was no early recurrence of effusion or tamponade. The iatrogenic intrapericardial clot resolved during a week.
▸ After chemotherapy, the patient lived for 16 months, dying of complications due to metastases.

Comments

▸ Pleural and pericardial effusions from lung cancer
▸ Injection of agitated saline during pericardiocentesis assisted in determining the position of the needle tip.
▸ Epicardial trauma was caused by the introducer needle but was not associated with ongoing or recurrent bleeding.

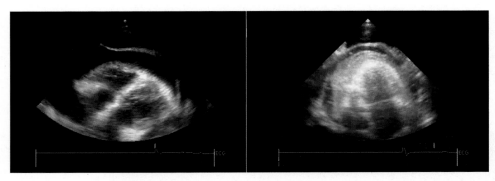

Figure 8-3. TTE views before (LEFT) and during (RIGHT) attempted pericardial tap. Before the tap, there are both pleural and pericardial effusions. During the tap, epicardial trauma resulted in formation of a clot over the epicardium, apparent by its bright specular echo texture.

CASE 3

History and Physical Examination

▸ A 45-year-old man, day 4 after aortocoronary bypass surgery
▸ An enlarging heart shadow was noted on the chest radiograph. Although there was venous distention, there was no hypotension, tachycardia, pulsus paradoxus, or pericardial rub.

Evolution

▸ There was no clinical evidence of tamponade or evolution to constriction.

▸ He was managed conservatively (without drainage).
▸ On serial follow-up scans during 6 weeks, it was seen that the hematoma had resolved.

Comments

▸ Intrapericardial thrombus without significant or specific cardiac chamber compression and without hemodynamic perturbation
▸ The lack of tachycardia in coronary patients who are assessed for tamponade is less meaningful when they are receiving beta-blocking medications.

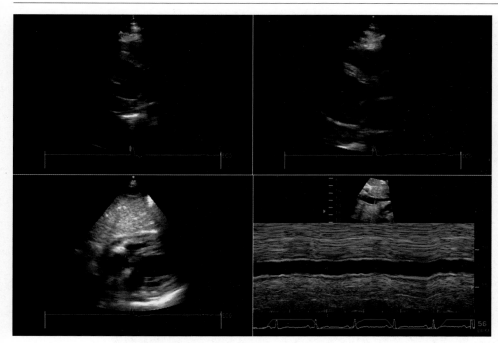

Figure 8-4. Parasternal long-axis deep chest view (TOP LEFT) and standard-depth view (TOP RIGHT). The cardiac chambers appear normal. There is a 2-cm rind of clot posterior to the left ventricle. BOTTOM LEFT, Subcostal view. There is no clot present inferior to the right ventricle and only a trivial-sized pericardial effusion. BOTTOM RIGHT, M-mode study of the inferior vena cava demonstrating dilation and no significant respiratory variation (note respirometry tracing along the bottom of the image).

8

CASE 4

History and Physical Examination

▸ A 65-year-old woman with prior aortocoronary bypass grafting, undergoing percutaneous coronary intervention (PCI) for an acute coronary syndrome, abruptly developed chest pain, severe hypotension, and transient but obvious dye extravasation after balloon inflation.

▸ No pulsus paradoxus

Evolution

▸ Volume infusion successfully resuscitated the blood pressure. There was no evidence of ongoing dye extravasation, and she remained stable. No further attempts were made to dilate the vessel.

▸ She remained stable through the hospital course and was managed conservatively.

Comments

▸ Fluid and clots often accumulate in unusual locations in patients who have previously undergone open heart surgery because of pericardial adhesions that formed after surgery.

▸ Pulsus paradoxus is commonly absent in intrapericardial clot cases. Tachycardia is also commonly absent in such cases, despite severely reduced output, because of widespread beta-blocker use in patients with coronary artery disease.

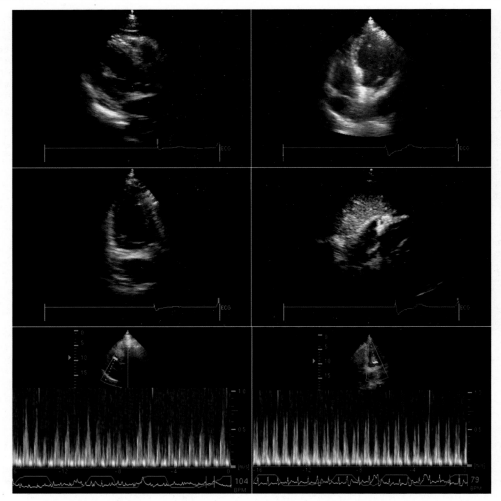

Figure 8-5. TOP LEFT, Parasternal long-axis view. The left ventricle appears to be unremarkable. The appearance of the left atrium is peculiar because there is a pericardial effusion posterior to it, displacing the posterior wall of the left atrium far anteriorly—toward the anterior mitral leaflet. TOP RIGHT, Apical 4-chamber view. There is a pericardial effusion or clot posterolateral to the left atrium, severely compressing the left atrial free wall inward, leaving a very small residual cavity. MIDDLE LEFT, Apical 2-chamber view revealing severe displacement of the left atrial posterior wall far anteriorly toward the mitral valve. MIDDLE RIGHT, Subcostal view revealing anterior displacement of the right atrial free wall and collapse. BOTTOM LEFT, Tricuspid inflow. There is significant increase in early diastolic inflow velocity with inspiration. BOTTOM RIGHT, Mitral inflow. There is no significant inflow velocity variation.

CASE 5

History and Physical Examination

▸ A 73-year-old man with a long history of COPD; before aortocoronary bypass surgery, he underwent PCI to RCA vein graft, complicated by perforation of graft. He was promptly and successfully treated with covered stent.

▸ BP 90/50 mm Hg, no tachycardia (on beta-blockers)

▸ Elevated neck veins; no pulsus paradoxus or pericardial rub

Evolution

▸ Because the accumulation of blood clot and left atrial compression were hemodynamically tolerated surprisingly well and the patient

had such severe COPD, he was managed conservatively and nonsurgically.

▸ 8 weeks later, the clot was no longer seen on repeated echocardiographic imaging.

Comments

▸ Fluid or clot often accumulates in unusual locations in patients who have previously undergone open heart surgery because of pericardial adhesions that formed after surgery.

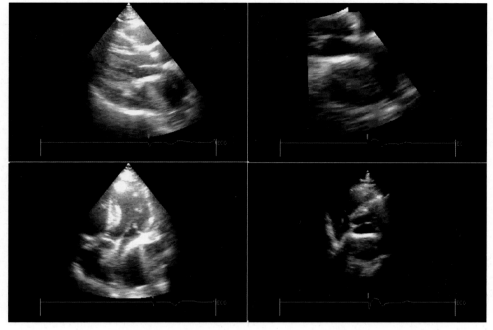

Figure 8-6. TOP LEFT, Parasternal long-axis view. There is a thick intrapericardial clot posterior to the left ventricle and left atrium. The left ventricular cavity is somewhat small; the left atrial cavity is difficult to understand. TOP RIGHT, Zoom parasternal long-axis view of the left atrium, which appears compressed, or filled, with clot. BOTTOM LEFT, Apical 4-chamber view. The posterolateral wall of the left atrium is severely compressed by a large bulk of thrombus. BOTTOM RIGHT, Parasternal short-axis view. The posterior wall of the left atrium has been severely compressed forward by a thick mass of material with the prominent specular appearance of thrombus.

CASE 6

History

▸ A 54-year-old man with mild hemophilia A and hepatitis C underwent aortocoronary bypass for severe triple-vessel disease. Postoperatively, there was higher than normal bleeding noted through chest tubes.

▸ On day 12 after aortocoronary bypass, there was the development of hypotension, tachycardia, and elevation of the central venous pressures but not of the pulmonary artery (PA) pressures. Despite use of high-dose inotropes and pressors, he worsened rapidly to the point of near cardiac arrest.

Evolution

▸ Emergency reopening of the chest and evacuation of large amount of clot and hemorrhagic fluid, with restoration of the circulation

▸ No obvious site of bleeding was noted.
▸ There was no recurrent bleeding or thrombus accumulation.

Comments

▸ Increased postoperative bleeding is associated with greater likelihood of fluid accumulation and tamponade or clot accumulation and compression. The hemophilia was a risk for bleeding.

▸ The large clot in this case extended well out onto the PA, as the parietal pericardium extends out to the PA bifurcation.

▸ Surgical evacuation was indicated because of the circulatory distress and the fact that the large majority of the compression of the heart (and PA) was by thrombus, not by fluid.

▸ TEE offered helpful images to delineate and to confirm the thrombus.

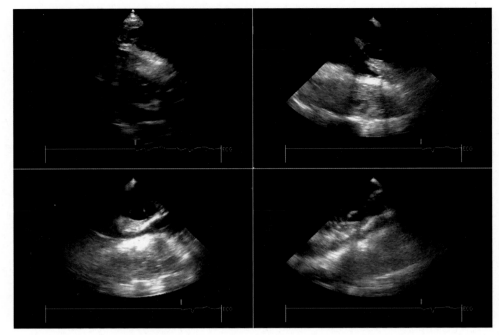

Figure 8-7. TOP LEFT, TTE view with unclear findings. TOP RIGHT, TEE horizontal 4-chamber view. There is a very thick intrapericardial clot anterior to the right atrium and right ventricle. On this plane, the right ventricle is severely compressed in its midsection and apex. BOTTOM LEFT, TEE vertical view of the right side of the heart. The intrapericardial clot, thicker than the entire heart, is tightly compressing the RVOT. BOTTOM RIGHT, TEE view of the RVOT and proximal pulmonary artery, which are both tightly compressed.

CASE 7

History and Physical Examination

▸ A 70-year-old man with severe mitral regurgitation and biventricular heart failure undergoing diagnostic right- and left-sided heart catheterization developed severe chest pain of a pleuritic nature during catheter manipulation in the right side of the heart.

▸ The BP fell to 100/60 mm Hg from 150/85 mm Hg. No pulsus paradoxus was seen. With volume infusion, the BP normalized.

Management and Outcome

▸ Because the BP normalized with volume and there were no clinical indices of low output, he was managed conservatively.

Comments

▸ RA or RV perforation from catheter manipulation probably caused transient bleeding into the pericardial space, resulting in pericarditic chest pain and mild (and manageable) tamponade.

▸ Although, as a general principle, soft tissue overlying the heart within the pericardial space may be thrombus, fat, or potentially a tumor, in this case it was most likely thrombus given the setting and gelatinous motion and appearance of it.

▸ As with many cases of mild or moderate tamponade, volume resuscitation to increase the RA pressure above the intrapericardial pressure stabilizes the patient.

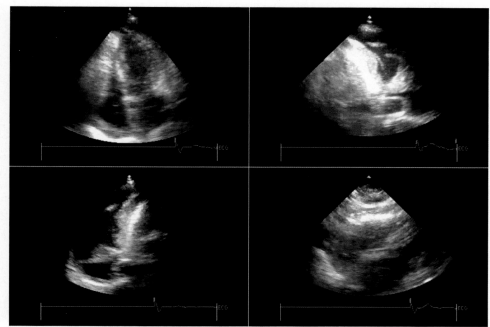

Figure 8-8. TOP LEFT, Apical 4-chamber view shows no definite abnormalities, although the right ventricular cavity is small on this plane. TOP RIGHT, RV inflow view shows the pacemaker lead. BOTTOM LEFT, There is a pericardial effusion to the right side of the heart and thrombus on the epicardial surface of the heart over the lateral right ventricle and right atrium. The pacer lead is not seen in the pericardial space. BOTTOM RIGHT, There is no pericardial effusion, or clot, inferior to the right ventricle.

References

1. Pierli C, Iadanza A, Del Pasqua A, Fineschi M: Acute superior vena cava and right atrial tamponade in an infant after open heart surgery. Int J Cardiol 2002;83:195-197.

2. Kochar GS, Jacobs LE, Kotler MN: Right atrial compression in postoperative cardiac patients: detection by transesophageal echocardiography. J Am Coll Cardiol 1990;16:511-516.

3. Ionescu A, Wilde P, Karsch KR: Localized pericardial tamponade: difficult echocardiographic diagnosis of a rare complication after cardiac surgery. J Am Soc Echocardiogr 2001;14:1220-1223.

4. Chan KW, Andrews J, Barrie M: Transesophageal echocardiography for assessing cause of hypotension after cardiac surgery. Am J Cardiol 1988;62:1142-1143.

Pericardial Constriction

KEY POINTS

▸ The causes of pericardial constriction are many, and presentations are often subtle.

▸ The diagnosis is often made late; therefore, heightened suspicion is appropriate.

▸ Physical diagnosis is useful.

▸ Echocardiography and catheterization now employ signs of ventricular interdependence as the better means of diagnosis of constrictive physiology.

▸ Advanced tomographic imaging modalities such as CT and CMR are complementary but should not be considered primary diagnostic tests.

▸ The key to diagnosis is understanding that the interaction of cardiac and pulmonary physiology results in observable manifestations of ventricular interdependence.

To constrict (kən-strikt′ v.t.) is "to compress, draw together; cramp or bind."[1] The implication is that the compression, cramping, or binding is extrinsically applied, and the term is well suited to the syndrome of pericardial constriction: extrinsic compression of the heart by noncompliant (fibrotic, occasionally calcified) pericardium that results in elevated, and typically equilibrated, diastolic filling pressures within the heart cavities (and thereby within the systemic and pulmonary veins), reducing diastolic filling and stroke volume and thereby cardiac output. The stiff and contracted pericardium resists deformation outward, severely restricting and often reducing overall filling, and also resists deformation inward by ventricular contraction such that on cessation of ventricular contraction, in very early diastole, there is an abnormally exaggerated recoil outward of the pericardium and myocardium.

The term *constriction* refers to pathophysiologic compression of the heart. Pericarditis is a common active or antecedent disease process that may result in constrictive physiology. These two entities are neither synonymous nor equivalent. Because many cases of constrictive physiology occur during or following pericarditis (especially when it is due to tuberculous disease), the term *constrictive pericarditis* remains popular, although most cases of pericarditis do not evolve to constrictive physiology, and many cases of constrictive physiology do not exhibit active clinical pericarditis or have a clear clinical history of it. The term *constriction* is suitable for describing the pathophysiologic state of equilibrated compression from diseased pericardium other than from pericardial fluid, independently of the degree of clinical or histologic pericarditis (inflammation).

PATHOPHYSIOLOGY OF PERICARDIAL CONSTRICTION

The increase in venous return produced by inspiration (as intrathoracic pressure falls relative to extrathoracic pressure) increases right-sided heart volume; but because of the noncompliance of the pericardium, the increase in right-sided heart filling occurs at the expense of a fall of left-sided heart filling, as the right and left sides of the heart competitively vie for filling space that is limited by the constrictive pericardium. Hence, inspiration-induced increase in right ventricular (RV) volume and systolic pressure (a function of the increased right ventricular diastolic volume or preload) occurs at the expense of left-sided heart filling (volume); lower left ventricular (LV) diastolic volume or preload results in lesser left-sided heart systolic pressures.

Unlike in pericardial tamponade, in which there is compression of the heart through the entire cardiac cycle by the pressurized fluid in the pericardial space, the compression imparted by the constrictive pericardium is reduced, is nullified, or becomes negative in early diastole because of the vigorous outward recoil of the constrictive pericardium. The deformed pericardium accrues potential energy as it is deformed inward by ventricular systole or contraction, such that on the release of the inward forces at the end of systole, there is outward recoil and accelerated early diastolic filling. Hence, constrictive physiology is notable for several diastolic phenomena: (1) abnormally rapid early filling, which is apparent as a prominent early diastolic dip of the zero point of a pressure (catheter) recording of ventricular pressure;

Table 9-1. Pathophysiologic Processes in Pericardial Constriction

Diastolic phenomenon

Noncompliance imparted to heart chambers by the noncompliant overlying pericardium

Compression by the constrictive pericardium uniformly elevates diastolic filling pressures.

Exaggerated recoil of the pericardium renders early diastolic pressure unusually low for the mean pressure ("early diastolic dip") and thereby filling is abnormally rapid.

Noncompliance of the pericardium rapidly arrests diastolic filling in early diastole.

Diastolic filling volumes determine the generated systolic pressure.

Systolic phenomenon

Ventricular interdependence results in directionally different effects on systolic pressures with inspiration.

Respiratory:cardiac interaction phenomenon

Isolation of the left-sided heart chambers from intrathoracic pressure variations

Inspiratory effort increases pulmonary capacitance, reducing left-sided heart venous return and pressure.

Inspiratory effort increases systemic venous return.

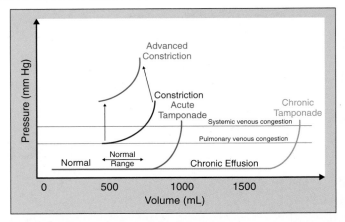

Figure 9-1. Diastolic pressure:volume relationships in pericardial disease. In constriction, the pressure:volume relationship of the pericardium is shifted upward and leftward; therefore, the diastolic pressures within the heart are elevated, resulting in venous congestion, even with ventricles of normal volume.

Table 9-2. Causes of Pericardial Constriction

Post–open heart surgery

Idiopathic

Postpericarditis

Posturemic

Tuberculous

Fungal

Post–myocardial infarction (Dressler syndrome)

Post-traumatic

Post–radiation therapy

Rare causes

Inflammatory diseases (systemic lupus erythematosus, progressive systemic sclerosis, dermatomyositis)

Sarcoidosis

Amyloidosis

Whipple disease

Mulibrey nanism (dwarfism and abnormalities of muscle, liver, brain, eyes)

(2) abruptly arrested diastolic filling commencing after the early diastolic dip, seen as a plateau of raised diastolic pressure; (3) elevated mean diastolic pressures; and (4) "equilibrated" diastolic filling pressures in different cardiac chambers (Table 9-1). Both intravascular depletion (from diuretics, illness, or bleeding) and severe volume overload (anasarca from constriction) may skew the hemodynamic findings of constrictive physiology.

Normally, the pericardium limits excessive cardiac filling, preserving the myocyte length:tension relationship and thereby systolic function. In constriction, the pericardium pathologically limits normal ventricular diastolic filling and initiates ventricular interaction or interdependence (competition for filling space in inspiration). The pericardium over the right ventricle free wall compromises the effective compliance of the right ventricle, and hence the right ventricle cannot receive the increased volume of venous return produced by inspiration without its diastolic pressure rising. The noncompliance of the right side of the heart is the basis of Kussmaul sign. Also occurring in inspiration is a reduction of pulmonary venous return to the left side of the heart due to increase in pulmonary venous capacitance from increased lung volume. The rise in right-sided heart volume and pressure, and the fall in left-sided heart venous return and pressure, accentuates the competition of filling within the constricted pericardial space such that the septum transiently shifts from the left to the right side as a result of change in LV:RV filling pressures and the change of the pressure gradient on the interventricular septum. Because developed ventricular systolic pressures are determined by the state of preload, as inspiration increases right ventricular diastolic filling, it increases right ventricular systolic pressure (RVSP); and conversely, as inspiration reduces left ventricular diastolic filling, it reduces left ventricular systolic pressure (LVSP). Thus, inspiration confers directionally opposite effects on the right and left ventricular diastolic volume-pressure and preload, systolic pressure, and stroke volumes (Fig. 9-1).

Hence, the nature of constrictive physiology is seen more strikingly through the respiratory cycle than through the cardiac cycle. Evaluation for the presence of constrictive physiology by bedside diagnosis, imaging, and catheterization should be attentive to findings both per cardiac cycle and per respiratory cycle (Tables 9-2 and 9-3).[2-5] Diagnostic testing requires use of electrocardiographic recording to associate findings to the cardiac cycle and of respirometry to associate findings to the respiratory cycle. Most commonly, cases of pericardial constriction present with dominant right-sided heart failure (Tables 9-4 and 9-5).

The nature of the referral population to a hospital heavily determines the observed causes of constrictive pericarditis. The past medical history and review of systems (and pathologic examination of pericardium) are an important means by which to establish the etiology of constrictive pericarditis. The etiology of

Table 9-3. Pericardial Constriction: Case Series

	Ling[2]	Cameron[3]	Vaitkus[4]	Bertog[5]	Combined
N	135	95	92	163	485
Idiopathic	33%	42%	15%	46%	31%
Postsurgical	18%	11%	39%	37%	27%
Post–radiation therapy	13%	31%	1%	9%	27%
Postinfectious	3%	6%	11%		5%
Other	33%	10%	34%	8%	22%

Table 9-4. Differential Diagnosis of Pericardial Constriction: Other Causes of Right-Sided Heart Failure

Tricuspid regurgitation, tricuspid stenosis

Cor pulmonale (RV diastolic failure and RV systolic failure)

Pulmonary airway and airspace diseases

Pulmonary vascular diseases

Cardiomyopathy

Congestive (dilated)

Restrictive (infiltrative)

Other pericardial diseases

Pericardial tamponade

Effuso-constrictive pericarditis

Masses within the pericardial space or pericardial encasement

Obstructive masses and lesions

Within the right-sided heart cavities

Pulmonary emboli

Pulmonic stenosis

Fluid overload

Simulating right-sided heart failure (SVC syndrome)

RV, right ventricular; SVC, superior vena cava.

Table 9-5. Approach to Resolving the Differential of Right-Sided Heart Failure

Basic testing

History and physical examination

Electrocardiography

Chest radiography

Echocardiography

± Catheterization

± Computed tomography, pulmonary function tests

Tricuspid regurgitation, tricuspid stenosis

Examination

Echocardiography

± Catheterization

Pulmonary hypertension

Lung causes (chronic obstructive pulmonary disease)

Physical examination

Chest radiography

Pulmonary function tests

Vascular causes

V:Q scanning

Spiral computed tomography

Angiography

Tamponade

Echocardiography

Fluid overload

Examination

Echocardiography

Cardiomyopathy

Congestive (dilated)

Echocardiography

± Catheterization

Restrictive (infiltrative)

Echocardiography

Catheterization

the constriction is relevant because it often indicates specific clinical issues. Constriction physiology develops in approximately 0.2% of open heart surgery cases, presenting a mean of 2 years postoperatively (but often much earlier), and it is notable for occurring with underlying abnormal hearts (due to residua of valve disease and infarction) and occurring in a localized manner in half of cases.[6,7] Radiation therapy–induced constriction almost always has concurrent fibrotic restrictive cardiomyopathy and fares far less well with surgical pericardiectomy than do other causes of constriction.

Hemodynamic Consequences of Pericardial Constriction

The application of pressure by the pericardium to the heart chambers results in elevation of the diastolic filling pressures. Because the applied pressure is fairly uniform, there is elevation and equil-

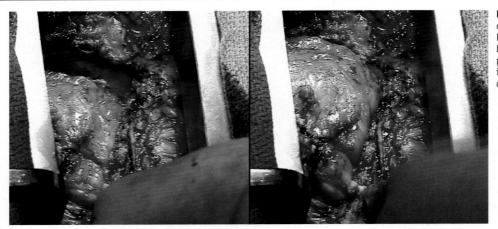

Figure 9-2. The pericardium has been opened anteriorly. LEFT, Systole. RIGHT, Diastole. Note how the right ventricle is bulging or herniating out through the partially resected constrictive pericardium in diastole because of the very high diastolic distending pressures.

ibration of the diastolic filling pressures (as long as the underlying heart is structurally normal). There is systemic and pulmonary venous congestion, with pressure elevations and waveforms similar to those of the corresponding atria. The constrictive pericardium limits diastolic filling, initially limiting stroke volume and later reducing stroke volume and cardiac output. The stroke volume in constriction is classically said to be of a "fixed" amount, as there is no ability to overfill the ventricles (although ventricular interdependence does vary filling volumes through the respiratory cycle). The fixed stroke volume makes cardiac output highly dependent on heart rate; bradycardia is therefore poorly tolerated. In constriction, diastole is notable; although diastolic filling is limited, the early filling component is actually abnormally rapid because of the early diastolic outward recoil of the constrictive pericardium, before it is violently arrested (Fig. 9-2). The cessation of filling is depicted on pressure tracings by the plateau. The end of the early diastolic dip, the beginning of the plateau, is the timing of the pericardial "knock" filling sound, supporting that arresting of rapid filling is the origin of the sound. Patients without a well-defined plateau do not have pericardial knock sounds because the ventricular filling is not abruptly arrested.[8]

Thickened pericardium, a common but not invariable finding in constriction, "isolates" the left-sided heart cavities more than the right-sided heart cavities from respiratory intrathoracic pressure changes. This is thought to be because the greater left ventricular wall thickness contributes to this phenomenon (Figs. 9-3 to 9-5).

The majority of the length of the pulmonary veins is extrapericardial; therefore, pulmonary veins are not isolated from intrathoracic pressure changes, and pulmonary venous pressure is influenced by variation in intrapleural pressure. Furthermore, pulmonary venous capacitance is prominently influenced by lung volume; hence, inspiration increases pulmonary venous capacitance and reduces pulmonary venous pressure by a second means. Inspiration therefore reduces pulmonary venous pressure, which reduces left ventricular filling in inspiration. Expiration causes intrathoracic pressure to rise and pulmonary venous capacitance to fall, thereby increasing pulmonary venous return and pressure, which normalizes left ventricle filling.

The pulmonary venous pressure normally falls in inspiration as a result of increase in lung capacitance and negative intrapleural pressure. The fall in pulmonary venous pressure may be

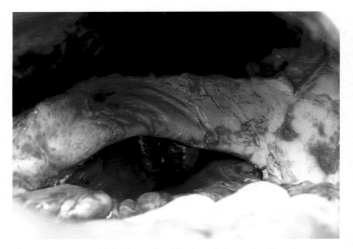

Figure 9-3. Gross thickening and stiffening of the pericardium in constrictive pericarditis. Note the thick (approximately 1 cm) segment of constrictive pericardium bridging over the heart.

accentuated in constriction as a result of the increased respiratory effort from pleural effusions or pulmonary venous congestion. The increase in inspiratory fall in pulmonary venous pressure simultaneously with reduced transmission of lower intrathoracic pressure to the left ventricle increases the pulmonary capillary wedge pressure (PCWP) to left ventricular diastolic pressure (LVDP) gradient variation in inspiration, typically more than 5 mm Hg.[9]

Ventricular Interdependence

Ventricular interdependence is a prominent pathophysiologic occurrence in pericardial constriction whereby spontaneous respiration-induced right-sided heart filling competes with left-sided heart filling within the space afforded by the constricting pericardium. Therefore, with inspiration, left-sided heart filling decreases by the amount that right ventricular filling increased.

The phenomenon of ventricular interdependence is a product of competition for limited available intrapericardial

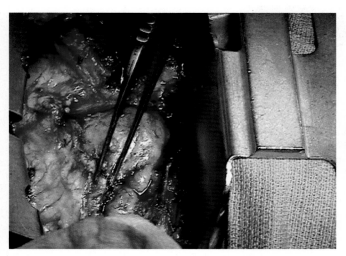

Figure 9-4. LEFT, Normal pericardium is seen during an aortocoronary bypass operation. Note saphenous vein grafts. The pericardium is seen between the arrows; it is 1 to 2 mm thick. The free edge of the pericardium has been thickened by the electrocautery cutting; it is actually thinner than this. Note as well the copious epicardial fat over the heart and under the parietal pericardium. This fat plane assists with imaging of the parietal pericardium because it has a different appearance by ultrasonography, CT, and MRI than the parietal pericardium does. RIGHT, In this patient with constrictive pericarditis, the pericardium is grossly thickened (12 mm—as thick as the sternum). Few cases of constrictive pericarditis are so obvious.

Figure 9-5. The pericardium has been opened anteriorly with a small triangular resection. Note how the right ventricle is frankly herniating out through the partially resected constrictive pericardium in diastole because of the very high diastolic distending pressures. Note as well the pericardial fat on the outside of the thickened pericardium, which assists with imaging of the thickening of the parietal pericardium, which in this case is about 4 mm. Note also the bleeding, an inherent risk of pericardiectomy.

The findings of ventricular interdependence require normal spontaneous respiration. Apnea, respiratory fatigue, and positive-pressure ventilation will not generate the findings of ventricular interdependence (Figs. 9-6 to 9-12).

DIAGNOSIS OF PERICARDIAL CONSTRICTION

Clinical, imaging, and hemodynamic assessments of constrictive pericarditis require the identification of findings and their timing to the respiratory cycle as well as to the cardiac cycle. This is critical with jugular venous pressure inspection to recognize Kussmaul sign; with echocardiography to identify 2-dimensional signs and Doppler signs of ventricular interdependence; and with catheterization to recognize Kussmaul sign, RVSP:LVSP discordance of ventricular interdependence, and an inspiratory increase in the PCWP:LVDP gradient. Hence, for echocardiography and catheterization, use of respirometry tracings is critical.

Diagnostic evaluation for suspected constrictive pericarditis includes a detailed history and physical examination, electrocardiography, chest radiography, echocardiography, computed tomography (CT) and cardiac magnetic resonance (CMR), and cardiac catheterization. Table 9-6 summarizes diagnostic signs of pericardial constriction. An algorithmic approach to the diagnosis and management of pericardial constriction is shown in Figure 9-13.

Medical History

Patients with pericardial constriction usually have complaints of right-sided failure that dominate their complaints of left-sided failure. Complaints attributable to low output are common (exertional fatigue or intolerance). The review of systems is important to establish possible causes of constriction (prior cardiac surgery, prior pericarditis, prior or recent tuberculosis or tuberculosis exposure, prior radiotherapy, prior trauma, and renal failure).

Pericardial constriction typically exhibits an insidious onset, of what are initially nonspecific complaints, often delaying

volume and limited pericardial compliance to accommodate increases in volume without increases in pressure. Ventricular interdependence is manifested in inspiration when the venous return to the right ventricle increases, resulting in a fall in available left ventricular volume, and the maximal effect of ventricular interdependence is seen in the first or second cardiac cycle of inspiration. Ventricular interdependence is also manifested as a pressure phenomenon: as right-sided heart filling or volume increases with inspiration, the right-sided heart diastolic pressures increase, and as right ventricular preload increases, so does the RVSP. However, left-sided heart diastolic and systolic pressures fall as left-sided heart filling is reduced by the combination of a greater PCWP to LVDP gradient and by the effect of interdependence. Hence, ventricular interdependence is manifested as directionally opposite left- and right-sided heart volume and pressure effects provoked by inspiration.

Text continued on p. 137.

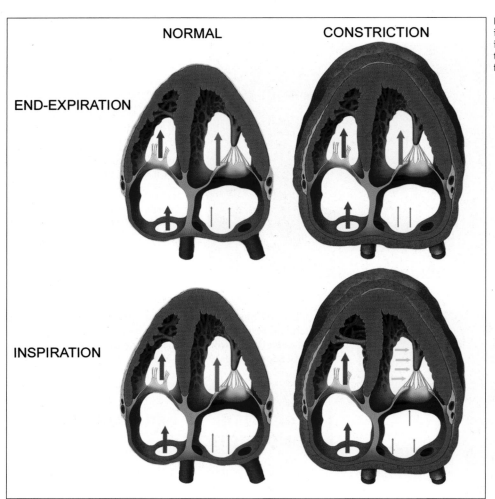

Figure 9-6. In the confined intrapericardial space of constriction, with inspiration, the septum shifts to the left as the RV filling increases and as the LV filling decreases.

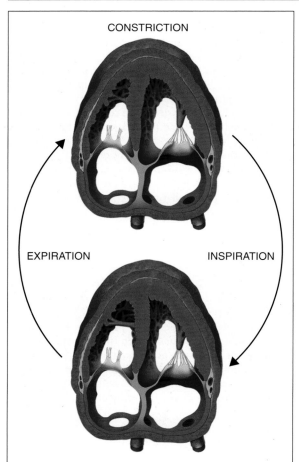

Figure 9-7. With inspiration, as the RV filling increases and as the LV filling decreases, the septum shifts to the left.

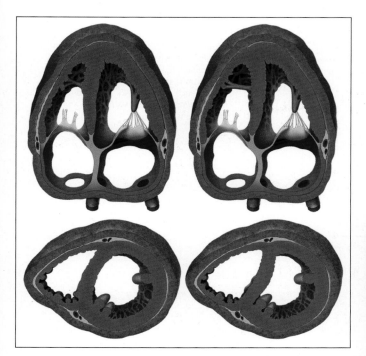

Figure 9-8. Another illustration of the transient septal shift to the left with inspiration, as the RV filling (volume and pressure) increases and as the LV filling (volume and pressure) decreases.

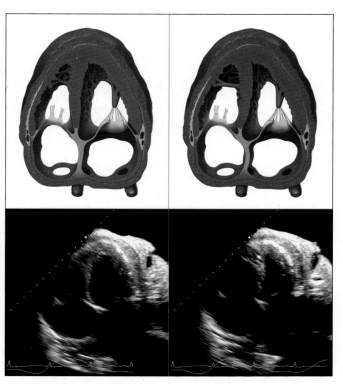

Figure 9-9. LEFT, Expiration. The septum is in its normal position. RIGHT, Inspiration. The septum is abruptly shifted toward the left side by the changes in RV and LV volume and pressure attributable to constrictive physiology. BOTTOM, Four-chamber echocardiographic views. Respirometry tracings along the bottom are superimposed over the ECG tracing of expiration (LEFT LOWER IMAGE), and inspiration (RIGHT LOWER IMAGE). Note upward deflection of respirometry tracing.

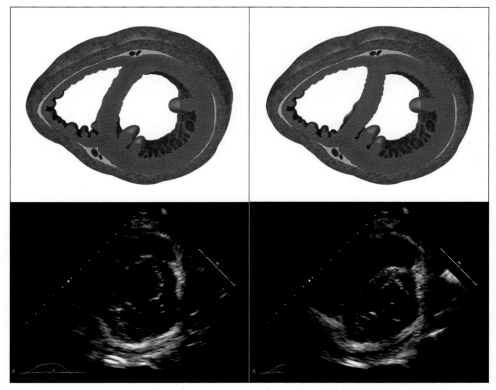

Figure 9-10. LEFT, Expiration. The septum is in its normal position. RIGHT, Inspiration. The septum is abruptly shifted toward the left side by the changes in RV and LV volume and pressure attributable to constrictive physiology. BOTTOM, Short-axis echocardiographic views. Respirometry tracings along the bottom are superimposed over the ECG tracing.

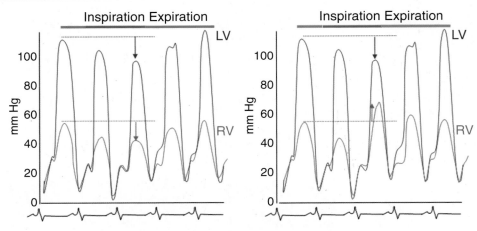

Figure 9-11. LEFT TRACING, normal; RIGHT TRACING, constriction. Normally, there is a concordant fall in LV and RV pressures in inspiration. In constriction, there is discordance of LV and RV pressure changes in inspiration: the LV pressure falls, and the RV pressure rises.

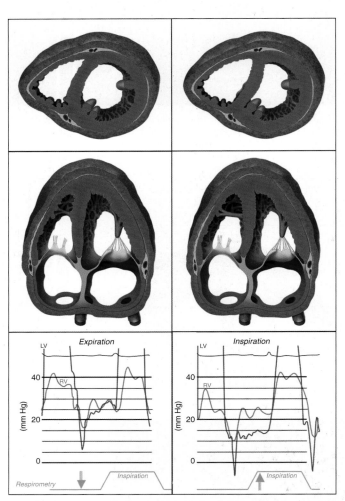

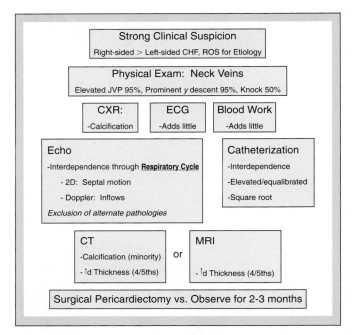

Figure 9-13. An overview of diagnostic and management steps in pericardial constriction. CHF, congestive heart failure; CT, computed tomography; CXR, chest radiography; ECG, electrocardiography; JVP, jugular venous pressure; MRI, magnetic resonance imaging; ROS, review of symptoms.

Figure 9-12. LEFT, Expiration. RIGHT, Inspiration. TOP, Parasternal short-axis views. MIDDLE, Apical 4-chamber views. BOTTOM, Simultaneous left (blue tracing) and right (red tracing) ventricular pressures. At expiration through mid and late diastole, the interventricular septum is in its normal position and has its normal curvature, as the diastolic pressure gradient across the septum is very little. At very early inspiration, as the left ventricular early diastolic pressure dip is often deeper than the right ventricular early diastolic pressure dip, there may transiently be a brief right-to-left ventricular pressure gradient resulting in an early diastolic (motion) dip of the septum to the left side. In the first or second beat of inspiration, the LVDP falls more than the RVDP, resulting in a pressure gradient that deflects the septum to the right side for that cardiac cycle.

Table 9-6. Diagnostic Signs of Pericardial Constriction

	Cause	Caveat
Physical diagnosis signs		
Elevated venous pressures	Noncompliance of the pericardium over the right side of the heart Volume overload from CHF state	Influenced by the degree of volume depletion from diuretics and disease and by volume overload from CHF state and impaired GFR
Exaggerated *y* descent	Augmented early diastolic recoil of the right side of the heart because the pericardium overlying it resists systolic deformation and recoils outward in early diastole	If venous column height exceeds the lowest extent of the *y* descent, it is too high to be seen. If the patient is supine, it may be too high to be seen. With severe volume contraction, it may be too low to be seen.
Kussmaul sign	Noncompliance of the pericardium over the right side of the heart manifested as an inability to accommodate the increased venous return of inspiration without a pressure rise	Difficult to assess if heart rate is irregular or breathing pattern is irregular
Pulsus paradoxus	Ventricular interdependence Increased inspiratory effort (more negative intrapleural pressure) Increased inspiratory effort (increased variation of pulmonary venous capacitance)	If blood pressure is measured too rapidly, pulsus is either missed or underestimated. Automated blood pressure cuffs do not detect
Pericardial knock	Abruptly arrested early diastolic filling	All heart sounds may be distant because of muffling from thickened pericardium, including extra heart sounds. Obesity, COPD, and thick pleural plaques will obscure
Apical retraction	Apex is displaced toward the base (rather than the base to the apex) because of pericardial adhesion to the chest cage	Obesity, COPD, and thick pleural plaques will obscure
Edema	Chronically elevated RAP Hypoalbuminemia from hepatic congestion or dysfunction State of renal function	Influenced by the degree of volume depletion from diuretics and disease and by volume overload from CHF state and impaired GFR
Electrocardiography signs—none is specific, but atrial fibrillation is common and important		
Chest radiography signs		
Pericardial calcification		Not present in most cases of constriction Not specific for constriction
Echocardiography signs		
2-Dimensional and M-mode signs		
Early diastolic dip	Magnitude difference of early diastolic pressure dips (LV >> RV) Temporal variation (LV later than RV) of early diastolic pressure dips	Requires use of high sweep speed M-mode study
Atrial septal notch	Atrial systole–augmented RVDP exceeds atrial systole–augmented LVDP	Requires use of high sweep speed M-mode study; lost in atrial fibrillation
Inspiratory septal shift	Inspiratory increase in RV diastolic filling Inspiratory decrease in LV diastolic filling due to isolation of LVDP from the thick pericardium Inspiratory increase in pulmonary venous capacitance	Heavily influenced by the respiratory mode and effort (poor respiratory effort will not generate the sign; exaggerated effort may falsely generate it) Not specific for constriction
Flattened LV posterior wall in mid-diastole	Limitation (plateauing) of LV filling imparted by pericardium arrests filling in early diastole	
Doppler signs		
Mitral E-wave variation	Inspiratory decrease in LV diastolic filling due to isolation of LVDP by the thick pericardium and inspiratory increase in pulmonary venous capacitance	Heavily influenced by the respiratory mode and effort
Pulmonary venous E-wave variation	Inspiratory decrease in LV diastolic filling due to isolation of LVDP by the thick pericardium and inspiratory increase in pulmonary venous capacitance	Heavily influenced by the respiratory effort Requires TEE sampling to yield clear profiles; respiration is seldom usual during TEE

Table 9-6. Diagnostic Signs of Pericardial Constriction—cont'd

	Cause	Caveat
Normal tissue Doppler findings	Absence of myocardial disease	Constrictive physiology may, if chronic, lead to myocardial abnormalities (atrophy).
		Concurrent pericardial constriction and myocardial processes or disease may occur.
Pulmonic valve presystolic opening	Atrial systole–augmented RVDP exceeds PA diastolic pressure, revealing the unusual state of high RVDP and low PA diastolic pressures	Lost in atrial fibrillation
Computed tomography signs		
	Intravenous administration of contrast material is not used to assess for calcification.	General limitations of and exclusions to CT scanning apply.
		Performed in breath-hold—will not reveal inspiratory septal shift
Thickened pericardium		One fifth of proven constriction cases have either normal or minimally thickened pericardium. The interface of the pericardium from the myocardium may be difficult to discern unless their attenuation coefficients contrast.
		Intravenous administration of contrast material in the RV generates artifacts over the right-sided pericardium.
		Older CT scanners overrepresented pericardial thickness because of inadequate temporal resolution.
Calcified pericardium		Most cases of constriction do not have calcified pericardium.
		Some cases of pericardial calcification do not have constrictive physiology.
Diastolic septal dips (cine CT, ECG gated)		May show early diastolic dip and atrial systolic dip; but because it is performed in breath-hold, it will not show inspiratory septal shift.
Cardiac magnetic resonance signs		
Thickened pericardium (T1-weighted black blood spin echo)		General exclusions to and limitations of CMR apply (need to breath-hold, need for regular cardiac rhythm)
		Performed in breath-hold—will not reveal inspiratory septal shift
Ventricular distortion		
Diastolic septal dips (SSFP)		
Delayed enhancement (IRGRE)		Unknown relevance
Cardiac catheterization signs		
Elevated and equilibrated (<5 mm Hg differences) diastolic pressures	Uniformly noncompliant and compressive pericardium over the heart	Asymmetric, localized constriction may occur.
		Assumes an underlying normal heart; poor specificity and PPV
RVDP > 1/3 RVSP	Noncompliance of pericardium over the right side of the heart	Limited specificity and PPV
PA pressures <55 mm Hg		Poor specificity and PPV
Dissociation of LVSP and RVSP (directionally opposite changes). On the first or second cardiac cycle of inspiration: rise in RVSP and fall in LVSP	Ventricular interdependence	May be difficult to discern with use of fluid-filled catheters
		Respiratory effort is relevant
		Need for respirometry
Inspiratory increase in PCWP:LVDP gradient (>5 mm Hg)	Isolation of left-sided heart diastolic pressures from intrathoracic pressures	May be difficult to discern with use of fluid-filled catheters
		Respiratory effort is relevant
		Need for respirometry

Table 9-6. Diagnostic Signs of Pericardial Constriction—cont'd

	Cause	Caveat
Right atrial pressure		
Kussmaul sign	Noncompliance of pericardium over the right side of the heart	Poor specificity and PPV
M pattern	Elevated filling pressure Exaggerated early diastolic recoil	M pattern may be seen in restrictive cardiomyopathies
W pattern	Elevated filling pressure, less prominent recoil	W pattern may be seen in restrictive cardiomyopathies
Pulsus paradoxus	Ventricular interdependence	
	Increased inspiratory effort (more negative intrapleural pressure)	
	Increased inspiratory effort (increased variation of pulmonary venous capacitance)	

CHF, congestive heart failure; CMR, cardiac magnetic resonance; CT, computed tomography; COPD, chronic obstructive pulmonary disease; ECG, electrocardiography; GFR, glomerular filtration rate; IRGRE, inversion recovery gradient echo; LV, left ventricle; LVDP, left ventricular diastolic pressure; LVSP, left ventricular systolic pressure; PA, pulmonary artery; PCWP, pulmonary capillary wedge pressure; PPV, positive predictive value; RAP, right atrial pressure; RV, right ventricle; RVDP, right ventricular diastolic pressure; RVSP, right ventricular systolic pressure; SSFP, steady-state free precession; TEE, transesophageal echocardiography.

the time until diagnosis. The average time from symptom onset to diagnosis ranges from 1 to 2 years. However, some cases follow within a couple of weeks of cardiac surgery. Commonly, patients with constriction are initially investigated for noncardiac problems that are secondary to constriction, such as congestion-related liver dysfunction or low output–related renal dysfunction. Atypical presentations of pericardial constriction abound, such as cough-syncope.[10]

Physical Examination Findings

Venous Contours

In constriction, venous pressure is elevated and venous contours are abnormal. The V-wave increase in constriction results from pericardial stiffness over the right atrium during ventricular systole when the tricuspid valve is closed; the pressure within the right atrium rises rapidly as the chamber is constricted by the noncompliant pericardium. The prominent or steep *y* descent results from the rapid outward recoil of the stiff pericardium in early diastole, allowing rapid ventricular filling and a rapid early fall in pressure of the atria. The prominent *y* descent is a cardinal finding of constriction and begins the distinction of constriction from tamponade at the bedside (Fig. 9-14). Although the mean right atrial/jugular venous pressure does not tend to fall with inspiration, the *y* descent typically accentuates with inspiration and the *x* descent may increase as well. If the mean venous pressure does not decrease with inspiration, a Kussmaul sign is present, indicating impaired right-sided heart diastolic function (ability to accommodate the increased venous return of inspiration) (Fig. 9-15). This noncompliance is imparted by the constrictive pericardium over the right side of the heart. A more obvious manifestation of Kussmaul sign is an actual mean pressure rise with inspiration, establishing severe impairment of right-sided heart compliance (Table 9-7).

Pericardial Knocks

Pericardial knocks are early diastolic filling sounds akin to the third heart sound (S_3), heard in the context of constriction,

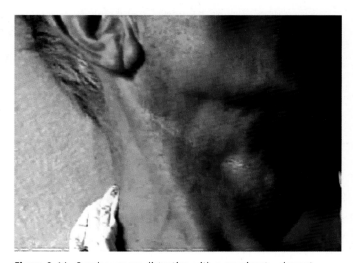

Figure 9-14. Jugular venous distention with a prominent *y* descent.

Table 9-7. Physical Examination Findings of Pericardial Constriction

Finding	Incidence
Edema	76%
Ascites	37%
Kussmaul sign	21%
Pulsus paradoxus	19%
Prominent *y* descent	94%
Elevated jugular venous pressure	93%
Pericardial knock	47%

From Ling LH, Oh JK, Schaff HV, et al: Constrictive pericarditis in the modern era: evolving clinical spectrum and impact on outcome after pericardiectomy. Circulation 1999;100:1380-1386.

produced by rapid inflow to the ventricles that is abruptly arrested by the noncompliant pericardium (Fig. 9-16). The inflow is particularly rapid because of the combination of elevated atrial pressure (pushing) and accentuated early ventricular filling due to rapid recoil of the constrictive pericardium (suction). Pericardial knocks occur 60 to 120 ms after S_2 and have been shown to occur simultaneously with the onset of the diastolic plateau. Pericardial knocks are appreciated in about half of constriction cases. They are more common in advanced and in calcific pericarditis.

Precordial Findings

Apical and right parasternal systolic retraction of the chest wall may occur. In a few patients, the constrictive process will focally distort or narrow the right ventricular outflow tract (RVOT), producing an ejection murmur, or the tricuspid or mitral annulus, producing a diastolic rumble of tricuspid or mitral stenosis.

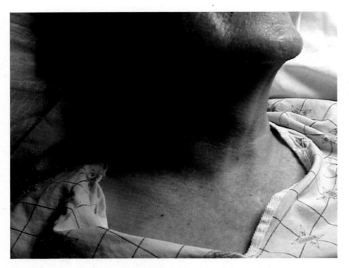

Figure 9-15. There is a "double descent" of the internal jugular venous column, conferred by the prominent *x* and *y* descents. The venous pressure is elevated, and with inspiration the venous pressure does not fall (Kussmaul sign).

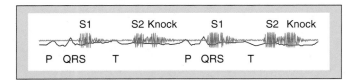

Figure 9-16. A pericardial knock in a 30-year-old woman with constrictive pericarditis.

Electrocardiographic Findings

There are no electrocardiographic (ECG) findings specific to the diagnosis of constriction. Atrial arrhythmias are common (atrial fibrillation, 20%; atrial flutter, 5%) and are due to atrial enlargement from elevated atrial pressures, with or without atrial involvement by the constrictive disease process. For patients in sinus rhythm, atrial abnormality (hypertrophy) is common due to the common finding of atrial enlargement. Ventricular voltages may be reduced (low voltages) if the pericardium is very thick and impairing surface recording of ECG voltages. Repolarization is usually abnormal. Pseudoinfarction Q waves may be seen, representing penetration of the fibrotic process into the pericardium. Right ventricular hypertrophy from RVOT narrowing and obstruction from focal constriction have been described. The ECG may represent the summation of abnormalities from constrictive lesions and from underlying structural heart disease.

Atrial Fibrillation

About 25% of patients with constriction have atrial fibrillation or flutter. Atrial fibrillation or flutter has a significant and often compromising impact on the hemodynamics of constriction cases and on several aspects of the diagnostic evaluation. The rhythm may be held responsible for the entire clinical picture and the diagnosis of constriction not considered or pursued (Fig. 9-17). The venous contours will lose the part of the *x* descents due to atrial relaxation, making the *y* descents predominant; the irregular R-R intervals will heavily influence and randomize the intracardiac flows and pressures, obscuring the influence of respiration—and the characteristic constriction findings seen per respiratory cycle. Overdrive pacing to regularize the rhythm may be used in the catheterization laboratory to eliminate the effect of the varying R-R intervals of atrial fibrillation on pressure.

Radiographic Findings

Mild enlargement of the cardiopericardial silhouette is usual. Left atrial enlargement is generally apparent and arises from increased atrial pressure (as a segment of the left atrium between the pulmonary veins is not intrapericardial and is prone to dilation despite the extrinsic constriction elsewhere). Atrial fibrillation also increases atrial size. Pericardial calcification is present in a minority of cases of constriction in North America; but when it is present and extensive, it establishes a high probability of constriction (Figs. 9-18 to 9-24). However, even if the adage that radiographically evident calcification is consistent with constriction is often true, there are some exceptions if the pericardial calcification thickening either is not sufficiently global or is frankly focal. A wide range of possible calcification may occur

Figure 9-17. Chronic constrictive pericarditis. Atrial fibrillation. Low voltages in the standard limb leads constitute nonspecific repolarization abnormalities.

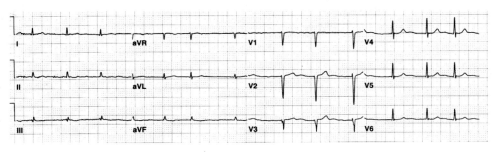

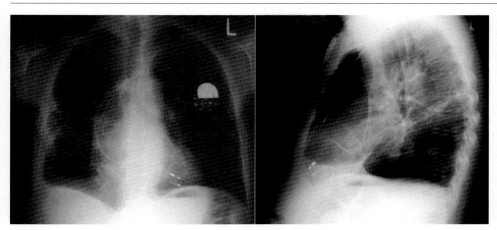

Figure 9-18. Pericardial calcification can be faintly seen on the posteroanterior view and well seen on the lateral view as thin plates over the RV anterior wall.

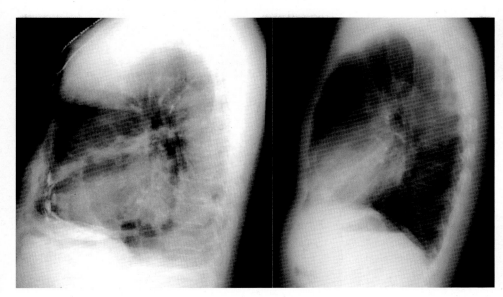

Figure 9-19. Pericardial calcification is seen well in these lateral views from different patients. The patient on the left also has calcified pericardium under the diaphragmatic surface of the heart. The thickness and distribution of the calcium are variable.

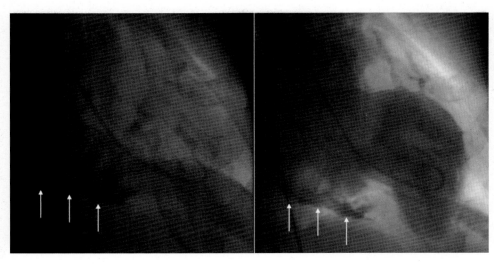

Figure 9-20. These fluoroscopic images of a contrast ventriculogram delineate dense pericardial calcification. As well, there is extreme distortion of the LV geometry due to the longitudinal shortening of the heart from the constrictive pericardium, which has "folded" the long axis of the LV.

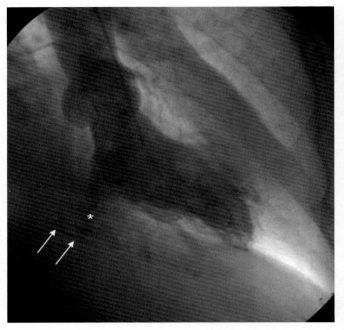

Figure 9-21. This RAO contrast ventriculogram delineates pericardial calcification extending along the right side of the heart. The plate of calcification is more easily seen when it is in-line *(arrows)* with the x-ray beam, as its attenuation effect is concentrated, than when it is en face *(asterisk)*, where its attenuation effect is dispersed and it appears as a smudge.

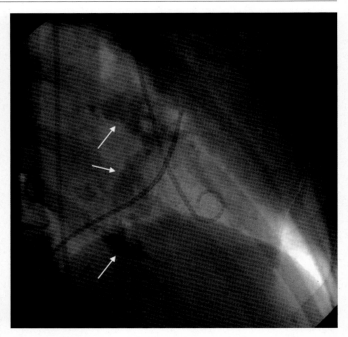

Figure 9-23. Extensive calcification is seen principally within the atrioventricular grooves.

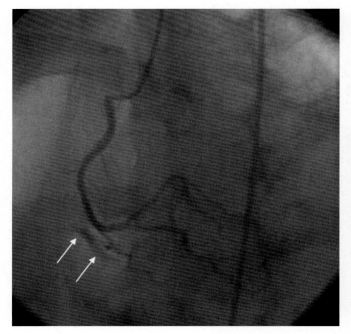

Figure 9-22. This right coronary injection localizes a plate of calcification near the right atrioventricular groove and extending over the RV free wall beside an acute marginal branch of the right coronary artery.

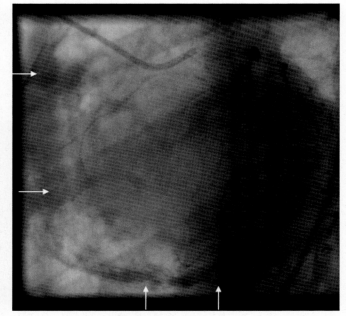

Figure 9-24. This LAO left coronary injection reveals nearly circumferential calcification, mainly within the atrioventricular grooves.

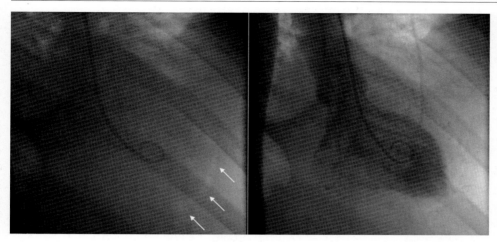

Figure 9-25. This RAO ventriculogram reveals a thick and lucent stripe around the apex of the heart—surgically proven pericardial thickening. There is no apparent calcification.

from none (most common) (Figs. 9-25 and 9-26) to massive (Figs. 9-27 and 9-28).

Vascular chest radiographic signs include azygos vein dilation or prominence and pulmonary venous dilation. The pulmonary arteries are not prominently dilated in constrictive physiology. The azygos and hemiazygos veins drain into the superior vena cava (SVC); therefore, elevated central venous pressure may render the azygos vein more prominent as it arches over the right main bronchus if it is tangentially depicted. Pleural plaques are sometimes seen. Pleural effusions are common and reflect either chronic elevation of the central venous pressure (as the right pleura drains through the azygos vein, and the left pleura drains through the hemiazygos vein) or concurrent pleural disease in some patients (e.g., tuberculosis) (Fig. 9-29).

Echocardiographic Findings

Echocardiography has several roles in the evaluation of patients with constriction:

- Exclusion of alternative pathologic processes that may be responsible (tamponade, valvular disease, and dilated cardiomyopathy). However, constriction may occur concurrently with other forms of structural heart disease, and the presence of a pericardial effusion with compression signs is consistent with both tamponade and effuso-constriction.
- Identification of usual morphologic findings
- Identification of physiologic signs of constriction on 2-dimensional and M-mode imaging and with Doppler interrogation
- Elimination of myocardial diastolic failure dysfunction (that would be consistent with restrictive cardiomyopathy) by establishing that the tissue Doppler velocities are normal[11]
- Evaluation of postoperative pericardiectomy patients for acute low-output, right ventricular dysfunction

Echocardiographic signs of constriction include the following:

- Septal motion per respiratory cycle (inspiratory septal shift)—a sign of ventricular interdependence (Fig. 9-30)
- Hepatic venous flow pattern per respiratory cycle (expiratory diastolic flow reversal increase) is 68% sensitive and 100% specific—a Kussmaul-like finding (Fig. 9-31).[12]

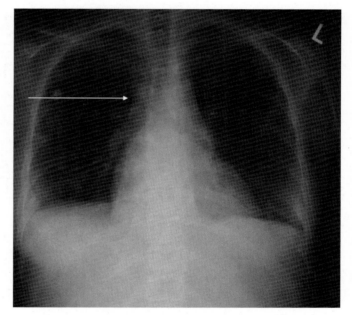

Figure 9-26. Normal cardiopericardial silhouette. No calcification. Arrow denotes large azygos vein, signaling elevated central venous pressure. Also evident are bilateral pleural effusions.

- Inspiratory increase in the tricuspid regurgitation velocity: mean increase in constriction, 13% ± 6% versus 8% ± 7% in controls—a Kussmaul-like finding (Fig. 9-32).[13] The technical challenge of this sign is to achieve and to maintain complete spectral profiles of the tricuspid regurgitation jet as the heart moves during respiration.
- Tissue Doppler: normal pattern militates against restrictive cardiomyopathy (Table 9-8)[14] but does not assist with the possible issue of concurrent constriction and ventricular dysfunction.
- An inspiratory fall of more than 25% of the early diastolic (E) transmitral flow is a sign of ventricular interdependence and increased PCWP:LVDP gradient finding (Fig. 9-33),[15] which is 88% sensitive for constriction (Figs. 9-34 and 9-35).[16] Although reversal of the pattern occurs during positive-pressure ventilation,[17] respiratory variation of mitral inflow

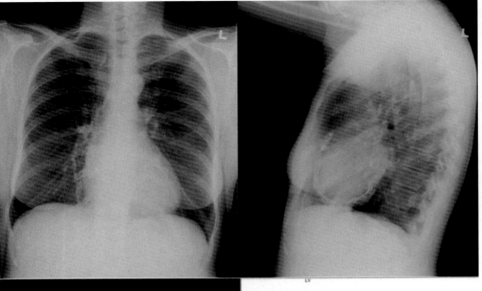

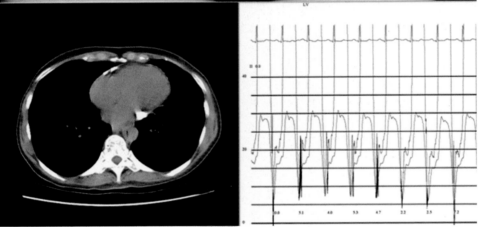

Figure 9-27. In this exceptional case, despite the extraordinarily obvious pericardial calcification, there was no clinical, echocardiographic, or hemodynamic evidence of constriction. To some extent, this is the exception to the rule that obvious pericardial calcification is predictive of constrictive physiology. The non–contrast-enhanced CT image (BOTTOM LEFT) localizes the calcification to the atrioventricular groove rather than over the cardiac chambers. The simultaneous LV:RV pressure recordings did not demonstrate convincing equilibration or most other signs of constriction physiology. Although the diastolic pressures were elevated, any limitation of filling imparted by the calcium may have been too localized to confer classic constrictive physiology to the heart.

Table 9-8. Distinguishing Restrictive Cardiomyopathy from Pericardial Constriction by Echocardiography

In Favor of Restrictive Cardiomyopathy	In Favor of Pericardial Constriction
2-Dimensional	2-Dimensional
LVH, RVH	Normal ventricles
Normal systolic function	Septal findings
No abnormal septal findings	Inspiratory septal shift (interdependence)
	Early diastolic dip
Doppler	Doppler
No variation of LV inflow velocities	LV inflow velocities fall by 25% with inspiration
No change in TR velocity	Hepatic venous flow reversal in expiration
Low tissue velocity	Normal tissue velocities

LV, left ventricle; LVH, left ventricular hypertrophy; RVH, right ventricular hypertrophy; TR, tricuspid regurgitation.

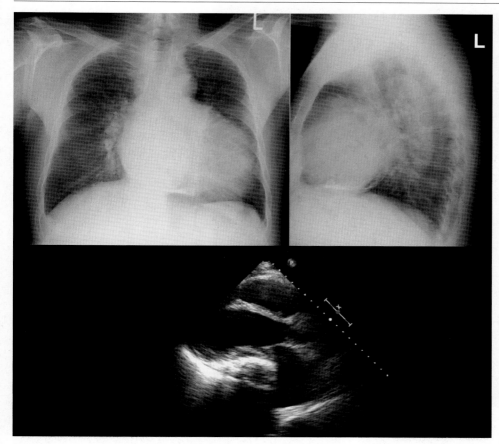

Figure 9-28. A prominently thick and large plate of calcium-containing material is seen along the diaphragmatic surface of the heart. This patient had remotely undergone pericardiectomy for tuberculosis; a large bleed had occurred postoperatively. It was assumed that the calcified mass, which was 3 cm thick, represented a calcified hematoma. It may also have represented severely thickened and calcified residual nonresected pericardium.

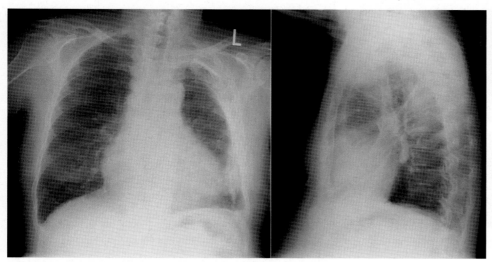

Figure 9-29. This patient was known to have had tuberculosis and to have undergone repeated left pleural drainage procedures. There are thick left pleural plaques that are seen to be calcified on the posteroanterior film. The restrictive effect has reduced the left hemithorax volume.

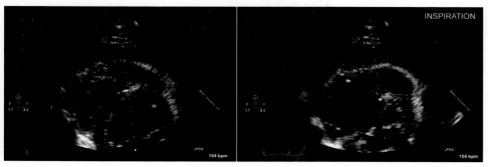

Figure 9-30. Parasternal short-axis view during expiration (LEFT) and inspiration (RIGHT). With inspiration, the septum shifts toward the left side, consistent with ventricular interdependence.

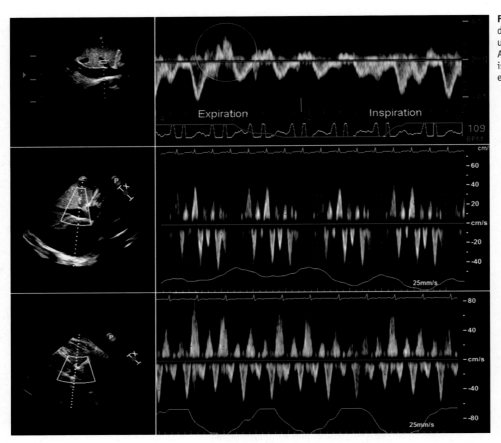

Figure 9-31. Expiratory increase in diastolic hepatic venous flow reversal is a useful sign of constrictive physiology. Although sampling of hepatic venous flow is difficult, the specificity of the sign of expiratory reversal justifies the effort.

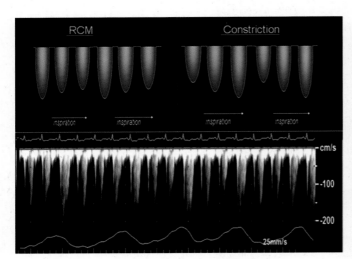

Figure 9-32. The influence of spontaneous respiration on RVSP is directionally different in cases of constriction and restriction. In restriction, the RVSP falls with inspiration; in constriction, the RVSP increases with inspiration. RCM, restrictive cardiomyopathy.

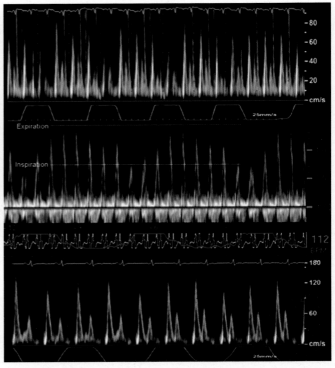

Figure 9-33. Mitral inflow profiles in constriction. With inspiration, there is a significant fall in early transmitral inflow velocities. At higher heart rates and at slower spectral display sweep speeds (TOP ROW), there is difficulty in distinguishing the early from the late transmitral inflows as summation of E- and A-wave profiles occurs. At faster sweep speeds, there is better dispersion of the E and A waves. The fall in E-wave height is greatest with the first beat of inspiration.

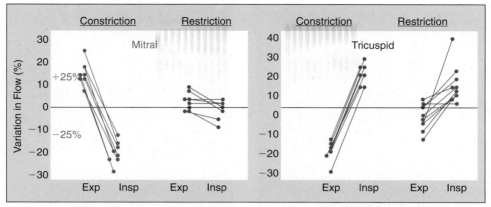

Figure 9-34. Mitral inflow (E wave) variation may help distinguish constriction from restrictive physiology. In constriction, during normal spontaneous respiration, mitral inflow variations are prominent and vary (fall with inspiration, rise with expiration) an average of ± 25% around apneic velocities. In restrictive physiology, mitral inflow variations through the respiratory cycle are less prominent. In both constrictive and restrictive physiologies, tricuspid inflow variations are the norm and do not assist with distinguishing the two types of physiology. With abnormal patterns of breathing or effort of breathing, and with mechanical ventilation, mitral inflow velocity variations are considerably less useful in distinguishing the two types of physiology. (From Hatle LK, Appleton CP, Popp RL: Differentiation of constrictive pericarditis and restrictive cardiomyopathy by Doppler echocardiography. Circulation 1989;79:370.)

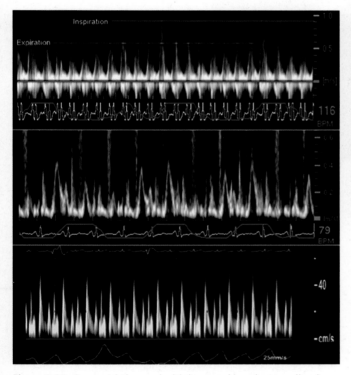

Figure 9-35. In constriction, and with innumerable pulmonary disorders, there is an increase in trans-tricuspid flow velocities. Note the lower spectral tracing: the respiratory pattern is as erratic as the respiration was ineffectual. Without regular respiratory cycles, the pattern of inflow velocities is inapparent.

velocities is still a useful but more difficult sign in the presence of atrial fibrillation.[18] Respiratory variation of mitral inflow is increased by preload reduction by changing the patient's position to reduce preload (sitting or head-up position).[19]

Other echocardiographic signs of constriction include the following:

• Marked (>40%) variation in trans-tricuspid valve flow early diastolic velocities is often seen in constriction cases but also

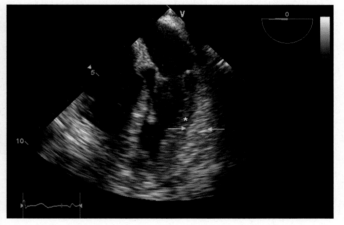

Figure 9-36. The pericardium is a centimeter thick over the LV lateral wall (*between arrows*). The myocardium is indicated by an asterisk.

may be seen in any cause of pulmonary disease or distress. Patients with constriction do not exhibit quite as prominent variations of SVC velocity as do COPD patients (see Fig. 9-35).[20]

• Pulmonic valve systolic preopening, seen with pulsed wave Doppler recording at the pulmonic valve level, demonstrates greatly elevated right ventricular end-diastolic pressure (RVEDP) that with atrial contraction rises above the low pulmonary artery diastolic pressure.[21] The sign is lost with atrial fibrillation.

• Septal motion per cardiac cycle (early diastolic dip and the atrial systolic notch)[22]

Frankly poor transthoracic echocardiographic signs include the following:

• Pericardial thickening. Transthoracic echocardiography is notoriously insensitive to the presence of pericardial thickness and highly limited in the anatomic field it can image. The better echocardiographic means by which to detect pericardial thickening is with transesophageal echocardiography (Figs. 9-36 to 9-39), and the best overall chance is with CMR or CT scanning.

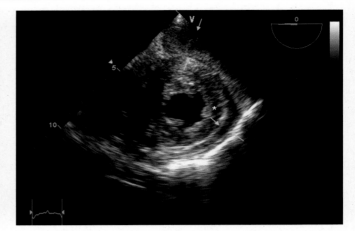

Figure 9-37. The pericardium lateral to the right atrium is nearly 2 cm thick (*between arrows*).

Figure 9-38. There is severe pericardial thickening, of different appearance by echocardiography (*between arrows*), seen posterior and lateral to the LV. The myocardium is indicated by an asterisk.

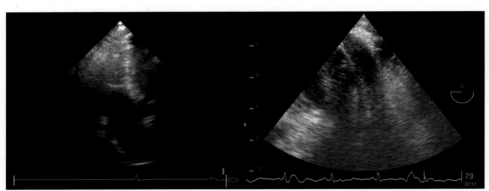

Figure 9-39. LEFT, Apical 4-chamber view: the RV wall and the pericardium over it are simply not seen. RIGHT, Transesophageal echocardiography short-axis view lateral to the LV; pericardial thickness is 1.4 cm.

- Flattened LV posterior motion in mid-diastole, due to limitation of diastolic filling by noncompliant pericardium. The sign is akin to the "plateau" of diastolic pressure.

All echocardiographic signs should be sought with simultaneous use of respirometry tracings.

Common problems encountered during the echocardiographic assessment of pericardial constriction include concurrent native valve disease and prosthetic valves, especially compounded by atrial fibrillation, that compromise velocity signs of constriction; underlying structural heart abnormalities that compromise 2-dimensional and M-mode signs of constriction; and abnormal breathing effort or mode.

The typical 2-dimensional findings of constriction consist of normal-sized ventricles with normal wall thickness and systolic function, normal or near-normal valves, some degree of atrial dilation, and absence of pericardial fluid. The absence of systolic dysfunction discounts dilated cardiomyopathy. The absence of left and right ventricular hypertrophy augers against the presence of restrictive or infiltrative cardiomyopathy. Enlarged atria support elevated diastolic pressures, as inferior vena cava (IVC) and hepatic vein dilation (plethora, blunted variation) support elevated central venous pressures. Ventricular interaction or interdependence signs suggest constriction but are not entirely specific and, if the respiratory effort is abnormal, do not appear sensitive (Table 9-9).[23]

There are three abnormal septal motion patterns that may be seen in constrictive physiology. None of the signs is perfect, but they are useful in context. The position of the interventricular (and interatrial) septum is determined by the pressure gradient across them and their own intrinsic stiffness.

1. The early diastolic (motion) dip. In early diastole, the interventricular septum rapidly moves a short distance toward the left side of the heart, then moves quickly back toward the right side of the heart. The sign is apparent on 2-dimensional imaging as a quick "dip" or jiggle, and it is best appreciated by M-mode display, on which it appears as a small beak-shaped deflection and correction (Figs. 9-40 to 9-42). The early diastolic dip reflects and results from the oscillations of early diastolic pressure (early diastolic pressure dip) that may transiently reverse the gradient on the septum and transiently shift the septum. The sign draws heavily from the catheterization sign of a prominent "early diastolic dip" due to brisk and forceful recoil of the constrictive pericardium over the left side of the heart. When the early diastolic pressure dip of the left ventricle significantly exceeds or precedes that of the right ventricle, the sign is likely to be present. It is seen per cardiac cycle, independently of the respiratory cycle.

2. The inspiratory septal shift. The inspiratory septal shift is a sign also borrowed from catheter studies that reveal LV:RV interaction or interdependence. The basis of it is not well described, but it is believed to arise from the directionally opposite pressure variations in the ventricles in inspiration provoked by LV:RV interaction or interdependence that displaces the septum from the right to the left side as the right ventricle briefly dominates the limited available space for filling (Fig. 9-43).

3. The atrial systolic notch. In some patients with constriction, after atrial contraction, the right ventricular diastolic pressure (RVDP) is initially greater than the LVDP, transiently displacing in late diastole the ventricular septum to the left side. It is

Table 9-9. Echocardiographic Signs of Constrictive Pericarditis

Parameter	Cutoff Value	Authorn (ref)	Sensitivity	Specificity	Comments
Mitral E-wave variation	>10%	Rajagopalan (23)	84%	91%	CP: n = 19 RCM: n = 11
	>25%	Hatle (15)	100%		CP: n = 7 RCM: n = 12
	>25%	Oh (16)	88%		CP: n = 25 RCM: n = 1 Normal pericardium: n = 2
	>25%, use of preload reduction maneuver	Oh (19)	75%		12 patients with proven constriction without initial E-wave variation subjected to head-up or sitting position; 75% developed >25% variation; mean variation rose from 5% ± 7% initially to 32% ± 28% with preload reduction
Pulmonary venous peak D-wave variation	>18%	Rajagopalan (23)	79%	91%	CP: n = 19 RCM: n = 11
Pulmonary venous peak D-wave variation, E-wave variation, on TEE					CP: n = 41 (31 patients in sinus rhythm, 10 patients in atrial fibrillation) Pulmonary venous D-wave variation: sinus rhythm, 25%; atrial fibrillation, 35% E-wave variation: sinus rhythm, 18%; atrial fibrillation, 15%
Pulmonary venous peak D-wave variation, E-wave variation on TEE	Combination of % E wave ≥40% and pulmonary venous systolic: diastolic flow ≥0.65%	Klein (28)	86% of patients classified correctly		CP: n = 14 RCM: n = 17
Tissue Doppler lateral mitral annulus (E_a)	>8.0 cm/s	Rajagopalan (23)	89%	100%	CP: n = 19 RCM: n = 11
	>8.0 cm/s	Garcia (11)	100%	100%	CP: n = 8 RCM: n = 7 Normals: n = 15 E_a normals: 14.5 ± 4.7 cm/s CP: 14.8 ± 4.8 cm/s RCM: 5.2 ± 1.4 cm/s
Increase in TR velocity with inspiration	>5% increase in TR peak velocity	Klodas (13)	100%	100%	CP: n = 5 CHF due to other causes: n = 12 CP: TR velocity increase 13% ± 6% CHF other causes: −8% ± 7%
Atrial septal notch		Tei (22)	88%	87%	CP: n = 13 RCM: n = 12
	Posterior septal motion after the P wave and before the QRS *when in sinus rhythm*	Engel (14)	34%	87%	
Early diastolic dip		Tei (22)	62%		CP: n = 13 RCM: n = 12 Seen in 25% of RCM patients as well
		Candell-Riera (38)	88%		CP: n = 8
	Abrupt change from gentle early diastolic posterior motion of the septum	Engel (14)	33%	100%	Anterior displacement of the septum was more specific than posterior displacement of the septum
Inspiratory septal shift		Unknown	Unknown		
Presystolic pulmonary valve opening		Wann (21)	Unknown	Low	1 of 6 cases of presystolic pulmonary valve opening 　Severe TR: n = 2 　Severe PI: n = 1 　Aorto–right atrial fistula: n = 1 　Löffler's endocarditis: n = 1 　CP: n = 1

Continued

Table 9-9. Echocardiographic Signs of Constrictive Pericarditis—cont'd

Parameter	Cutoff Value	Authorn (ref)	Sensitivity	Specificity	Comments
		Tanaka (37)	Unknown	Low	Of 2 cases of constriction that underwent M-mode interrogation, both had deep a-dips
	Premature opening on M-mode before QRS	Engel (14)	14%	0%	
Pericardial thickness on TEE	>4 mm	Hutchison (24)	85%		CP: n = 13
	≥3 mm	Ling (26)	95%	86%	CP: n = 11 Normals: n = 21 Mean normal thickness was 1.2 ± 0.8 mm; no normals exceeded 2.5 mm
	>3 mm (transgastric view)	Izumi (27)	100%		CP: n = 7
		Engel (14)	53%	100%	
Diastolic flattening of the posterior wall	<1 mm motion	Voekel (29)	92%	100%	CP: n = 12 Normals: n = 10
	<1 mm posterior motion in mid and late diastole	Engel (14)	85%	86%	
		Gibson (39)	40%		

CHF, congestive heart failure; CP, constrictive pericarditis; PI, pulmonary insufficiency; RCM, restrictive cardiomyopathy; TEE, transesophageal echocardiography; TR, tricuspid regurgitation.

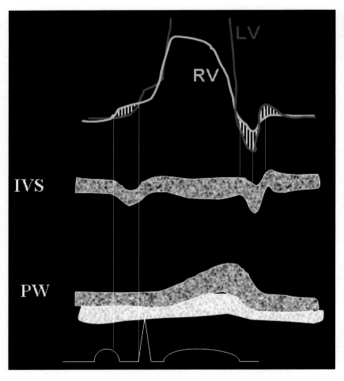

Figure 9-40. An atrial systolic dip (from the right to the left side) of the interventricular septum (IVS) is seen in some cases of constriction (that are in sinus rhythm), as an early diastolic dip (from the left to the right side) may also be. LV, left ventricle; PW, posterior wall; RV, right ventricle.

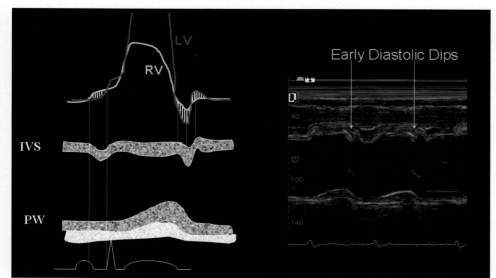

Figure 9-41. A prominent early diastolic dip of the interventricular septum (IVS), seen in many cases of constriction, is due to falling of early diastolic left ventricular (LV) pressure more than of early diastolic right ventricular (RV) pressure. Other M-mode signs are inconstant and subjective. PW, posterior wall.

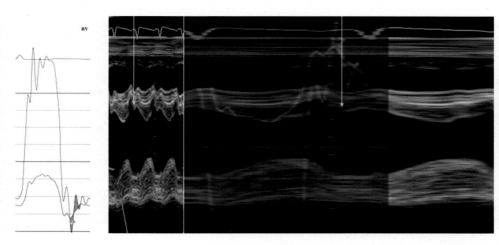

Figure 9-42. LEFT, Simultaneous LV and RV pressure tracings. The early diastolic RV and LV pressures oscillate, and transiently, the RV pressure exceeds the LV pressure. RIGHT, M-mode study of the septum at low speed and at high speed, with a prominent early diastolic dip. The LV and RV pressure tracings are superimposed (and inverted) to lie over the respective ventricle. The oscillations of early diastolic pressure and the transient inversion of the LV:RV pressure differential are seen temporally associated with the early diastolic septal dip (motion oscillation).

Figure 9-43. Inspiratory septal shift is a sign of pericardial constriction.

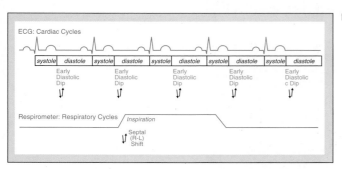

seen per cardiac cycle, independently of the respiratory cycle.[22] The atrial systolic notch is absent in atrial fibrillation and presumably in atrial failure. It is best appreciated by M-mode imaging. Distinguishing an early diastolic septal dip from an atrial systolic notch may be difficult at higher heart rates and with longer PR intervals.

Elevated central venous pressure, a hallmark of constriction physiology, is indicated by dilation and lack of respiratory collapse and spontaneous contrast within the IVC (Fig. 9-44).

Transesophageal Echocardiography for Pericardial Constriction

Transesophageal echocardiography (TEE) offers little more than transthoracic echocardiography (TTE) for the assessment of constriction, with the exception of affording some means by which to assess pericardial thickness over the right ventricular and atrial anterolateral walls from a lower esophageal view[24] and under the left and right ventricles from a transgastric view.[25] There is good correlation of TEE and electron beam CT assessment of pericardial thickness, and there is low interobserver variability and high positive predictive value for detection of pericardial thickening in constriction (with use of a cutoff of 3 mm) with sensitivity of 95% and specificity of 86%.[26] However, CMR and CT scanning have become the standard tests to assess pericardial thickness.

Positive-pressure ventilation (e.g., in intraoperative TEE) will attenuate or reverse the Doppler findings and septal motion pattern of ventricular interdependence.[27] Left-sided heart flow velocity patterns as recorded by TEE are predictive of the presence of constrictive physiology: a pulmonary venous systolic: diastolic flow ratio of 0.65 and mitral E-wave percentage of 40% are 86% predictive of constrictive physiology.[28]

Computed Tomography for Pericardial Constriction

Chest CT now also includes cardiac CT through several advances in image acquisition (gating), ECG gating, slice number or coverage, and software. Contemporary CT scanners and systems have 64 slices and very high spatial and temporal resolution and the opportunity to ECG gate acquisition. Contemporary equipment represents a significant improvement over older equipment; but older equipment is almost without exception what is represented in the literature of CT imaging. Other limitations of CT literature in addition to not reflecting contemporary equipment capabilities include the small size of studies and that most were single-center studies (the same limitations apply to CMR literature). Although nongated chest CT is able to image the pericardium well, gated cardiac CT is better for the cardiac details but does not offer the wide field of imaging of chest CT.

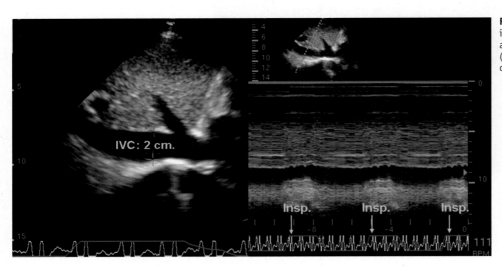

Figure 9-44. The inferior vena cava (IVC) is grossly dilated (as are the hepatic veins) and fails to collapse during inspiration (which is recorded as the upward deflection of the respirometry tracing).

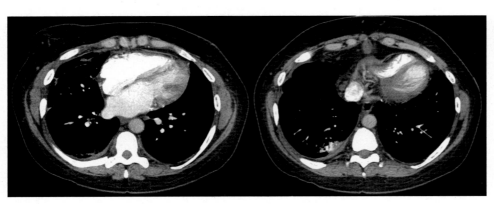

Figure 9-45. Patient with proven constriction yet minimally thickened pericardium. The right image demonstrates that there is distortion of the right ventricle consistent with some extrinsic phenomenon, in this case constriction.

Normal pericardium is anatomically 1 mm thick (Fig. 9-45). By ECG-gated cardiac CT, "normal" pericardial thickness is 1 to 1.5 mm; by non–ECG-gated chest CT, it is 2 mm or less; and by CMR, it is less than 3 mm (Figs. 9-46 to 9-49). CT is an excellent means of detecting pericardial calcification and the distribution of calcification; however, most cases of constriction in North America are noncalcified. CT does not depict the complex physiology of constriction and reflects only basic hemodynamic disturbances. For example, the sign of raised central venous pressure is simply reflux of intravenous contrast material (when it is injected into an arm vein) into the IVC in the presence of dilation of the systemic veins. Cine CT imaging is able to depict septal motion patterns per cardiac cycle but not per respiratory cycle because acquisition is not performed over a respiratory cycle.

In a retrospective study of 29 patients with constriction after cardiac surgery, the sensitivity of older generation CT scanning systems for the detection of "constriction" was 78% and the specificity 100%.[29] In a very small series, cine CT correctly identified, on the basis of pericardial thickness, all 5 constriction cases (mean pericardial thickness, 10 ± 2 mm) among 7 restrictive cardiomyopathy cases (mean pericardial thickness, 2 ± 1 mm) and 7 normal controls (mean pericardial thickness, 1 ± 1 mm).[30] Furthermore, the filling fraction (volume − ESV/stroke volume ×

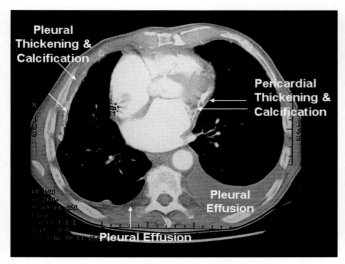

Figure 9-46. This nongated contrast-enhanced chest CT image depicts extensive chest abnormalities, at the expense of optimal resolution of cardiac detail. However, it is still clear that the pericardium is thickened, and there is a plate of calcification over the LV lateral wall on this plane.

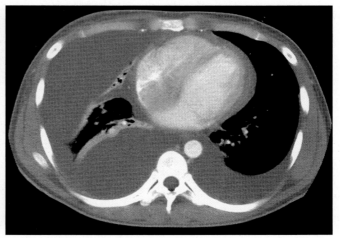

Figure 9-47. This nongated chest CT image shows a very large left pleural effusion and a smaller right-sided one. There is pericardial thickening and layering, but it is difficult to resolve what is what. Because of a lack of gating, there is prohibitive motion artifact of the heart.

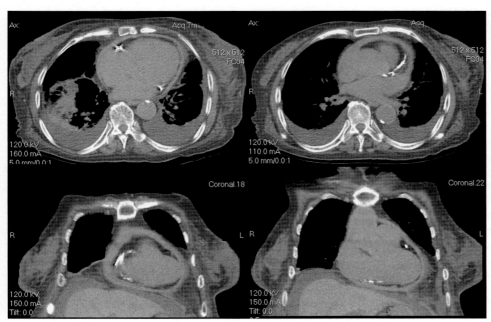

Figure 9-48. A nongated, non–contrast-enhanced CT image of a patient with renal insufficiency. Pericardial thickening is circumferential and seen on the axial images (TOP) and coronal images (BOTTOM). The myocardium is seen as a lower attenuation plane, similar to chest cage muscle. The calcification is not pericardial, but coronary, and extremely extensive. Although pericardial calcification in constriction commonly involves the atrioventricular and interventricular grooves, the coronaries also reside there. The motion of the atrioventricular plane is suggested by the two lines of right coronary artery calcification in the bottom left image.

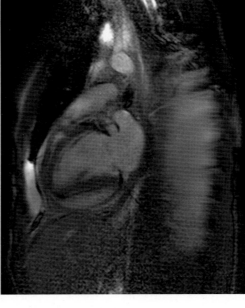

Figure 9-49. LEFT, This nongated CT image demonstrates the myocardium and its boundary from the pericardium, the pericardial thickening, and a layering within the pericardium, but it is not optimal in defining tissue planes. RIGHT, The MRI image (steady-state free precession) gives a better but imperfect delineation of myocardium:visceral pericardium and intrapericardial material: parietal pericardium.

100% for all slices) also appeared to distinguish the three groups: constriction, 83% ± 6%; restrictive cardiomyopathy, 62% ± 9%; normals, 44% ± 5%.[30]

In up to 20% of patients with surgically proven constriction, preoperative imaging shows normal pericardial thickness. Potential reasons for this include the subset of constriction cases with normal or minimally thickened (but stiff) pericardium and that epicardial constriction rather than parietal pericardial constriction is predominant.[31]

Potential contrast nephropathy risk is an issue for patients with renal insufficiency or renal failure associated with constriction.

Cardiac Magnetic Resonance for Pericardial Constriction

CMR has multiple techniques and sequences that may be used to evaluate suspected constrictive pericardium. The most common are T1-weighted black blood spin echo sequences for pericardial thickness, steady-state free precession (SSFP) cine imaging for ventricular function and septal motion, and gadolinium contrast delayed hyperenhancement.

T1-weighted black blood spin echo sequences are used to assess for pericardial thickening, which is most easily assessed over the right ventricle and is dependent on available fat planes. The parietal pericardium appears on spin echo imaging as low signal tissue between high signal epicardial and pericardial fat. Epicardial thickening, lacking an underlying fat plane, may be difficult to image if its signal does not contrast from that of myocardium. Thickened pericardium by CMR is greater than 3 mm. T1-weighted black blood spin echo sequences and other CMR sequences are unable to reliably distinguish pericardial calcification from fibrosis. In a study of 29 patients with suspected constrictive pericarditis, using spin echo CMR criteria for thickened pericardium greater than 4 mm, the sensitivity was 88% and specificity was 100%. CMR was unable to detect pericardial calcification.[32]

The inversion recovery gradient echo gadolinium delayed enhancement contrast technique is not well validated to identify constriction or to distinguish it from pericarditis without constriction, but it may prove helpful (Fig. 9-50). The actual cause of delayed enhancement in constrictive pericarditis is not well understood. Whether it reflects a more pericarditic cause (increased interstitial space from edema, increased interstitial space from inflammation) or a more scar-like cause (increased interstitial space from collagen) has not been established, nor has its predictive value. Similar to CT, CMR does not depict the complex hemodynamics of constriction well, although septal motion patterns per cardiac cycle may be clearly depicted, not per respiratory cycle, as acquisition is not gated to the respiratory cycle.

Tagged cine imaging may also have a role in constriction to show adhesion of the pericardium (lack of normal slippage of the parietal pericardium over the heart) in suspected constriction cases, but it has not been extensively validated.[33]

Real-time imaging may be used to depict the abnormal septal motions, including inspiration-induced septal motion.

Technical issues that are relevant to obtaining good-quality CMR scans include the need for breath-holding (an issue if there are large pleural effusions) and the adverse effect of an irregular cardiac rhythm on image acquisition.

Limitations of Computed Tomography and Cardiac Magnetic Resonance for the Evaluation of Pericardial Constriction

Both CT and CMR are useful to support the diagnosis of constriction by identifying the usual substrate of thickened pericardium, but there are limitations to both techniques. The finding of thickened pericardium is seen in only 80% of cases. Thickened pericardium in a nonselected population of patients is not necessarily associated with constriction. Neither technique establishes enough of the specific physiologic changes of constriction or is able to

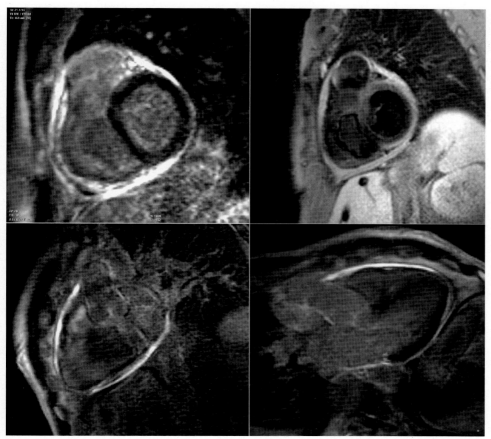

Figure 9-50. Constrictive pericarditis. The parietal pericardium is clearly thickened and is enhancing after gadolinium infusion.

identify associated myocardial dysfunction or restrictive cardio-myopathy. Existing studies are small, limited, and dated with respect to existing technologies and are representative of a high pretest probability (the published numbers of 80% to 100% sensitivity for the detection of pericardial thickening or constrictive pericarditis by CT or CMR seem to exceed the 80% incidence of pericardial thickening).

The contribution of CT and CMR to the evaluation of constriction is principally for the detection of pericardial thickening and calcification that would support the diagnosis. However, for the subset of patients with near-normal thickness of the pericardium, CT and CMR will not be able to support the diagnosis because their principal sign supportive of constriction is pericardial thickening.

CT and CMR can delineate the distribution of pericardial disease to assist with surgical planning. The finding of ventricular distortion is useful because it infers extrinsic compression of the cardiac chambers rather than intrinsic restriction. CT and CMR are not the principal tests to establish the physiologic consequences of constriction, such as ventricular interdependence (Table 9-10).

Cardiac Catheterization

Cardiac catheterization retains an important role in the evaluation of suspected constrictive pericarditis. The advantages of cardiac catheterization are as follows:

- Newer hemodynamic signs have high predictive value.
- Catheterization enables coronary angiography.
- Catheterization enables several maneuvers to optimize diagnostic testing by addressing confounding factors: pacing to regularize rhythm; volume infusion to unmask constrictive physiology in volume-contracted patients (patients given diuretics); and nitroprusside to lower filling pressures to unmask constrictive physiology in grossly volume-overloaded patients.
- Catheterization enables endomyocardial biopsy.[34]
- Catheterization is the surest means to identify pressures and waveforms.

New hemodynamic signs of ventricular interdependence and PCWP:LVDP gradients require use of respirometry to associate findings to the phase of the respiratory cycle.[9] A simultaneous and discordant change in the right ventricular and left ventricular pressures in the first or second beat of inspiration (increase in the RVSP and decrease in the LVSP) establishes interdependence of filling and is a useful sign. Irregular heart rhythm and poor or variable inspiratory effort may obscure the finding. An inspiratory increase in the PCWP:LVDP gradient of more than 5 mm Hg is another useful sign. Catheter whip and other artifacts of fluid-filled catheters, irregular heart rhythm, and poor or variable inspiratory effort may obscure the finding. Ideally, micromanometer-tipped catheters are used (Figs. 9-51 and 9-52).

In a study of 15 patients with surgically proven constrictive pericarditis and 21 patients with heart failure but without constrictive pericarditis (7 of 21 had restrictive cardiomyopathy),

Table 9-10. Limitations of Computed Tomography and Cardiac Magnetic Resonance for the Evaluation of Pericardial Constriction

Limitations of Computed Tomography (CT)	Limitations of Cardiac Magnetic Resonance (CMR)
Chest CT delineates a wide range of potential pathologic changes relevant to the diagnosis of constriction but does not offer the same cardiac anatomic detail as does gated cardiac CT.	CMR requires ECG gating; atrial fibrillation is a problem and is seen in about one quarter of patients with constriction.
Gated cardiac CT offers the highest cardiac anatomic detail but does not delineate the chest in its entirety, as does chest CT.	Pacers and implantable cardioverter defibrillators are currently contraindications.
Contrast material is nephrotoxic; many sicker and older patients with constriction have renal insufficiency.	Breath-holding is necessary, and it is more difficult for patients with large pleural effusions resulting from the right-sided heart failure of their constriction. The timing of cardiac CMR should be optimized so that the patient is as comfortable and participative as possible.
Radiation risk	Claustrophobia is an issue for several percent of patients, accentuated by lying supine if they are dyspneic.
	Calcium is poorly represented by CMR.
	The utility of the gadolinium contrast technique is neither well understood nor developed.
	The utility of the cine tagged technique is neither well understood nor developed.

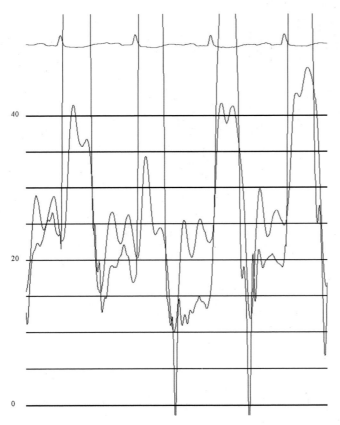

Figure 9-51. Simultaneous right and left ventricular pressure tracings in constriction. The timings of the different hemodynamic diagnostic signs of constriction are not simultaneous. In this example, with inspiration, the diastolic pressure fall in the left ventricle, which times with the variation in PCWP:LVDP gradient, precedes the increase in RVSP by one cardiac cycle.

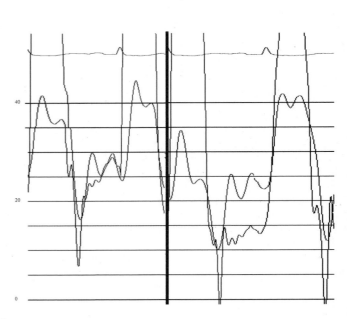

Figure 9-52. Simultaneous right and left ventricular pressure tracings in constriction. LEFT, Expiration. RIGHT, Inspiration. There is near-perfect equilibration of the RVDP and LVDP in expiration. With inspiration, a 5- to 10-mm right-to-left ventricular gradient has developed from a fall in the LVDP.

thermistor respirometry and high-fidelity micromanometer-tipped catheters were used to record dynamic respiratory changes in left and right ventricular pressures. If the patient was in atrial fibrillation, temporary pacing during hemodynamic recording was used to regularize the rhythm and to avoid the effect of R-R interval differences on pressures.[9] The PCWP:LVDP gradient variation and discordant RVSP and LVSP in inspiration signs had excellent predictive value. Use of fluid-filled catheters, especially without respirometry, can yield unclear depiction of the PCWP:LVDP gradient variation (Table 9-11 and Figs. 9-53 to 9-56; see also Fig. 9-11).

Older traditional hemodynamic signs include elevated RVDP ($\geq^1/_3$ of the RVSP), pulmonary artery pressure of less than 50 mm Hg, LVEDP:RVEDP difference of less than 5 mm Hg, and the "dip-and-plateau" configuration of the diastolic pressure tracing. These older signs are useful, but other than elevated RVDP ($\geq^1/_3$ of the RVSP), they lack predictive value. The dip-and-plateau sign is difficult to see at higher heart rates when diastole is shortened (Figs. 9-57 to 9-59).

Kussmaul sign is readily appreciated from the right atrial recording, especially when the mean pressure and not the waveform is recorded. If the y descent is greatly dominant, an M pattern is present. If the x and y descents are similar, the waveform has a W pattern (Fig. 9-60).

Fluoroscopy is able to depict pericardial and other cardiac calcification. Endomyocardial biopsy may be used to exclude or to include the diagnosis of restrictive cardiomyopathy.

Catheterization (combined with imaging) is also the best means to unravel the findings of unusually complicated cases of constriction, such as those with localized gradients or obstructions that result from deep fibrotic bands over either the RVOT or tricuspid annulus, resulting in RVOT gradients or tricuspid stenosis. Fluid challenge (1 L during 5 to 10 minutes) may unmask

constriction (this is especially useful if the patient has low filling pressures and is plausibly volume depleted, e.g., from use of diuretics). Although thought to be useful, the technique is not well validated. Conversely, sodium nitroprusside can lower severely elevated pressures and render them more typical of constriction. Pacing to regularize the cardiac rhythm rendered irregular by atrial fibrillation may be useful to eliminate the effect of R-R interval variation on volume and pressure phenomena.

Text continued on p. 159.

Table 9-11. Catheterization Findings of Pericardial Constriction

Criteria	Sensitivity (%)	Specificity (%)	PPV	NPV
Traditional				
LVEDP − RVEDP < 5 mm Hg	60	38	4	57
RVEDP/RVSP > 1/3	93	38	52	89
PASP < 55 mm Hg	93	24	47	25
New				
PCWP/LV respiratory gradient > 5 mm Hg	93	81	78	94
LV/RV interdependence	100	95	94	100

LV, left ventricle; LVEDP, left ventricular end-diastolic pressure; NPV, negative predictive value; PASP, pulmonary artery systolic pressure; PCWP, pulmonary capillary wedge pressure; PPV, positive predictive value; RV, right ventricle; RVEDP, right ventricular end-diastolic pressure; RVSP, right ventricular systolic pressure.
From Hurrell D, Nishimura RA, Higano ST, et al: Value of dynamic respiratory changes in left and right ventricular pressures for the diagnosis of constrictive pericarditis. Circulation 1996;93:2007-2013.

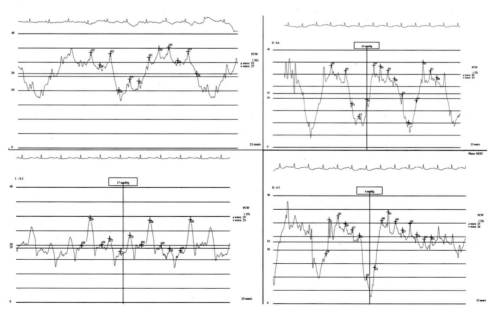

Figure 9-53. Pulmonary capillary wedge pressure tracings in proven constriction cases. TOP, The mean pulmonary capillary pressures are all elevated. The prominent inspiratory fall in pressure due to increased inspiratory effort is due to lung compliance increasing with increased lung volume and superimposition of negative intrapleural pressure during inspiration. BOTTOM LEFT, V waves are present and due to poor left atrial compliance conferred by the constrictive pericardium over the left atrium. As venous return to the left atrium varies through the respiratory cycle, so does the magnitude of the V wave. BOTTOM RIGHT, On the left half of the tracing, there are two respiratory cycles; on the right half of the tracing, there is a long shallow inspiration.

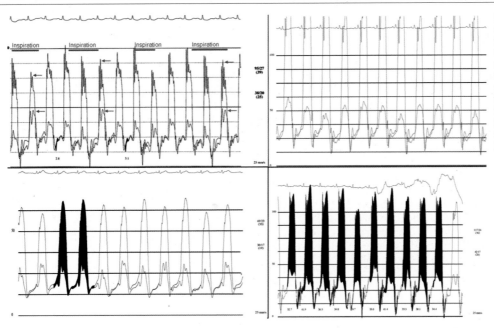

Figure 9-54. Simultaneous left ventricular and pulmonary capillary wedge pressure tracings in proven constriction cases during respiration, seeking the LV-RV discordance sign of ventricular interdependence. A respirometry tracing would help prove the phase of the respiratory cycle. The upper tracings and the right lower tracing are fairly convincing for a simultaneous rise in the RVSP and fall in the LVSP. Discordance of pressures is possibly present in the left lower tracing.

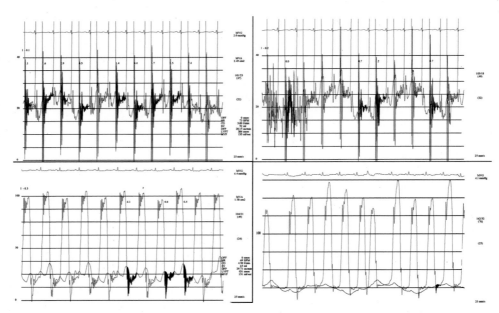

Figure 9-55. Simultaneous LV and PCWP tracings in proven constriction cases. Revealing the inspiratory increase of PCWP:LVDP gradient is difficult with fluid-filled catheters. TOP LEFT, At low scale, the whip motion artifact is more apparent and obscuring interpretation. There is phasic variation in pressures, suggesting that the respiratory effort is regular. TOP RIGHT, Augmented respiratory effort (greater fluctuations in pressure) still has not revealed the sign. BOTTOM LEFT, At lower scale and with less whip artifact, the inspiratory increase in gradient is present although difficult to appreciate and to measure. With inspiration, there is a fall of both the pulmonary capillary and left ventricular diastolic pressures, but a greater fall of the pulmonary capillary pressure. The V wave also decreases in inspiration because of lesser venous return to the left side of the heart. BOTTOM RIGHT, At a larger scale and with the pulmonary capillary tracing on mean, the inspiratory increase in gradient is more reliably depicted.

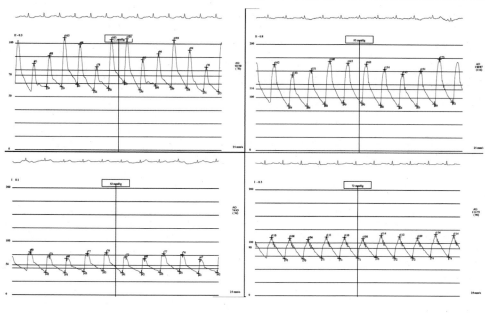

Figure 9-56. Aortic pressure tracings in proven constriction cases. TOP LEFT, There is hypertension, with a pulsus paradoxus, although the variation in pulse pressure is less. TOP RIGHT, There is hypotension and a prominent pulsus paradoxus (with an inspiratory fall in both systolic pressure and pulse pressure). BOTTOM LEFT, There is severe hypotension due to low output. The pulsus paradoxus is less apparent although present. BOTTOM RIGHT, Normotensive, no pulsus paradoxus versus breath-hold.

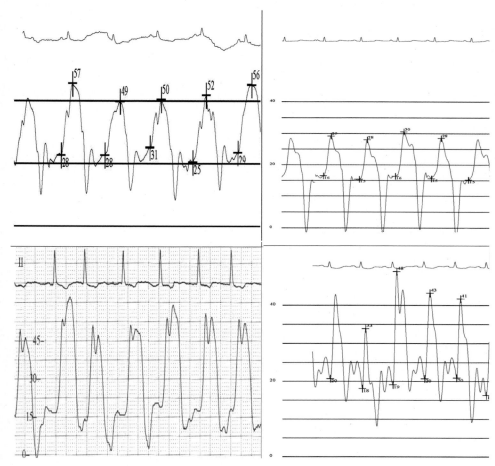

Figure 9-57. RVP tracings in proven constriction cases. TOP, Typical tracings (in different patients) show marked elevation of the diastolic pressure, a prominent early diastolic dip, and an absence of substantial hypertension (systolic pressure <55 mm Hg). BOTTOM LEFT, The tracing reveals an elevation of the diastolic pressure and an early diastolic dip of variable depth, depending on the phase of the respiratory cycle. The systolic pressure, though, is mildly high for an average constriction case. The underlying heart in this case was abnormal (aortic stenosis). BOTTOM RIGHT, The mean diastolic pressure is elevated, and the systolic pressure is not. The early diastolic dip is variable. The tracing may actually be a PA tracing with the catheter intermittently falling into the RV to record the early diastolic dip.

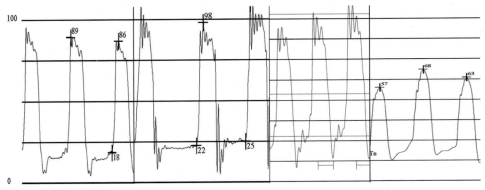

Figure 9-58. Left ventricular pressure tracings in proven constriction cases. The two tracings on the left are typical for the square-root sign of an early diastolic dip, elevated diastolic pressure that is steady (a plateau). The far left tracing is from a patient in sinus rhythm; the middle left tracing is from a patient in atrial fibrillation. The atrial contraction confers a late diastolic bump to the plateau, which is otherwise steady in atrial fibrillation. The two tracings on the right are less typical; neither has a plateau, and the far right tracing lacks an early diastolic dip. The diastolic pressures are elevated.

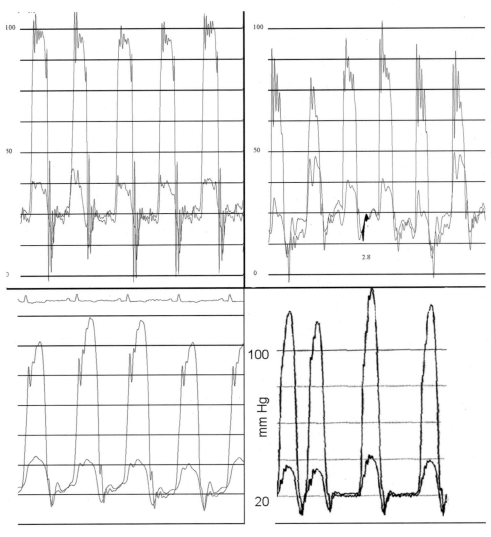

Figure 9-59. Simultaneous left and right ventricular pressure tracings in proven constriction cases. There is equilibration (<5 mm Hg difference) of LV and RV diastolic pressures in all tracings. Catheter whip artifact is plaguing the tracings of the left upper image. Respiratory influence is partially confounding the assessment of equilibration in the left upper and also the right lower images. Inspiration, denoted by the fall in LVSP, also lowers the LVDP. Equilibration should be sought with breath-holding. The tracings in the bottom right image are from a patient in atrial fibrillation. At shorter R-R intervals, neither the square-root sign nor equilibration can be appreciated. With longer R-R intervals and thereby longer diastole, the square-root sign and equilibration are revealed.

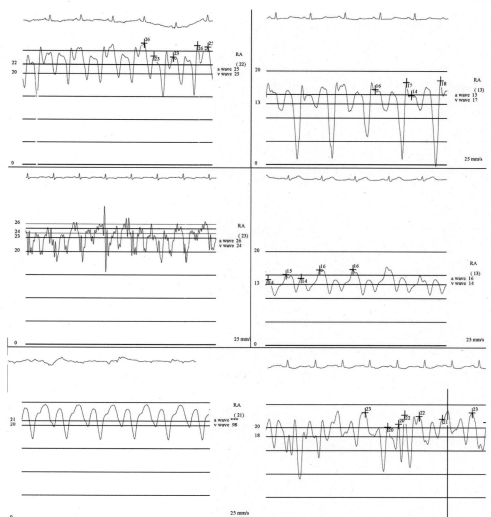

Figure 9-60. RAP tracings in proven constriction cases. The mean pressures are all elevated. Although the x and y descents are all exaggerated, it can be seen how variable the depth of the x and y descents may be. In most cases, the magnitude of the x and y descents are similar, producing an M or W pattern. In the right upper tracing, the y descents are greatly dominant because of unusually vigorous recoil of the constrictive pericardium. In the right lower image, the inspiratory increase in x and y descents is depicted over two respiratory cycles. In later inspiration, the mean pressure rises as the right-sided heart compliance is exceeded by increased venous return and the pressure increases—Kussmaul sign. It is better appreciated by a mean pressure tracing.

The Paradigm of Constrictive Pericarditis Versus Restrictive Cardiomyopathy

Although distinguishing constrictive pericarditis from restrictive cardiomyopathy is a classic paradigm in cardiology, this paradigm has some misleading features in that it suggests that these two diagnoses are dichotomous and may not occur concurrently, as they do commonly after radiotherapy and as they may rarely with amyloidosis. As well, myocardial dysfunction (systolic or more commonly diastolic) may be present in constriction cases that develop myocardial atrophy, that are older and had preexistent hypertension, or that are post–open heart surgery and previously had aortic stenosis or a prior infarction. Tissue Doppler findings would likely be abnormal in patients with concurrent restrictive cardiomyopathy, with severe atrophy, with left ventricular hypertrophy, and with prior infarction; but the few published tissue Doppler studies that compared findings in patients who were normal, who had restrictive cardiomyopathy, and who had constrictive pericarditis did not include another group with constriction and myocardial dysfunction.

Ventricular Interdependence Signs and Constrictive Physiology

The application of the concept of ventricular interdependence to the diagnosis of constrictive physiology is currently validated for pressure recording, not 2-dimensional imaging. Ventricular interdependence does occur in other disease states, including pericardial tamponade and right ventricular infarction; therefore, ventricular interdependence is not pathognomonic of constriction. Furthermore, septal inspiratory shift may be seen in other pulmonary disease states and is not alone diagnostic of constrictive physiology (Fig. 9-61).

PERICARDIECTOMY FOR PERICARDIAL CONSTRICTION

Relief of compressive physiology is most reliably afforded by resection of sufficient constrictive pericardium. Pericardiectomy

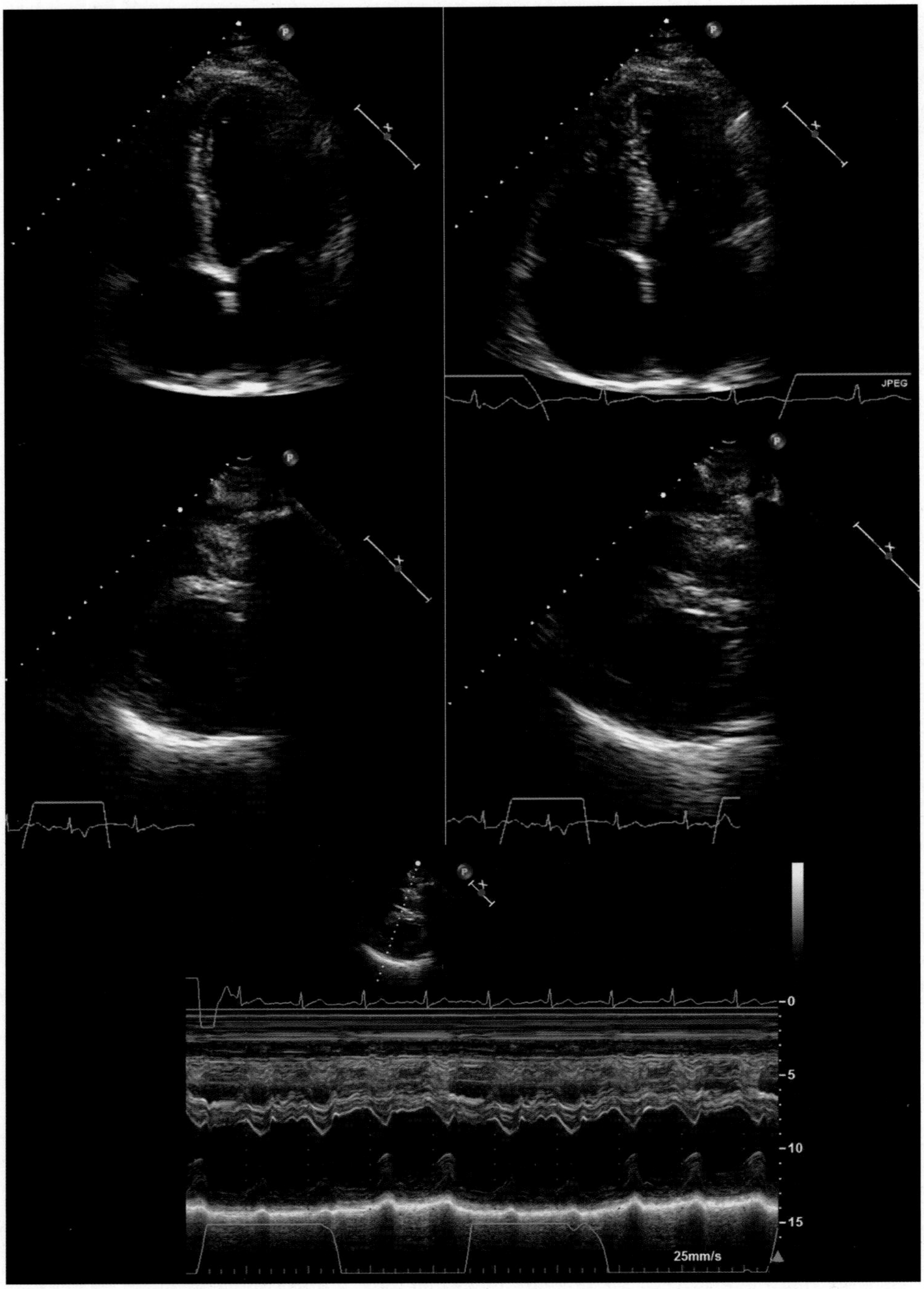

Figure 9-61. This 78-year-old man was admitted with pneumonia and respiratory distress. He had severe mitral regurgitation and probably an element of left-sided heart failure. With inspiration (clearly increased effort—hyperpnea), there is septal shift to the left side. There was no clinical evidence of constriction.

to different degrees may be performed. "Complete" pericardiectomy involves the resection of the parietal pericardium, actually leaving strips where the phrenic nerves run and some pieces at the reflections. The visceral pericardium is also removed if it is found to be thickened. One of the most common forms of pericardiectomy is resection of the parietal pericardium between the two phrenic nerves ("phrenic to phrenic"), leaving the pericardium posteriorly.

Incomplete pericardiectomy occurs in all cases of phrenic to phrenic resection, when the pericardium over the sleeves of the great vessels is left, when constrictive serosal pericardium is left, and when resection engenders too much bleeding.

The usual perioperative mortality of pericardiectomy for constriction is 5% to 15%. Perioperative mortality is heavily influenced by the preoperative right atrial pressure (RAP) and RVEDP (which may be substantially influenced by diuretic use). The mortality is higher with greater heart failure class, worst if there is shock, and well predicted by the RAP: 15 mm Hg, 5% mortality; 20 mm Hg, 10% mortality; 30 mm Hg, 30% mortality.[35] As would be expected, the presence of comorbidities increases perioperative mortality (Table 9-11).[5]

The three most common complications are bleeding, low-output syndrome, and incomplete pericardiectomy. Bleeding is common, especially if the dissection of the pericardium was difficult for the surgeon and traumatic to the heart, as it often is when fibrosis extends into the myocardium or when there is calcification. Bleeding is generally apparent by excessive chest tube drainage. Low-output syndrome is a high-risk occurrence. The effect of surgically releasing the constrictive pericardium from the right ventricle may be that the right side of the heart acutely dilates, and its systolic function thereby fails. Factors that may compound acute (early) postoperative right-sided heart failure are poor myocardial protection, myocardial atrophy from the chronicity of the constriction process, loss of tricuspid competence from the acute right ventricular dilation, and concurrent radiation-induced restrictive cardiomyopathy. Low-output syndrome accompanied by acute right-sided heart failure is recognized by bedside echocardiography (Fig. 9-62). The treatment is inotropes and hemodynamic support (intra-aortic balloon counterpulsation). Incomplete pericardiectomy is to some extent, in most cases, inevitable, as the pericardium that underlies the phrenic nerves must be left intact. In some cases, dissection of the pericardium is so traumatic to the heart that continuing the dissection is unwise. The failure to eliminate a sufficient proportion of the constrictive physiology diminishes the chances

of surviving the physiologic stresses of the perioperative period.

Factors predictive of a worse long-term prognosis include radiotherapy-induced constrictive pericarditis (typically, there is concurrent myocardial fibrosis and restrictive cardiomyopathy, leaving many patients with incomplete benefit or progressive congestive heart failure) and possibly calcification (Figs. 9-63 and 9-64).[2,5]

A large series of patients (n = 135; mean age, 56 years) undergoing pericardiectomy at a highly experienced center between the years 1985 and 1995, with a mean follow-up of 3.9 years, illustrates the encountered early perioperative and late postoperative results. Perioperative mortality was 6%; half of perioperative deaths were related to low output, and half were related to incomplete pericardiectomy. The survival was estimated to be 71% at 5 years and 52% at 10 years.[2] Long-term outcome was predicted by age, NYHA class, and post–radiation therapy etiology (the most powerful predictor) (Fig. 9-65). Of long-term survivors, 83% were free of symptoms.[2,5] During a mean follow-up of 4 years, the post–radiation therapy subgroup mortality was 77%, and the incidence of mortality or NYHA class IV congestive

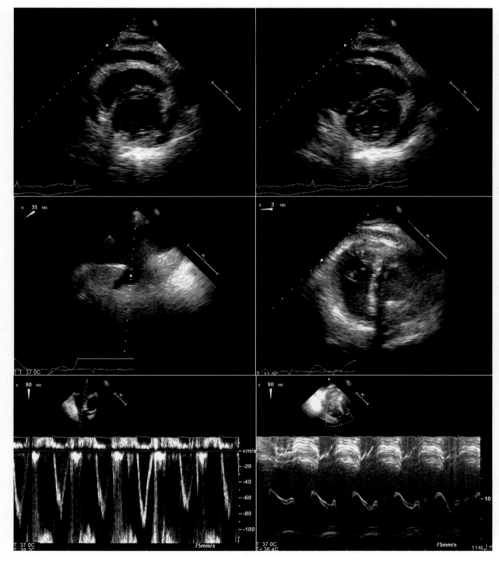

Figure 9-62. Postpericardiectomy low output. An 80-year-old man underwent pericardiectomy for effuso-constrictive pericarditis. TOP, Preoperative echocardiography during expiration (LEFT) and inspiration (RIGHT). Note the inspiratory septal shift consistent with ventricular interdependence. Only the anterior pericardium was resected. The effusion anteriorly made the resection straightforward. The pericardium was fused posteriorly. Immediately postoperatively, there was a low-output state, characterized by hypotension and anuria and marked venous congestion. The right ventricle was dilated and severely hypokinetic, as was the right atrium, and high-dose inotropes were needed. MIDDLE, TEE views. The IVC is massively dilated (LEFT). Seen on the transgastric short-axis view (RIGHT), the right ventricle is severely enlarged. There is more than 1 cm of thick pericardium on the underside of the heart. The right ventricle has dilated. BOTTOM, TEE pulsed wave and M-mode imaging of the pulmonic valve. There is no presystolic flow or opening. The acute atrial dilation and akinesis may have obviated this sign of constriction. The patient died 4 days postoperatively of a combination of acute right-sided heart dilation and incomplete pericardiectomy.

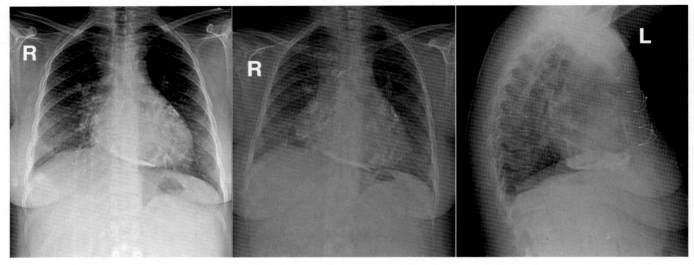

Figure 9-63. Chest radiographs before pericardiectomy (LEFT) and 4 years after incomplete pericardiectomy (MIDDLE AND RIGHT). The patient returned with severe right-sided heart failure and cirrhosis. The chest radiographs both before and after pericardiectomy demonstrate a marked amount of calcification.

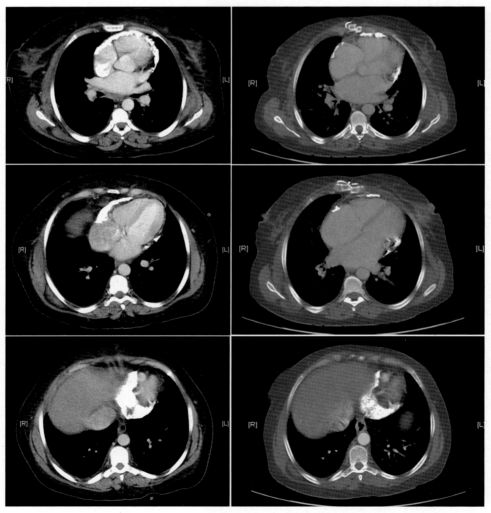

Figure 9-64. CT scan in the same patient as in Figure 9-63. LEFT, Before pericardiectomy. RIGHT, Four years after incomplete pericardiectomy. Segments of calcified anterior pericardium were resected, but not lateral or inferior calcified pericardium.

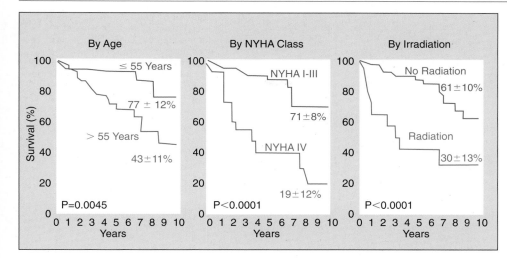

Figure 9-65. Postpericardiectomy mortality by New York Heart Association (NYHA) class. (From Ling LH, Oh JK, Schaff HV, et al: Constrictive pericarditis in the modern era: evolving clinical spectrum and impact on outcome after pericardiectomy. Circulation 1999;100: 1380.)

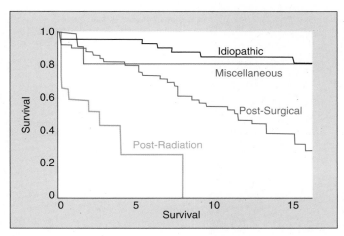

Figure 9-66. Cause-specific survival after pericardiectomy. (From Bertog SC, Thambidorai SK, Parakh K, et al: Constrictive pericarditis: etiology and cause-specific survival after pericardiectomy. J Am Coll Cardiol 2004;43: 1445.)

heart failure was 88% (Fig. 9-66). None of the radiation therapy cohort died of recurrent malignant disease, establishing that this tragic subset, saved from their malignant disease, subsequently died of the curative treatment of their malignant disease. Calcific pericarditis also predicts greater perioperative mortality but not greater long-term mortality. Diastolic filling abnormalities may persist postoperatively, as may symptoms, and imaging findings correlate with the duration of symptoms preoperatively, thereby engendering the argument that prompt pericardiectomy may alleviate persistence of postoperative symptoms.[36]

CASE 1

History

▸ A 74-year-old woman with no significant past medical history was diagnosed with constrictive pericarditis 1 year previously after an episode of atrial fibrillation. Pericardial calcification noted on chest radiograph and CT scan. A 6-cm ascending aortic aneurysm was identified at this time.

▸ Initial medical management during 12 months failed, with increasing complaints of dyspnea and signs of right-sided heart failure.

Physical Examination

▸ Elevated venous pressure with prominent *y* descent
▸ No Kussmaul sign
▸ Normal heart sounds with pericardial knock

▸ II-IV early peaking SEM at the base of the heart without diastolic murmur of aortic insufficiency
▸ Pedal edema

Evolution

▸ Referred for surgical pericardiectomy and graft replacement of ascending aorta

▸ Surgical findings: extensive calcification of visceral pericardium extending into epicardium on diaphragmatic surface of both ventricles

▸ Cardiopulmonary bypass is required for full pericardiectomy from left to right phrenic nerve. Minor residual areas of calcified epicardium were unable to be resected.

▸ Successful recovery and discharge from hospital. Symptomatic improvement with resolution of heart failure symptoms and findings during 6 months

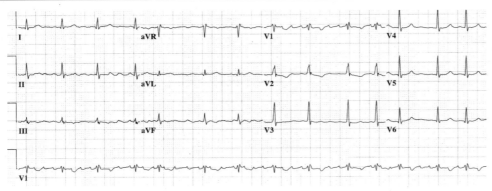

Figure 9-67. TOP, ECG shows atrial flutter with variable block, normal voltages, incomplete right bundle branch block, and mild nonspecific repolarization abnormalities. Atrial flutter is seen in 5% of constriction cases and atrial fibrillation in 20%.

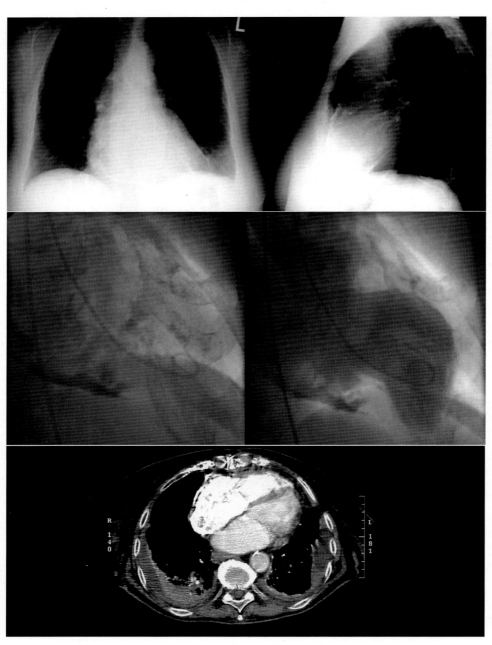

Figure 9-68. TOP, Chest radiographs show clear lungs and cardiomegaly. Thick calcification of the pericardium is seen on the diaphragmatic surface on the posteroanterior film and anterior to and over the RV/RVOT on the lateral view. MIDDLE, RAO ventriculography and fluoroscopy images show calcification of the pericardium, especially the diaphragmatic surface. Marked distortion of the LV cavity by presumed axial compression of the LV by the constricting pericardium is present. BOTTOM, Contrast-enhanced axial CT scan shows pericardial calcification over the right atrium, atheromatous calcification of the aorta, small bilateral pleural effusions, and no pleural plaques.

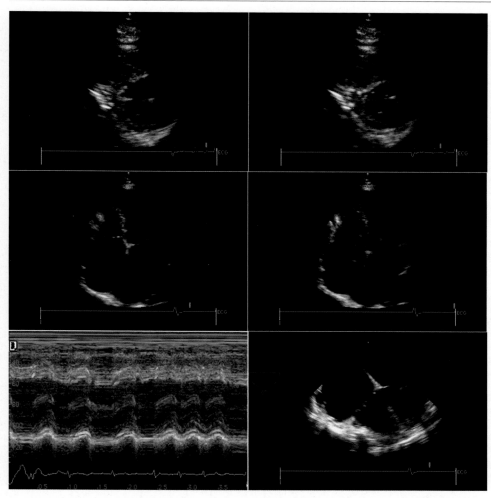

Figure 9-69. TTE parasternal short-axis (TOP ROW) and apical 4-chamber (MIDDLE ROW) views depict a single cardiac cycle; the left images are from end-diastole, and the right images are from early diastole. There is a prominent early diastolic dip, which is also delineated on the M-mode recording (BOTTOM LEFT) and best seen in the third and fourth cardiac cycles. BOTTOM RIGHT, TEE shows large atria and small ventricles. The appearance of the pericardium is difficult to assess.

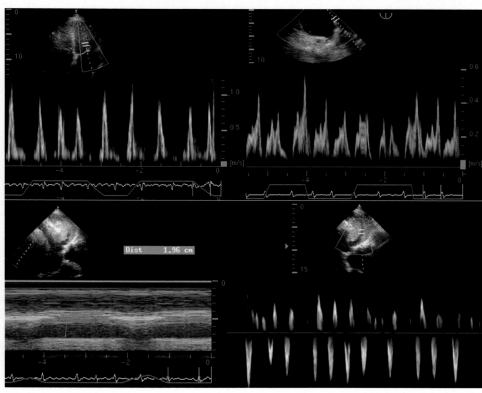

Figure 9-70. Mitral inflow (TOP LEFT) and pulmonary venous flow (TOP RIGHT). The irregularity of the cardiac rhythm (variable R-R intervals) confounds convincing assessment of the influence of the respiratory cycle on the inflow pattern, but there does appear to be a significant fall with inspiration. BOTTOM LEFT, The IVC is dilated and does not collapse with inspiration (denoted by the respirometry tracing), consistent with elevation of the central venous pressure. BOTTOM RIGHT, Hepatic venous flow. The hepatic venous spectral pattern is difficult to interpret because of the irregularity of the rhythm and the lack of the respirometry tracing on it.

Pathology Findings

▸ Chronic inflammatory changes and nodular calcification
▸ No granulomas seen, and stain and cultures negative for acid-fast bacilli
▸ No evidence of aortitis in ascending aortic specimen

Comments

▸ Most typical features of constriction were present.
▸ Pericardial knocks are more common in advanced and calcific cases, such as this.
▸ Atrial fibrillation is present in 20% of constriction cases and atrial flutter in 5%. Irregular cardiac cycle length due to atrial dysrhythmia confounds assessment of interdependence. Overdrive pacing during catheterization would have regularized the cardiac cycles, eliminating one aspect of difficulty in indentifying signs of interdependence.
▸ The catheterization findings included all of the traditional pressure abnormalities seen in constriction, and fluoroscopy showed the pericardial calcification better than any other test did in her case.
▸ Despite the pericardial calcification, the surgery was uneventful, and bleeding was not a problem, nor was low output postoperatively from (unrestrained) chamber dilation.
▸ The LV was very distorted by the constriction. This was well depicted by the ventriculogram (depicting long-axis shortening of the left ventricle) and hinted at by the echocardiogram (suggesting indentation of the right ventricle by a plaque). Fibrocalcific plaques can compress or constrict focally as well as globally, leading to local gradients within the heart and valve dysfunction.
▸ Constriction is traditionally, and correctly in some regards, thought of as a disorder that globally and uniformly affects the heart. Although this is true in most cases in terms of diastolic pressures, constriction may also lead to focal disturbances due to greater constriction by thicker plaques and bands, and the plaques may be very different over (and into) different parts of the heart. Often at surgery, the heterogeneous involvement of the pericardium by the constriction process finally becomes apparent.
▸ As with many cases undergoing surgery, removal of all of the pericardium proved difficult. If pericardiectomy is substantially incomplete, improvement is also incomplete.

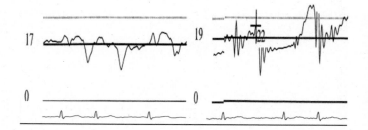

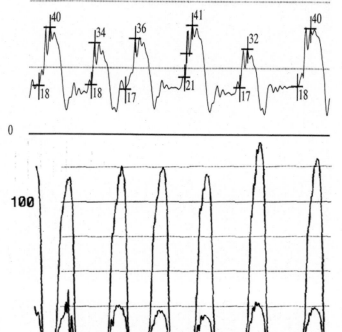

Figure 9-71. TOP, RAP and PCWP tracings show irregular rhythm, elevation and equilibration of the RAP and PCWP, prominent y descent of the right atrial tracing, and prominent catheter whip artifact of the PCWP tracing. MIDDLE, RV pressure tracing shows elevation of the RVDP ($\geq^1/_3$ of the RVSP) as well as square-root pattern of RVDP. BOTTOM, Simultaneous LV and RV pressure tracings show elevation and equilibration of the LVDP and RVDP. The RVDP is more than one third of the RVSP. There is considerable variation in cardiac cycle length (R-R intervals). Although this assists with recognition of the square-root pattern when the R-R interval is longer, it also confounds interpretation of LVSP:RVSP changes due to ventricular interdependence as the RVSP and LVSP increase with longer cardiac cycles. Again, the lack of respirometry tracing renders interpretation assumptive. Overdrive pacing would have regularized the cardiac cycles, eliminating one aspect of difficulty in indentifying signs of interdependence.

CASE 2

History

▸ A 70-year-old man with a tentative diagnosis of constrictive pericarditis made 15 years previously, on the basis of findings of pericardial calcification on chest radiography and symptomatic atrial fibrillation. He had been treated medically during this time (rate control of atrial fibrillation, anticoagulation, and diuretics) with reasonable symptom control (NYHA class II); but during the last 6 months, he developed increasing symptoms of dyspnea on exertion (NYHA class IV) and peripheral edema.

Physical Examination

▸ BP 140/80 mm Hg; no pulsus paradoxus
▸ Venous pressure elevated 10 cm with prominent *y* descent; no Kussmaul sign
▸ Normal heart sounds with no pericardial knock or rub
▸ Bilateral pedal edema ++

Surgical Findings

▸ Marked pericardial thickening and calcification, particularly at the apex, with calcium extending into myocardium
▸ Subtotal pericardiectomy performed, with minor areas of calcified pericardium remaining on diaphragm

Pathology Findings

▸ Severe fibrotic changes with extensive calcification; no granulomas or acid-fast bacilli seen in pericardial specimen
▸ Occasional granuloma seen in mediastinal lymph node, but no acid-fast bacilli detected by staining
▸ Possibility of old tuberculosis raised but never confirmed by acid-fast bacilli stains or cultures

Outcome

▸ Uneventful operative and postoperative course
▸ Improvement of heart failure symptoms (NYHA class IV to II-III)

Comments

▸ Classic case of calcific pericarditis
▸ The suspicion of tuberculosis was never confirmed by culture or acid-fast bacilli staining from cardiac tissue or from noncardiac source. No specific cause was ever detected, and he was not prescribed empirical antituberculous treatment.
▸ Atrial fibrillation is present in 20% of constriction cases and atrial flutter in 5%. Irregular cardiac cycle length due to atrial dysrhythmia confounds assessment of interdependence. Overdrive pacing during catheterization would have regularized the cardiac cycles, eliminating one aspect of difficulty in indentifying signs of interdependence.
▸ Calcific pericarditis renders pericardiectomy more technically difficult and increases the likelihood of incomplete pericardiectomy (as in this case), excessive bleeding (which did not occur in this case), and early right-sided heart dilation and low output postoperatively (which also did not occur).
▸ The pericardial knock was the only classic bedside finding of constriction that was not present. In long-standing cases, especially calcific constrictive pericarditis, it usually is present.
▸ The force of the early diastolic recoil of the thickened and stiff constrictive pericardium in this case was seen in the negative pressure of the zero point of the early diastolic pressure dip and the extremely short deceleration time, indicating rapidity of early diastolic filling.

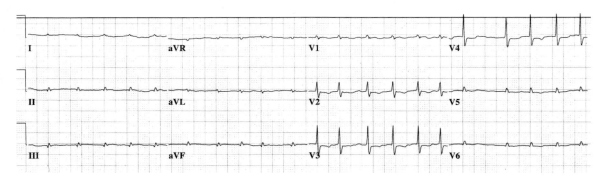

Figure 9-72. ECG shows atrial fibrillation with a rapid ventricular response, RV hypertrophy, nonspecific repolarization abnormalities, and low voltages.

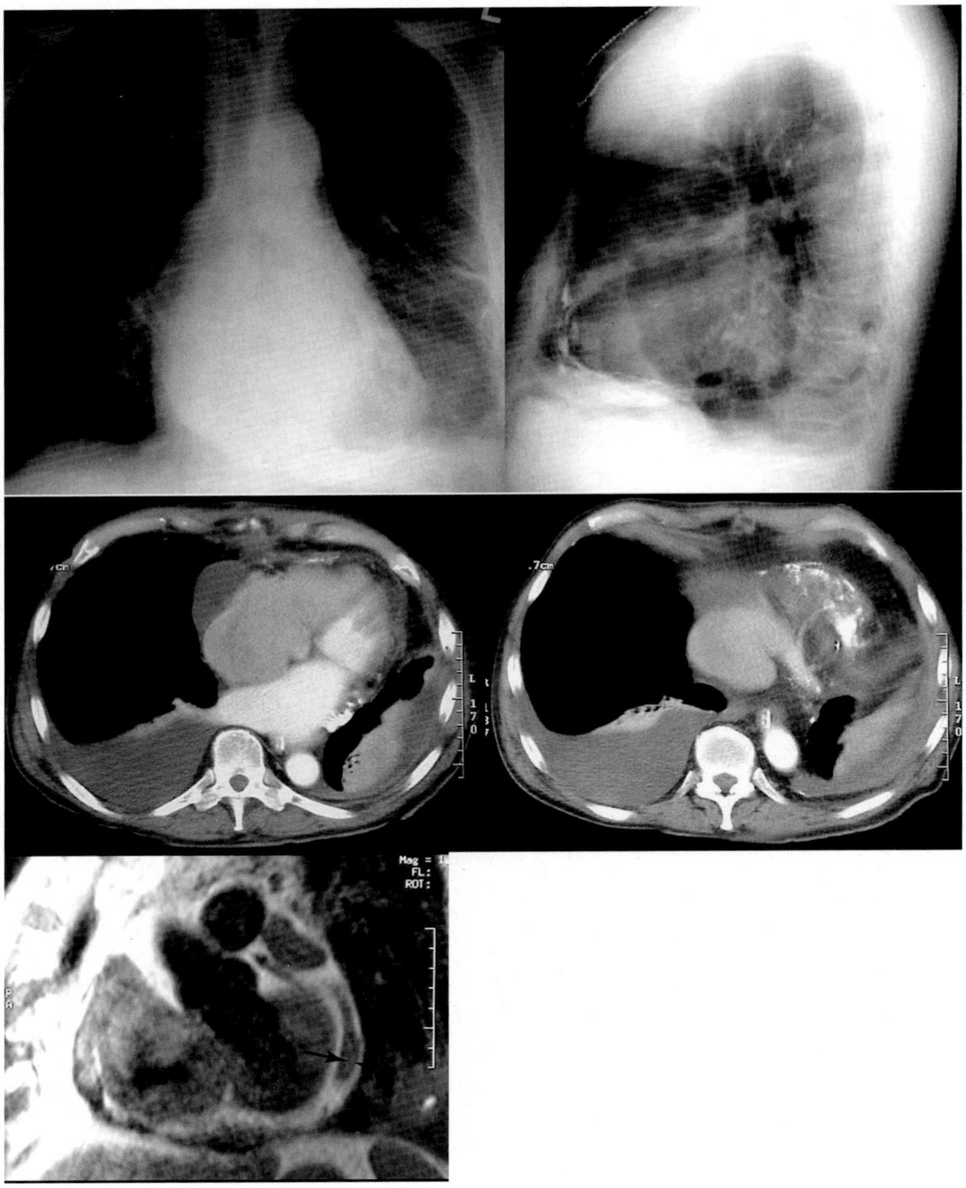

Figure 9-73. TOP, Chest radiographs show clear right lung field, infiltrates at the left base versus pleural plaques, mild cardiomegaly, and left pleural effusion versus left pleural fibrotic disease. Calcified pericardial plaques are best seen on the lateral view over the RV anterior wall and diaphragmatic surface. MIDDLE, Contrast-enhanced axial CT scan shows pericardial thickening and calcification anterior to the right ventricle and left ventricle and posterolateral to the left atrium. There is marked thickening anterolateral to the right atrium. This view shows contrast material opacifying the left side of the heart more than the right, bilateral pleural effusions, and no calcified pleural plaques. BOTTOM, CMR T1-weighted spin echo black blood sequence. Note pericardial thickening posterior to the left ventricle *(arrows)*, between the epicardial fat (bright stripe) and the pericardial fat (bright stripe). Note the varying pericardial thickness.

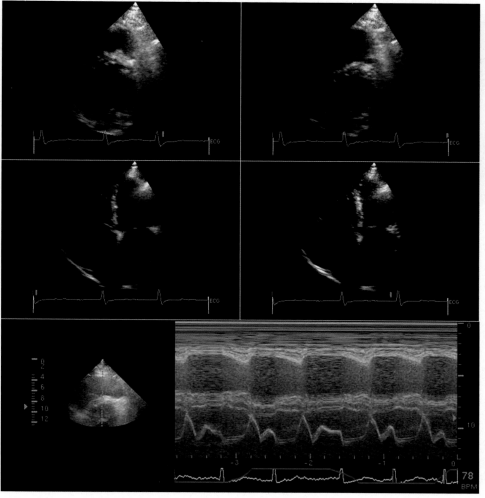

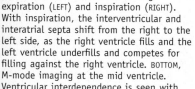

Figure 9-74. TOP AND MIDDLE, TTE parasternal short-axis views during expiration (LEFT) and inspiration (RIGHT). With inspiration, the interventricular and interatrial septa shift from the right to the left side, as the right ventricle fills and the left ventricle underfills and competes for filling against the right ventricle. BOTTOM, M-mode imaging at the mid ventricle. Ventricular interdependence is seen with the shift of the septum from the right to the left side, during the third cardiac cycle, with inspiration (upward deflection of the respirometry tracing), as the right ventricle fills and the left ventricle underfills.

Figure 9-75. TOP LEFT, TTE recording of mitral inflow. TOP RIGHT, TEE recording of mitral inflow. There is a very rapid inflow time (deceleration time) consistent with elevated left atrial pressure and restrictive filling due to the constriction physiology. BOTTOM LEFT, M-mode image of the IVC showing dilation and lack of respiratory variation—signs of elevated central venous pressure. BOTTOM RIGHT, Hepatic venous flow pattern shows a phasic variation in diastolic flow reversal, although in this case in inspiration.

169

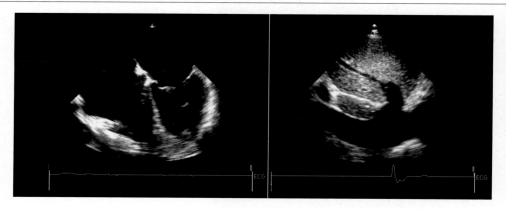

Figure 9-76. Echocardiography images. TEE 4-chamber view (shown on the left) presents typical findings of biatrial dilation and small ventricles. There is pericardial thickening best seen anterior to the right ventricular free wall. The IVC is severely dilated as is the superior hepatic vein. Hepatic venous distention assists with pulsed wave Doppler sampling.

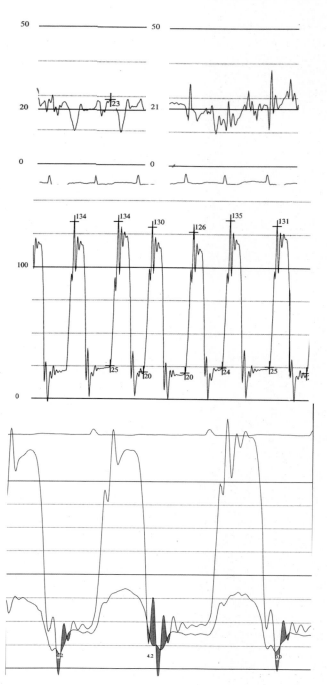

Figure 9-77. TOP, RAP and PCWP tracings show a near-equilibration of the RAP and PCWP (20 and 21 mm Hg, respectively). Prominent *y* descent of the RAP contour. Underdamping (catheter whip artifact) of the PCWP tracing is typical for fluid-filled catheters. MIDDLE, LV pressure tracing shows normal LVSP and LVDP with dip-and-plateau or square-root sign. Despite the elevation of diastolic pressure, the zero point of the early diastolic pressure dip reaches zero or even below, indicative of the force of the recoil of the constrictive pericardium. BOTTOM. Simultaneous LV and RV pressure tracings. Elevated diastolic pressure with dip-and-plateau sign of both the left and right ventricular pressure tracings. There is less than a 5 mm Hg difference between the LVDP and RVDP. The RVDP is more than one third of the RVSP. Again, the left ventricular early diastolic pressure dip reaches below zero.

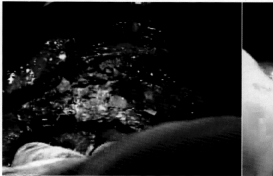

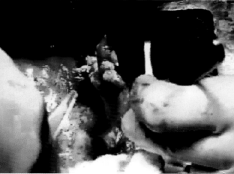

Figure 9-78. Surgical findings. Thick, stiff, and crusty calcific pericardium over the right ventricular free wall and elsewhere.

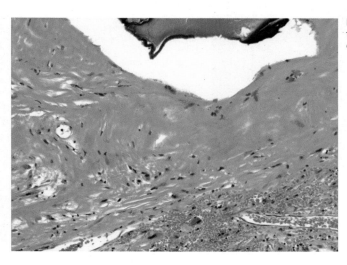

Figure 9-79. Pathologic findings. Collagenous material and fibroblasts throughout the thickened pericardial tissue. (Other sections showed calcification.)

CASE 3

History

▸ 77-year-old man with exertional fatigue and dyspnea
▸ Underwent aortocoronary bypass grafting 4 years previously, has a dual-chamber pacer and paroxysmal atrial fibrillation

Physical Examination

▸ BP 120/60 mm Hg, HR 65 bpm (irregular)
▸ Elevated jugular veins with prominent *y* descent, mild edema
▸ Heart sounds distant, early diastolic filling sound (S_3/knock)
▸ Apex displaced, enlarged, and remote; no retraction
▸ Dullness to percussion and reduced air entry at left base

Impression

▸ Probable diagnosis of post–aortocoronary bypass pericardial constriction, given the traditional catheterization findings and the CT evidence of pericardial calcification

Surgical Management

▸ Surgery found moderately and irregularly thickened pericardium with calcified areas and left pleural thickening and effusion.
▸ Complete pericardiectomy was obtained, initially off bypass but eventually with use of bypass to complete the resection. Most of the pericardium was removed without difficulty; some, though, was densely adherent to the myocardium.
▸ Postoperative bleeding was moderate but manageable.
▸ Low output developed within 12 hours because of acute dilation of the heart (especially the RA and RV), with moderate tricuspid regurgitation as well.

Evolution and Outcome

▸ Protracted ICU and hospital course, with eventual recovery and discharge but incomplete symptom relief

Comments

▸ Post–aortocoronary bypass grafting constriction
▸ Elevated neck veins with obvious *y* descent strongly suggested the diagnosis.
▸ Interdependence findings were not present on echocardiography or catheterization; traditional catheterization findings were more obvious.
▸ Surprisingly calcified pericardium
▸ Several adverse markers to a good outcome: need for concurrent revascularization, calcification, postoperative bleeding, and acute chamber dilation

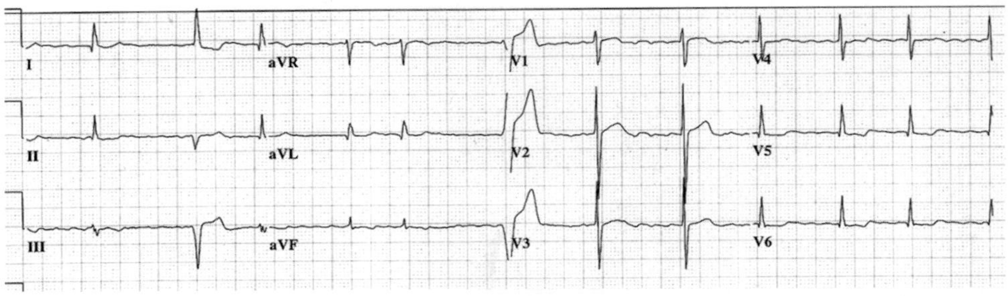

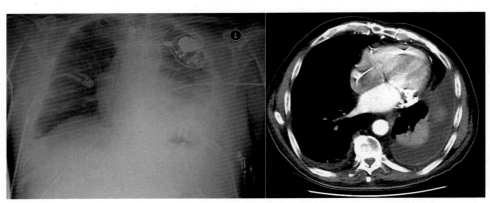

Figure 9-80. ECG shows atrial fibrillation with aberrantly conducted or ventricular ectopic beats and nonspecific repolarization abnormalities.

Figure 9-81. LEFT, Chest radiograph shows cardiomegaly, left pleural effusion, pacer, and wires. No calcification seen on this view. RIGHT, Contrast-enhanced CT axial scan shows cardiomegaly, pleural effusions (left >> right), pacer wires, fine calcification at the apex and heavy calcification in the left atrioventricular groove, and streak artifacts from pacer wires in the right side of the heart.

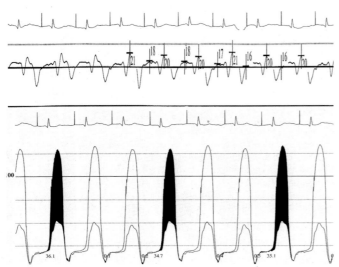

Figure 9-82. TOP, RAP tracing shows elevated RAP (mean, 16 mm Hg), prominent y descent, and Kussmaul sign (failure to descend with inspiration). BOTTOM, LV and RV pressure tracings show no pulsus paradoxus, regularized rhythm from atrial pacing, and equilibration and elevation of the ventricular diastolic pressures.

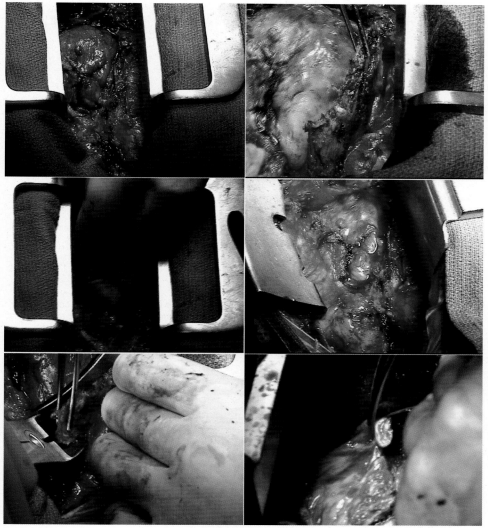

Figure 9-83. Surgical findings. Through resection of a small amount of the thickened and stiff anterior pericardium, the heart was bulging outward as a result of the high diastolic pressures. Cutting of the calcified pericardium by strong scissors produces a gritty sound. In some places, the pericardium was too unyielding to be cut by scissors, and bone cutters were needed. Bleeding, one of the most common and significant risks to pericardiectomy, regularly occurred.

CASE 4

History

▸ 76-year-old woman with a 5-year history of peripheral edema and shortness of breath, initially on exertion but over time worsened to NYHA class IV
▸ Past history of hypertension, poorly treated

Physical Examination

▸ Profoundly weak, anasarcic, gross ascites
▸ BP 90/50 mm Hg, pulsus paradoxus <15 mm Hg; weak, shallow breathing; HR 100 bpm
▸ Markedly elevated venous pressure, with prominent *y* descent
▸ No pericardial knock or rub
▸ Tense ascites and severe leg edema
▸ There was moderate to severe renal insufficiency.

Management and Outcome

▸ The patient underwent total pericardiectomy converted to bypass. Surgery revealed thickened, leather-like pericardium.
▸ Pathology findings included fibrous thickening without calcification and negative stains and cultures for tuberculosis.

▸ Postoperative course was poor and accompanied by acute low-output syndrome of acute right-sided heart dilation and failure.
▸ She died within 8 hours.

Comments

▸ Terminal constrictive pericarditis with low output and renal insufficiency
▸ Past history of hypertension probably contributed to the abnormal LV diastolic properties and may have been responsible for the attenuated early diastolic dip seen at the time of cardiac catheterization (myocardial stiffness opposing pericardial recoil). The past long history of hypertension probably set the stage for renal insufficiency.
▸ The respiratory effort was failing against the work of breathing against the ascites, which was repeatedly tapped for palliation. The lack of consistent respiratory effort probably explained the variable manifestation of interdependence signs. Lying flat for the cardiac catheterization appeared to increase the inspiratory effort, as seen on the PCWP tracing.
▸ Neither echocardiography nor catheterization was robust for presence of signs of interdependence, but each offered some.
▸ Early perioperative death from acute low-output (acute right ventricular dilation) syndrome

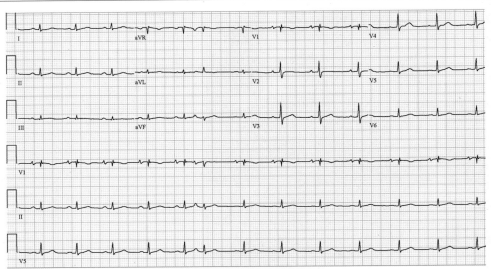

Figure 9-84. ECG shows sinus rhythm with premature atrial contractions and low voltages in the standard limb leads.

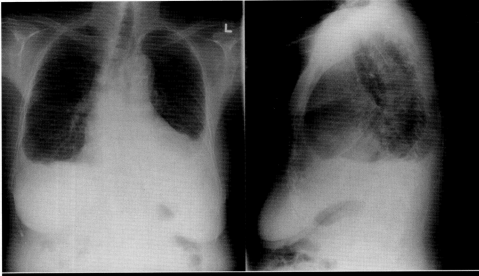

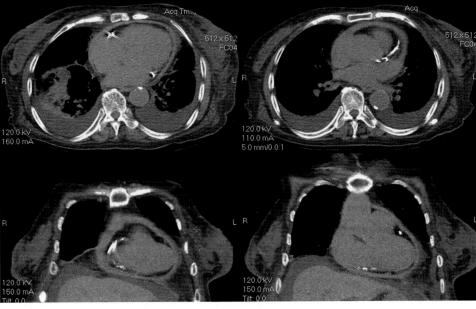

Figure 9-85. TOP, Chest radiographs show cardiomegaly, but the extent of the pleural effusions renders cardiac assessment limited. There is interstitial pulmonary edema as well as atherosclerotic plaques in the aortic arch. MIDDLE AND BOTTOM, Non-contrast-enhanced chest CT scans in the axial (MIDDLE) and coronal (BOTTOM) orientation show circumferential pericardial thickening. There is no pericardial calcification but rather remarkably severe coronary calcification. Bilateral pleural effusions and ascites are evident. The nongated nature of the images is responsible for motion artifact of the coronary calcium.

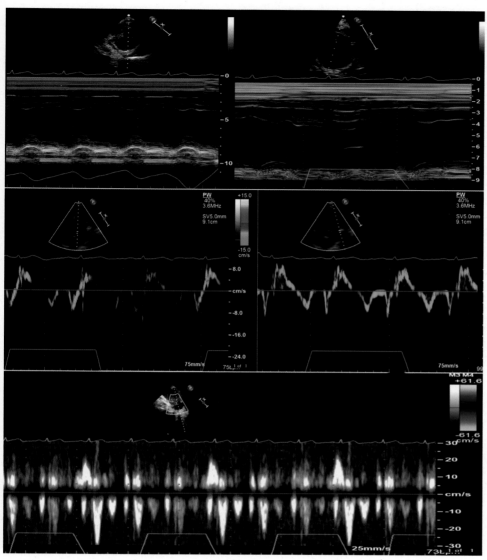

Figure 9-86. TTE. TOP, M-mode study of the interventricular septum. The respiratory effort is weak and rapid, and there is no septal shift with inspiration (LEFT). With a better inspiration, there is some evidence of inspiratory septal shift (RIGHT). MIDDLE, Tissue Doppler study of the mitral annulus. The tissue Doppler tracing shows reduced E' velocities, consistent with diastolic (myocardial) dysfunction, plausibly from the borderline left ventricular hypertrophy and prior history of chronic hypertension. BOTTOM, Hepatic venous flow shows augmented reversal of hepatic vein diastolic flow in expiration, consistent with constrictive physiology.

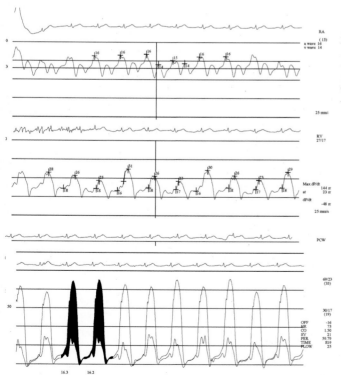

Figure 9-87. TOP, RAP tracing shows elevation of the mean RAP and prominent *x* and *y* descents with a W or M pattern. The mean pressure does not decrease with inspiration (presence of Kussmaul sign). MIDDLE, RV pressure tracing shows normal RVSP, elevated RVDP ($\geq^1/_3$ RVSP), and possible dip-and-plateau (square-root) pattern. BOTTOM, Simultaneous left and right ventricular pressure tracing shows a near-equilibration of the LVDP and RVDP, although LVDP is consistently higher. The tracing lacks the dip-and-plateau pattern. Without a respirometer, it is impossible to see if there is ventricular interdependence.

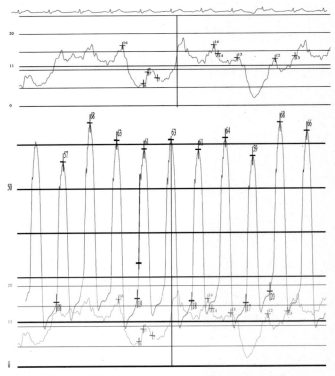

Figure 9-88. TOP, PCWP tracing. The mean PCWP at end-expiration is 13 mm Hg. There is a significant fall in pressure with inspiration, consistent with increased respiratory effort. BOTTOM, PCWP:LVDP gradient. The tracings are superimposed. There is a significant inspiratory increase in the PCWP:LVDP gradient.

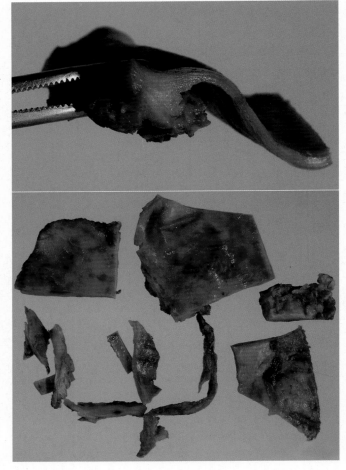

Figure 9-89. Surgical pathology. The pericardium is 3 mm thick and leather-like in most places.

CASE 5

History

▸ 55-year-old woman with an episode of pericarditis associated with renal failure 5 years before

Physical Examination

▸ BP 110/70 mm Hg, with a pulsus paradoxus of 10 to 15 mm Hg
▸ Elevated venous pressures with strikingly exaggerated *y* descents, possible Kussmaul sign
▸ Pericardial knock, no rub
▸ Mild ankle edema

Management and Outcome

▸ Diagnosis of constrictive pericarditis by supportive imaging; referred to surgery

▸ Surgery revealed mildly thickened but stiff pericardium tightening especially over the right ventricular free wall.
▸ Slow and incomplete symptom resolution

Comments

▸ Idiopathic or posturemic constrictive pericarditis
▸ Thickened pericardium, but not strikingly
▸ Deformation of the right ventricle cavity produced from the constriction
▸ Most findings on examination, by imaging, and by hemodynamic study were present.
▸ Surgery was survived, but the symptom relief was disappointing.

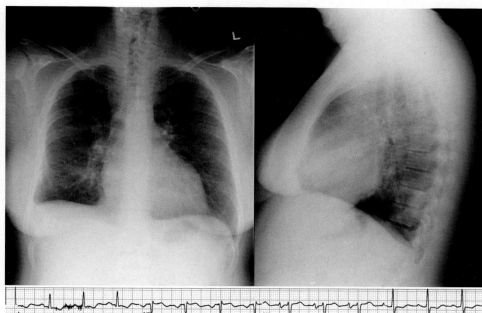

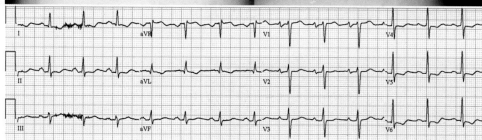

Figure 9-90. TOP, Chest radiographs show cardiomegaly, left atrial enlargement, and increased vascular markings. BOTTOM, ECG shows sinus rhythm, nonspecific repolarization abnormalities, and normal voltages.

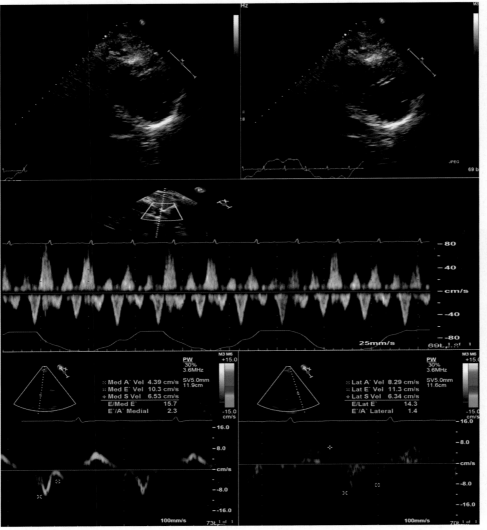

Figure 9-91. TOP, TTE parasternal short-axis views during expiration (LEFT) and inspiration (RIGHT). Note the inspiratory septal shift (with inspiration, the RV dimension increases and the LV dimension decreases), consistent with ventricular interaction or interdependence. MIDDLE, Hepatic venous flow. There is an expiratory increase in diastolic flow reversal consistent with constriction. BOTTOM, TTE tissue Doppler study shows normal myocardial relaxation, excluding restrictive cardiomyopathy.

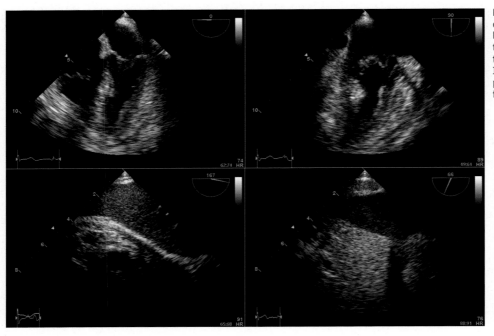

Figure 9-92. TOP, TEE images show a plane of pericardial thickening as thick as the left ventricular wall. BOTTOM LEFT, TEE transgastric view shows pericardial thickening. BOTTOM RIGHT, Hepatic veins and IVC. The veins are dilated, and there is prominent spontaneous contrast due to low flow.

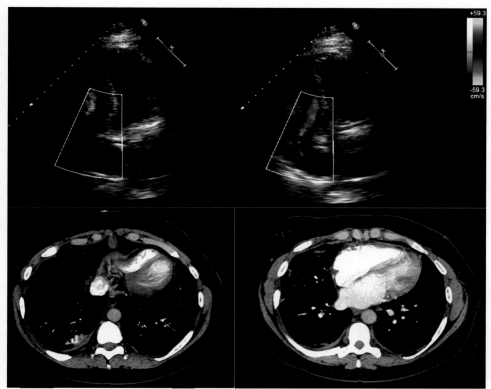

Figure 9-93. Echocardiography and CT comparison. TOP, TTE apical 4-chamber view shows a distortion (indentation) of the mid right ventricular free wall. BOTTOM, Contrast-enhanced axial CT scan shows no calcification of the pericardium. The parietal pericardium is seen over the right ventricular free wall and does not appear thickened. There is prominent distortion of the right ventricular free wall, a possible sign of pericardial constriction with a local effect on the right ventricle.

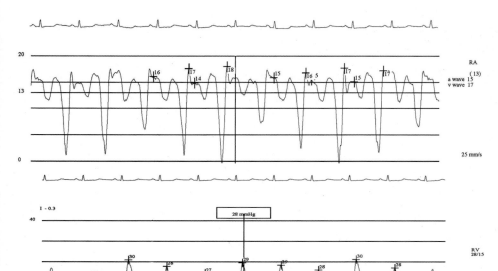

Figure 9-94. TOP, RAP tracing shows elevation of the mean RAP, with a prominent x descent and a very prominent and dominant y descent. There is no variation of the mean RAP with the respiratory cycle, but the y descents appear to accentuate with inspiration. BOTTOM, RV pressure tracing shows that RVSP is normal and RVDP is elevated (RVDP $\geq \frac{1}{3}$ RVSP). There is a prominent dip-and-plateau (square-root) pattern.

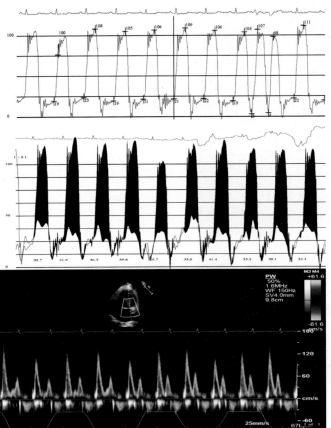

Figure 9-95. TOP, Left ventricular pressure tracing shows elevated diastolic pressure, dip-and-plateau or square-root sign. Prominent early diastolic dip with a low zero point that becomes negative with inspiration is indicative of prominent recoil of the pericardium and myocardium. MIDDLE, Simultaneous left and right ventricular pressure tracings. Elevation and equilibration of the LVDP and RVDP, and the dip-and-plateau pattern of both. There is inspiratory discordance of the LVSP and RVSP—ventricular interdependence. BOTTOM, Mitral inflow recording shows a 25% variation in inflow velocity—fall with inspiration.

CASE 6

History

▸ An 18-year-old man presented with dyspnea and edema developed during 3 months; fevers had been intermittent through this time.
▸ He has had a tuberculosis contact in the past.

Physical Examination

▸ BP 105/70 mm Hg, pulsus paradoxus of 20 mm Hg; HR 110 bpm
▸ Markedly elevated venous pressure, without appreciable contours
▸ No pericardial knock or rub
▸ Edema of both legs and the right arm

Evolution and Management

▸ The etiology was unclear and tuberculosis was suspected, given the contact history.
▸ Bronchoscopy, though, was negative for acid-fast bacilli.
▸ To drain the pleural cavities and to obtain pericardial tissue for histology, staining, polymerase chain reaction (PCR) analysis, and culture, the patient underwent surgery. Bilateral chest tubes were inserted, and a pericardial specimen was resected. The tissue specimen was negative for granuloma, stains, and PCR for tuberculosis or other pathogens.
▸ Antituberculous treatment and steroids were started, with the outlook of pericardial resection in 6 to 8 weeks.
▸ Diagnosis of constrictive pericarditis was made by supportive imaging.
▸ The patient was referred to surgery.

Management

▸ The patient underwent successful radical pericardiectomy that revealed thickened and calcified pericardium and localized purulent foul-smelling yellow material in the inferior margin of the pericardial space.
▸ Pathology findings were acute inflammation and lymphocytic inflammation, acid-fast bacilli negative (no granuloma).
▸ The yellow liquid was gram-negative and had a positive growth of *Fusobacterium* (gram-negative anaerobic bacillus).
▸ The patient was treated with antimicrobials. The cardiovascular function postoperatively was not a problem, but multiple comorbidities complicated the course.

Outcome

▸ Uneventful postoperative course
▸ Well at follow-up

Comments

▸ Pericarditis in this case was initially solely constrictive and then evolved into pericardial effusion with associated central venous thrombosis due to *Fusobacterium* (Lemierre syndrome).
▸ The unexpected finding of purulence in one area of the pericardium underscores the undeniable diagnostic role of surgery.
▸ The right upper extremity deep venous thrombosis may have been associated with the low-flow state of the constrictive physiology and possibly with pericardial narrowing (pinching) of the upper SVC. Thrombosis of the internal jugular vein has been described in Lemierre syndrome.

Text continued on p. 185.

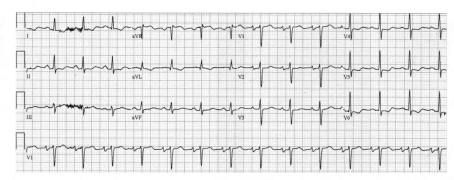

Figure 9-96. ECG shows sinus tachycardia, atrial abnormality, and nonspecific repolarization abnormalities.

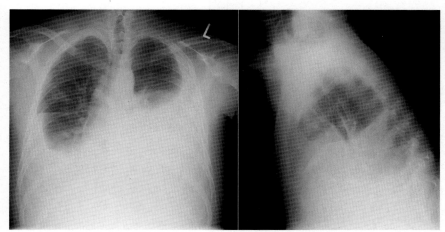

Figure 9-97. Chest radiography. The heart size and contours are unreadable, given the size of the pleural effusions. There is midline shift from the left-sided pleural effusion.

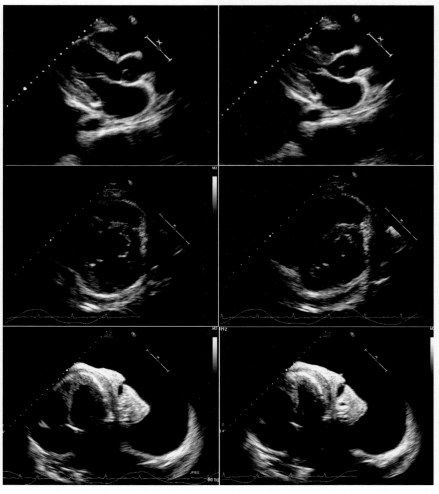

Figure 9-98. TTE views during expiration (LEFT) and inspiration (RIGHT). Note the inspiratory septal shift, the RV dimension increases, and the left ventricular dimension decreases. There is a very large left pleural effusion. The pericardium is grossly thickened. There is atelectatic lung against the left lateral aspect of the pericardium.

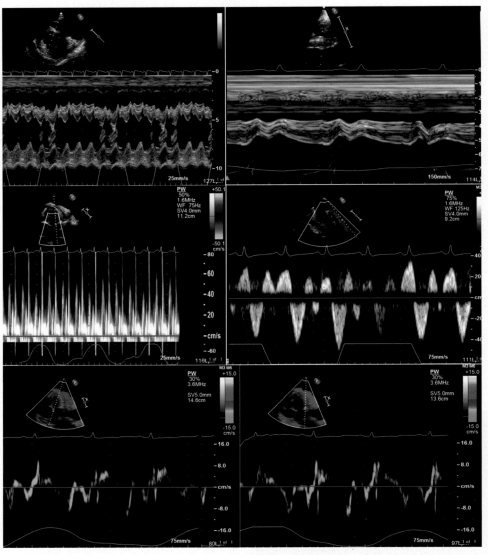

Figure 9-99. TTE M-mode imaging of the interventricular septum. TOP LEFT, Slow-speed recording shows the ventricular interdependence findings of an inspiratory septal shift. TOP RIGHT, High-speed recording shows the atrial systolic notch on the interventricular septum. MIDDLE LEFT, Left ventricular inflow. Note the significant fall in left ventricular early diastolic inflow velocity with inspiration. MIDDLE RIGHT, There is an increase in diastolic flow reversal in expiration. BOTTOM, Mitral annular tissue Doppler study. The early diastolic (E') velocity is normal, consistent with normal myocardial function.

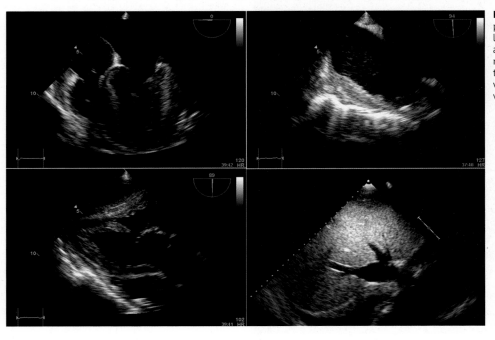

Figure 9-100. TOP, TEE views show prominent pericardial thickening, especially lateral to the left ventricle and to the right atrium. BOTTOM LEFT, TEE transgastric view reveals that the pericardium is almost as thick as the myocardium. BOTTOM RIGHT, TTE view of the liver showing IVC and hepatic venous dilation and prominent ascites.

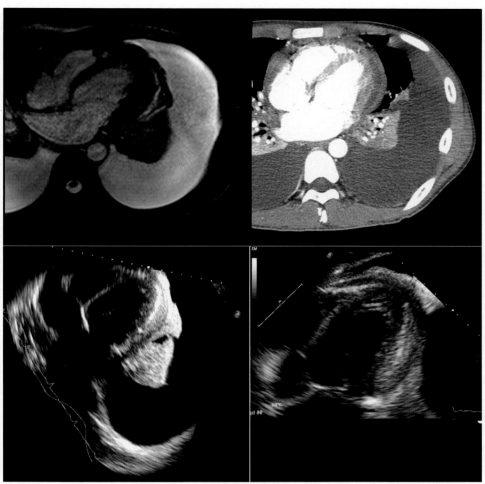

Figure 9-101. CMR, CT, and TTE apical views. TOP LEFT, CMR SSFP sequence. TOP RIGHT, Contrast-enhanced CT scan. BOTTOM, TTE images. The appearance of the pericardial thickening is different by each modality, and none of the techniques allows definitive delineation of serosal versus parietal thickening.

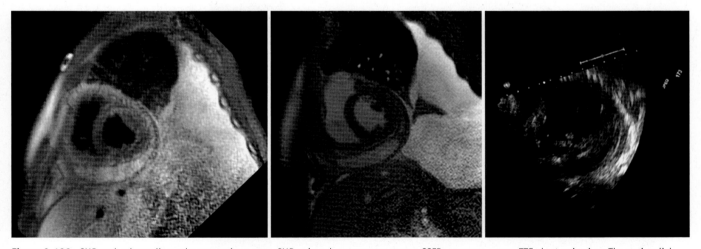

Figure 9-102. CMR and echocardiography comparison. LEFT, CMR spin echo sequence. MIDDLE, SSFP sequence. RIGHT, TTE short-axis view. The pericardial thickening and the underlying pericardial effusion are apparent by each modality. The anatomic extent of depiction by echocardiography is considerably more limited than by CMR.

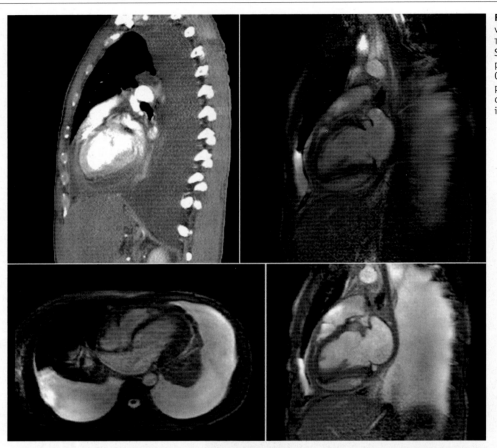

Figure 9-103. CMR, CT, and CMR apical views. TOP LEFT, Contrast-enhanced CT scan. TOP RIGHT, CMR SSFP sequence. BOTTOM, CMR SSFP sequences. The nature of the inferior pericardial thickening is better resolved by CMR as the high signal is consistent with a pericardial effusion. The lower attenuation coefficient of the effusion by CT scanning is ambiguous.

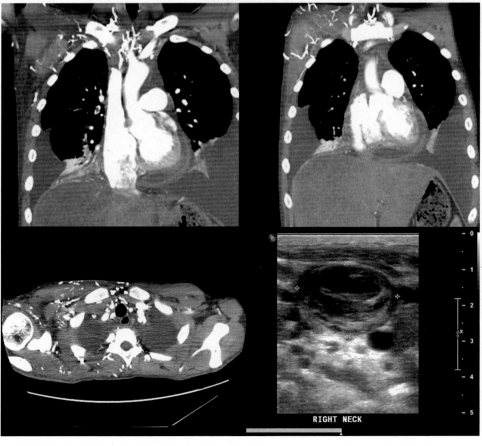

Figure 9-104. Right subclavian vein and internal jugular vein thrombosis. TOP, Contrast-enhanced coronal CT images showing pericardial thickening, right distal internal jugular thrombosis, and extensive collateralization. BOTTOM LEFT, Note collateral vessels. BOTTOM RIGHT, Ultrasound cross-sectional view of the internal jugular vein showing thrombosis.

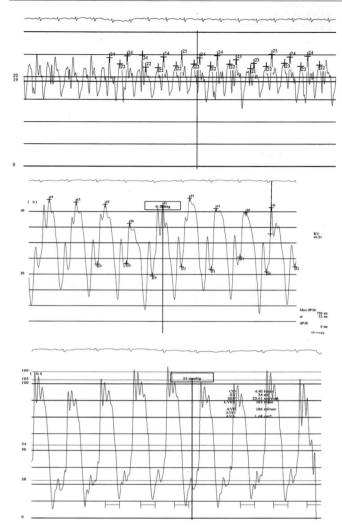

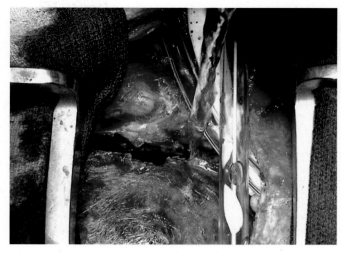

Figure 9-106. Surgical findings. The parietal pericardium has been opened. It is more than 1 cm thick anteriorly.

Figure 9-105. TOP, RAP tracing. Note the elevation of the RAP and the very prominent *x* and *y* descents with a W or M pattern. MIDDLE, Right ventricular pressure tracing shows normal RVSP and elevated RVDP (RVDP nearly two thirds of the RVSP). Note a dip-and-plateau square-root pattern.

References

1. Funk & Wagnalls Standard Dictionary of the English Language, 2nd ed. New York, HarperCollins, 2003.
2. Ling LH, Oh JK, Schaff HV, et al: Constrictive pericarditis in the modern era: evolving clinical spectrum and impact on outcome after pericardiectomy. Circulation 1999;100:1380-1386.
3. Cameron J, Oesterle SN, Baldwin JC: The etiologic spectrum of constrictive pericarditis. Am Heart J 1987;113:354-360.
4. Vaitkus PT, Kussmaul WG: Constrictive pericarditis versus restrictive cardiomyopathy: a reappraisal and update of diagnostic criteria. Am Heart J 1991;122:1431-1441.
5. Bertog SC, Thambidorai SK, Parakh K, et al: Constrictive pericarditis: etiology and cause-specific survival after pericardiectomy. J Am Coll Cardiol 2004;43:1445-1452.
6. Killian DM, Furiasse JG, Scanlon PJ, et al: Constrictive pericarditis after cardiac surgery. Am Heart J 1989;118:563-568.
7. Thomas WJ, Steiman DM, Kovach JA, Vernalis MN: Doppler echocardiography and hemodynamic findings in localized pericardial constriction. Am Heart J 1996;131:599-603.
8. Tyberg TI, Goodyer AV, Langou RA: Genesis of pericardial knock in constrictive pericarditis. Am J Cardiol 1980;46:570-575.
9. Hurrell D, Nishimura RA, Higano ST, et al: Value of dynamic respiratory changes in left and right ventricular pressures for the diagnosis of constrictive pericarditis. Circulation 1996;93:2007-2013.
10. Dhar R, Duke RJ, Sealey BJ: Cough syncope from constrictive pericarditis: a case report. Can J Cardiol 2003;19:295-296.
11. Garcia MJ, Rodriguez L, Ares M, et al: Differentiation of constrictive pericarditis from restrictive cardiomyopathy: assessment of left ventricular diastolic velocities in longitudinal axis by Doppler tissue imaging. J Am Coll Cardiol 1996;27:108-114.
12. von Bibra H, Schober K, Jenni R, et al: Diagnosis of constrictive pericarditis by pulsed Doppler echocardiography of the hepatic vein. Am J Cardiol 1989;63:483-488.
13. Klodas E, Nishimura RA, Appleton CP, et al: Doppler evaluation of patients with constrictive pericarditis: use of tricuspid regurgitation velocity curves to determine enhanced ventricular interaction. J Am Coll Cardiol 1996;28:652-657.
14. Engel PJ, Fowler NO, Tei CW, et al: M-mode echocardiography in constrictive pericarditis. J Am Coll Cardiol 1985;6:471-474.
15. Hatle LK, Appleton CP, Popp RL: Differentiation of constrictive pericarditis and restrictive cardiomyopathy by Doppler echocardiography. Circulation 1989;79:357-370.
16. Oh JK, Hatle LK, Seward JB, et al: Diagnostic role of Doppler echocardiography in constrictive pericarditis. J Am Coll Cardiol 1994;23:154-162.
17. Abdalla IA, Murray RD, Awad HE, et al: Reversal of the pattern of respiratory variation of Doppler inflow velocities in constrictive pericarditis during mechanical ventilation. Am Soc Echocardiogr 2000;13:827-831.
18. Tabata T, Kabbani SS, Murray RD, et al: Difference in the respiratory variation between pulmonary venous and mitral inflow Doppler velocities in patients with constrictive pericarditis with and without atrial fibrillation. J Am Coll Cardiol 2001;37:1936-1942.
19. Oh J, Tajik AJ, Appleton CP, et al: Preload reduction to unmask the characteristic Doppler features of constrictive pericarditis: a new observation. Circulation 1997;95:796-799.
20. Boonyaratavej S, Oh JK, Tajik AJ, et al: Comparison of mitral inflow and superior vena cava Doppler velocities in chronic obstructive pulmonary disease and constrictive pericarditis. J Am Coll Cardiol 1998;32:2043-2048.
21. Wann LS, Weyman AE, Dillon JC, Feigenbaum H: Premature pulmonary valve opening. Circulation 1977;55:128-133.
22. Tei C, Child JS, Tanaka H, Shah PM: Atrial systolic notch on the interventricular septal echogram: an echocardiographic sign of constrictive pericarditis. J Am Coll Cardiol 1983;1:907-912.

23. Rajagopalan N, Garcia MJ, Rodriguez L, et al: Comparison of new Doppler echocardiographic methods to differentiate constrictive pericardial heart disease and restrictive cardiomyopathy. Am J Cardiol 2001;87:86-94.

24. Hutchison SJ, Smalling RG, Albornoz M, et al: Comparison of transthoracic and transesophageal echocardiography in clinically overt or suspected pericardial heart disease. Am J Cardiol 1994;74:962-965.

25. Oh JK, Hatle LK, Seward JB, et al: Diagnostic role of Doppler echocardiography in constrictive pericarditis. J Am Coll Cardiol 1994;23:154-162.

26. Ling LH, Oh JK, Tei C, et al: Pericardial thickness measured with transesophageal echocardiography: feasibility and potential clinical usefulness. J Am Coll Cardiol 1997;29:1317-1323.

27. Izumi C, Iga K, Sekiguchi K, et al: Usefulness of the transgastric view by transesophageal echocardiography in evaluating thickened pericardium in patients with constrictive pericarditis. J Am Soc Echocardiogr 2002;15:1004-1008.

28. Klein AL, Cohen GI, Pietrolungo JF, et al: Differentiation of constrictive pericarditis from restrictive cardiomyopathy by Doppler transesophageal echocardiographic measurements of respiratory variations in pulmonary venous flow. J Am Coll Cardiol 1993;22:1935-1943.

29. Voekel AG, Pietro DA, Folland ED, et al. Echocardiographic features of constrictive pericarditis. Circulation 1978;58:871-875.

30. Oren RM, Grover-McKay M, Stanford W, Weiss RM: Accurate preoperative diagnosis of pericardial constriction using cine computed tomography. J Am Coll Cardiol 1993;22:832-838.

31. Nishimura RA: Constrictive pericarditis in the modern era: a diagnostic dilemma. Heart 2001;86:619-623.

32. Masui T, Finck S, Higgins CB: Constrictive pericarditis and restrictive cardiomyopathy: evaluation with MR imaging. Radiology 1992;182:369-373.

33. Kojima S, Yamada N, Goto Y: Diagnosis of constrictive pericarditis by tagged cine magnetic resonance imaging. N Engl J Med 1999;341:373-374.

34. Schoenfeld MH, Supple EW, Dec GW Jr, et al: Restrictive cardiomyopathy versus constrictive pericarditis: role of endomyocardial biopsy in avoiding unnecessary thoracotomy. Circulation 1987;75:1012-1017.

35. Seifert FC, Miller DC, Oesterle SN, et al: Surgical treatment of constrictive pericarditis: analysis of outcome and diagnostic error. Circulation 1985;72:264-273.

36. Senni M, Redfield MM, Ling LH, et al: Left ventricular systolic and diastolic function after pericardiectomy in patients with constrictive pericarditis: Doppler echocardiographic findings and correlation with clinical status. J Am Coll Cardiol 1999;33:1182-1188.

37. Tanaka C, Nishimoto M, Takeuchi K, et al: Presystolic pulmonary valve opening in constrictive pericarditis. Jpn Heart J 1979;20:419-425.

38. Candell-Riera J, Garcia del Castilo H, Permanyer-Miralda G, Soler-Soler J: Echocardiographic features of the interventricular septum in chronic constrictive pericarditis. Circulation 1978;57:1154-1158.

39. Gibson TC, Grossman W, McLaurin LP, et al: An echocardiographic study of the interventricular septum in constrictive pericarditis. Br Heart J 1976;38:738-743.

Pericardial Constriction Variants

KEY POINTS

▶ The classic paradigm of constrictive pericarditis has been expanded to include the following:

  ▶ Constriction caused by pericardium with normal thickness

  ▶ Transient pericardial constriction

  ▶ Coexisting constriction and restriction

▶ Partial or localized constriction

▶ Constriction of an underlying abnormal heart

▶ Such cases require a greater degree of diagnostic suspicion and proficiency and are real clinical challenges.

Although the majority of pericardial constriction cases are fairly typical, there are important variants and permutations of pericardial constriction, such as constriction with "normal" pericardial thickness, transient constriction, effuso-constriction, localized constriction, constriction with concurrent myocardial restriction, and constriction with an underlying abnormal heart.

PERICARDIAL CONSTRICTION WITH NORMAL OR MINIMALLY THICKENED PERICARDIUM

The finding of normal pericardial thickness (by imaging) in a case thought to have pericardial constriction is often perturbing to the clinician because classically pericardial constriction was associated with gross abnormalities (thickening and calcification) of the pericardium. However, there is a minority subset of pericardial constriction cases that have normal or nearly normal pericardial thickness, in which the problem is sheer stiffness of the pericardium.

Detection of some measure of pericardial thickening has been a standard—and reassuring to the clinician—aspect of the diagnostic evaluation of suspected constriction cases. The poor temporal resolution of older generation computed tomography (CT) scanners systematically and artifactually resulted in the appearance of increased pericardial thickness, sometimes dubiously—and dubiously reassuringly. The low temporal resolution of older generation CT scanners, and the lack of electrocardiography (ECG) gating in particular, caused translational motion of the pericardium and the heart through the time of image acquisition, resulting in the appearance of more extensive pericardial thickness than was anatomically true. True normal anatomic pericardial thickness is less than 1 mm. Given the current limits of temporal and spatial resolution, the thickness of normal pericardium images by non–ECG gated CT and cardiac magnetic resonance (CMR) is generally held to be 1 to 2 mm. Older publications and statements that normal pericardial thickness is less than 4 mm (this number reflected the limited accuracy of older equipment, not true anatomic thickness) engendered considerable misunderstanding and confusion as to what true normal parietal pericardial thickness is among nonsurgeons and nonpathologists who knew better.

It has been demonstrated that among five cases of constriction, only four have pathologically thickened pericardium; therefore, one case of five will not appear thickened on imaging (Fig. 10-1). Among 143 cases of constriction seen at the Mayo Clinic from 1993 to 1999, 26 patients had pericardial thickness less than 2 mm and 117 patients had pericardial thickness greater than 2 mm. There were few differences in clinical features, presumed causes, or relief by pericardiectomy depending on pericardial thickness.[1] Thus, overt thickening is seen in only about 80% of cases of constriction by current imaging. A caveat concerning this study is that 2-mm thickness is not actually normal; therefore, the subset may be better described as constriction with normal pericardial thickness or minimally thickened pericardium. The stiffness of the pericardium is the primary determinant of constrictive physiology; pericardial thickness is an indirect determinant of constrictive physiology. Furthermore, a finding of pericardial thickening is not specific for compressive physiology from constriction.

Transient Constriction

Classically, pericardial constriction has been viewed as a progressive disorder, with a variable rate of progression. An interesting

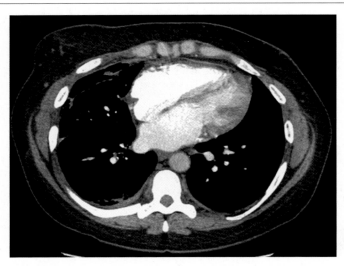

Figure 10-1. This case was proven at surgery to be constrictive, and pericardiectomy afforded prominent clinical relief. On CT scanning, the parietal pericardial layer shows thickness in the normal range (≤2 mm). The surgeon observed only mild thickening of the pericardium but noted that it was tough to the touch.

and important subset of pericardial constriction cases, most commonly an average of 8 weeks after open heart surgery, are transient in nature (Figs. 10-2 to 10-6).[2,3] With what is currently known, it does not seem possible to accurately predict which cases are transient; hence, a short trial of medical therapy and observation may be warranted in some cases to allow transience to declare itself. The long-term outcome of initially transient constriction cases is also unknown (Fig. 10-7).

EFFUSO-CONSTRICTIVE PERICARDITIS

Some cases of compression or constriction of the heart occur with both pericardial fluid and pericardial stiffness ("effuso" and "constrictive") contributing to the compression. In effuso-constrictive pericarditis, after the pericardial fluid is removed and the intrapericardial pressure is reduced to 0 mm Hg or less, evidence of compression of the heart remains (elevated right atrial pressure with a prominent *y* descent, elevated end-diastolic left and right ventricular pressures with an early diastolic dip or square-root pattern), excluding that the tamponade was responsible for all of the compression.[4] Thus, effusive and constrictive pericardial processes may be concurrent. When compression of the heart persists after pericardial fluid is drained, the constrictive physiology is conferred by either the visceral pericardium[4] or areas of pericardium where the visceral and parietal pericardium are fused (Fig. 10-8).

Residual significant signs of compression after drainage of the pericardial fluid are diagnostic of effuso-constrictive pericarditis and may also assist with identifying the etiology of the disorder, as may surgical resection of pericardial tissue.

In effuso-constrictive pericarditis, the underlying heart may be compressed by the following:

- An underlying constrictive visceral pericardial layer
- Pericardial fluid under pressure
- Overlying constrictive parietal pericardium
- Areas of fused and constrictive parietal and visceral pericardium
- The interaction of the distending pericardial fluid with the enclosing and stiffened parietal pericardium

Each effuso-constrictive heart will have different degrees of these. Thus, drainage of the pericardium may afford a variable amount of relief of compressive physiology and will change the nature of the compression toward constrictive findings. The optimal intervention—drainage alone and observation; parietal pericardiectomy and drainage of fluid; or parietal pericardiectomy, drainage of fluid, and resection of serosal pericardium—will depend on the individual heart and must be weighed against the small risks of fluid drainage, the usually low risk of open chest surgical resection of parietal pericardium or drainage, and the higher risk of resection of the serosal pericardium as well (which confers higher risk of bleeding).

CMR has a significant role to play in the evaluation of patients with effuso-constrictive pericarditis. It is able to determine the presence and extent of pericardial fluid accumulation and the extent and distribution of pericardial thickness.

LOCALIZED CONSTRICTION

To cardiologists, the notion of constriction comes with the concept of global compression of the heart, achieving equilibration of diastolic pressures in all chambers. Although in typical cases this is true, cardiac surgeons have a different knowledge of constriction, that is, that the disease process is *variable* in its distribution of thickening, calcification, and adherence to the heart chambers. The constrictive process may also be variable to the degree that it is indenting or constricting portions of the underlying chamber.[5] Some cases of constriction involve extreme variation of disease over the heart chambers, leading to compression of some but not all chambers or of some chambers more than others. Nonuniform belt-like indentation into the heart from pericardial constriction may result in gradients in underlying right-sided heart (lower pressure, more easily compressed) cavities, usually at the tricuspid valve level or right ventricular outflow tract level.

CONSTRICTION WITH COEXISTING MYOCARDIAL RESTRICTION

Although, classically, constrictive pericarditis and restrictive cardiomyopathy are dichotomized pathologic processes, a few rare cases concurrently have both pathologic conditions. Such cases would be expected to engender confusion and in general to fare poorly with relief of the constrictive component, as underlying myocardial dysfunction would persist. Disease states that may have concurrent pericardial constriction and myocardial restriction include almost all post–radiation therapy cases of constriction and occasional amyloidosis restrictive cardiomyopathy cases that experienced prior amyloidosis-associated pericarditis.

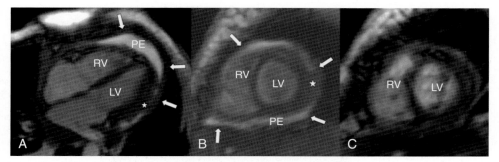

Figure 10-2. CMR imaging (steady-state free precession) end-diastolic 4-chamber (**A**) and short-axis (**B** and **C**) views demonstrate the presence of a pericardial effusion (PE) with epicardial fibrin strands *(asterisk)* and pericardial thickening *(arrows)* at presentation. Follow-up after 3 months of antituberculous chemotherapy shows resolution of the pericardial effusion. RV, right ventricle; LV, left ventricle. (Courtesy of Jan-Peter Smedema, MD, Cape Town, South Africa.)

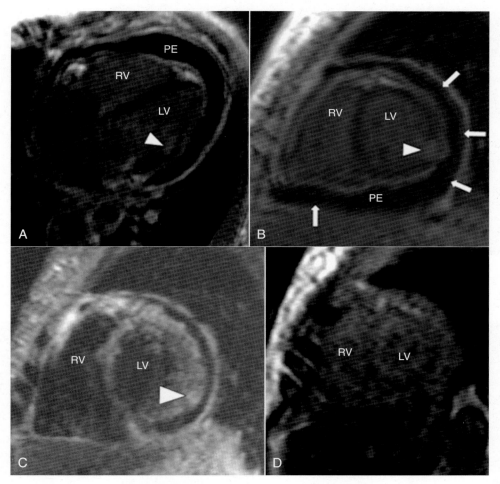

Figure 10-3. CMR imaging (inversion recovery gradient echo sequence) 10 minutes after the administration of 0.1 mmol/kg gadolinium-DTPA (**A, B, D**) and T2-weighted short T1 inversion recovery sequence (**C**) demonstrate a protein-rich pericardial effusion (PE). Pericardial thickening (**B**, *arrows*) and a myocardial tuberculoma in the posterolateral left ventricular wall (**B** and **C**, *triangle*) at presentation. Follow-up after 3 months (**D**) of antituberculous chemotherapy shows resolution of the pericardial effusion and myocardial tuberculoma. RV, right ventricle; LV, left ventricle. (Courtesy of Jan-Peter Smedema, MD, Cape Town, South Africa.)

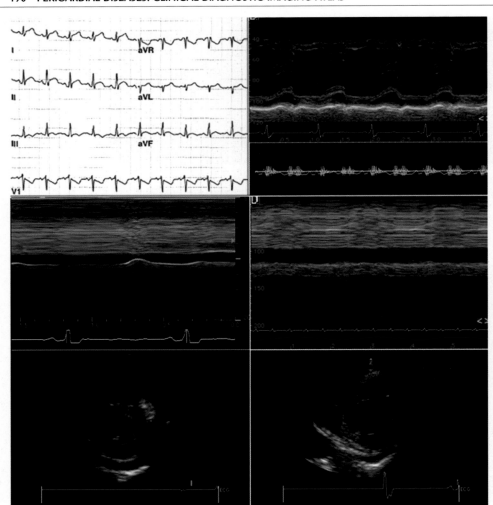

Figure 10-4. LEFT IMAGES, Acute pericarditis phase. RIGHT IMAGES, Constrictive pericarditis phase. A 30-year-old woman with scleroderma developed clinical and electrocardiographic evidence of pericarditis, including a triphasic rub, diffuse ST elevation, and PR elevation in aVR (TOP LEFT). Her neck veins were not elevated, and the venous pressure contours were normal; correspondingly, the inferior vena cava was only mildly dilated (MIDDLE LEFT) but had preserved collapse with inspiration or sniff. BOTTOM LEFT, Small pericardial effusion that the patient had while having a pericardial rub is evident. Two months later, she presented with anasarca and liver failure. Her neck veins were strikingly elevated, the y descent predominated, and there was a loud pericardial knock. TOP RIGHT, The M-mode interrogation reveals an early diastolic dip of the septum, and phonocardiography documents the pericardial knock. MIDDLE RIGHT, M-mode study of the inferior vena cava reveals marked dilation and a complete absence of respiratory motion, consistent with very elevated central venous pressure. BOTTOM RIGHT, The effusion had nearly completely resolved by this time when constriction developed. Three weeks later, she experienced complete clinical normalization and has remained well since.

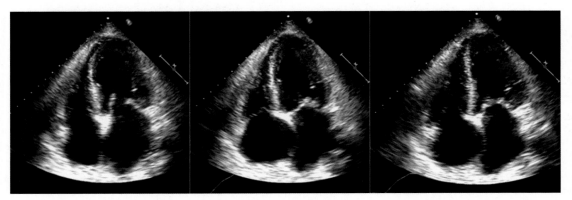

Figure 10-5. This 77-year-old woman had undergone aortic valve replacement for aortic stenosis 2 weeks previously and had persistently elevated neck veins, even after diuresis and elimination of volume overload. The y descent predominated. There was neither a rub nor a pericardial knock. Echocardiography reveals the absence of pericardial fluid and striking right:left heart interaction findings (note the respirometry tracing on each panel). LEFT, Expiration: normal interatrial and interventricular septal position. MIDDLE, Onset of inspiration. There is a marked deviation of the interatrial septum from the right to the left side as venous return increases to the right side of the heart. RIGHT, Second cardiac cycle of inspiration. Now the increased venous return to the right side of the heart has deviated the interventricular septum, despite its hypertrophy, to the left side, consistent with ventricular interaction or interdependence.

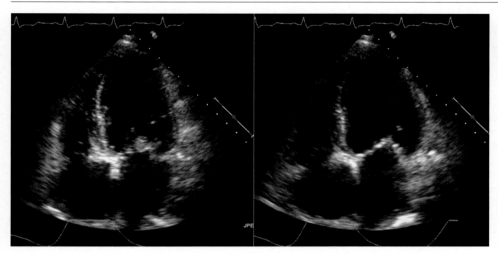

Figure 10-6. The same patient as in Figure 10-5. Ten days later, all clinical and echocardiographic findings had normalized. Note septal positions in expiration (LEFT) and in inspiration (RIGHT).

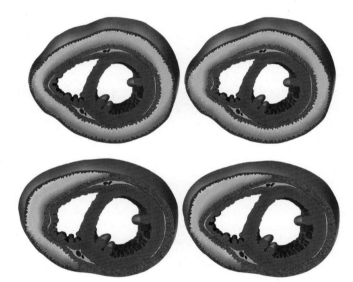

Figure 10-8. Effuso-constrictive pericarditis may occur with several permutations that depend on the distribution of pericardial fluid, the compressiveness and resistance of thickened serosal pericardium, and the intrapericardial pressure. TOP LEFT, Generalized fluid distribution; no right-sided heart collapse is present as the raised intrapericardial pressure is not sufficient to compress or to collapse the right-sided heart cavities. TOP RIGHT, Generalized fluid distribution; right-sided heart collapse is present as the raised intrapericardial pressure is sufficient to compress or to collapse the right-sided heart cavities. BOTTOM LEFT, Localized fluid distribution; right-sided heart collapse is present as the raised intrapericardial pressure is sufficient to compress or to collapse the right-sided heart cavities. BOTTOM RIGHT, Localized fluid distribution; no right-sided heart collapse is present as the raised intrapericardial pressure is not sufficient to compress or to collapse the right-sided heart cavities. By echocardiographic imaging, the finding of right-sided heart collapse in the presence of an effusion will engender the recognition of tamponade compressive physiology; however, the case may be effuso-constrictive— only observing the effect of fluid removal will generalize fluid distribution, no right-sided heart collapse as the raised intrapericardial pressure is not sufficient to compress or to collapse the right-sided heart cavities. Localized pericardial fluid accumulations with right-sided heart compression similarly are likely to initially be understood as localized tamponade but may actually be part of effuso-constrictive syndromes with the segments of the obliterated pericardial space, or the serosal layer under the pericardial fluid, compressing the underlying heart cavities.

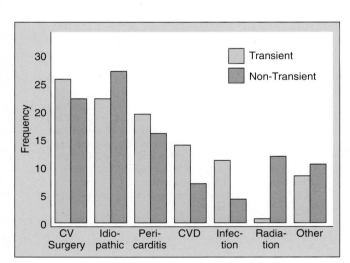

Figure 10-7. Transient pericardial constriction occurs in 20% of cases. CV, cardiovascular; CVD, cardiovascular disease. (From Haley JH, Tajik AJ, Danielson GK: Transient constrictive pericarditis: causes and natural history. J Am Coll Cardiol 2004;43:271-275.)

CONSTRICTION WITH AN UNDERLYING HEART ABNORMALITY

The classic case of constrictive pericarditis has underlying normal myocardium, underlying normal valves, underlying normal coronary arteries, underlying normal electrical conduction, and underlying normal cardiac rhythm; hence, the constrictive findings are not muddied by other abnormalities. The more the underlying heart is normal, the more straightforward the diagnosis, and the better the chance of significant improvement with pericardiectomy. However, the underlying heart may be abnormal, entering atypicality into the physical diagnosis, imaging, and hemodynamic findings. Patients who had undergone previous open heart surgery (for coronary bypass or valve replacements) often have myocardial residua of their coronary disease or valve disease that may affect hemodynamic findings and increase the diagnostic challenge.[6]

Tissue Doppler assessment of myocardial relaxation has proved very useful to distinguish suspected constriction cases (normal early diastolic relaxation) from suspected restriction cases (abnormal early diastolic relaxation). The use of tissue Doppler indices in this way inherently assumes, first, that constriction and restriction are not concurrent, and second, that there are no other myocardial disorders in patients with constrictive pericarditis. However, older patients with constrictive pericarditis may have had antecedent hypertension or coronary artery disease (CAD), rendering tissue Doppler findings abnormal. Post–open heart surgery cases, especially valve cases (mitral valve disease cases having undergone surgery have a higher incidence of atrial fibrillation) and aortic valve disease (especially aortic stenosis) cases, are likely to have diastolic dysfunction yielding abnormal tissue Doppler findings. CAD cases with ventricular dysfunction may have diastolic dysfunction yielding abnormal tissue Doppler findings from prior infarction, from ischemia, or from hypertension. Further confusion may arise from the fact that lesser degrees of pericardial thickening are common after open heart surgery, lessening suspicion of constriction. Furthermore, transient constriction is well described after open heart surgery, increasing suspicion.

CASE 1

History

- 41-year-old male construction worker with a past history of asthma and sinusitis; no history of tuberculosis, irradiation, or other disorders
- 2-month history of dyspnea and progressive pedal edema

Physical Examination

- Pulsus paradoxus of 20 mm Hg
- Elevated venous pressure; no Kussmaul sign or prominent *y* descent
- Normal heart sounds
- No pericardial knock or rub
- Mild pedal edema

Management

- Effuso-constrictive pericarditis was suspected on the basis of the following findings: effusion on echocardiography and CT scanning; pericardial thickening on transesophageal echocardiography and CT; and calcification on chest radiography, transesophageal echocardiography, and CT (Figs. 10-9 to 10-13).
- Surgical drainage of pericardial effusion and pericardial biopsy were performed; findings were negative for tuberculosis.
- Evidence of constrictive physiology remained after drainage of the fluid-elevated neck veins with a now prominent *y* descent and ventricular interaction or interdependence by 2-dimensional and Doppler signs.
- The patient was referred for angiography (which was normal) and cardiac catheterization, with the view to surgery (Figs. 10-14 to 10-16).

Surgical and Pathologic Findings

- Surgical procedure (total pericardiectomy off bypass) was performed and found thickened parietal and visceral pericardium with focal calcifications (Fig. 10-17).

- Fibrous thickening with focal calcification
- Nonspecific perivascular chronic inflammatory cell infiltrate
- Stains and cultures negative for tuberculosis

Outcome

- Postoperatively, the heart failure symptoms resolved.
- The septal motion of interdependence improved during several months but not immediately.

Comments

- Cardiac compression after drainage of pericardial fluid (normalization of intrapericardial pressure) resulted in effuso-constrictive pericarditis.
- Both the parietal and visceral layers were extensively diseased and contributed to compression of the underlying heart. The visceral layer accounted for some of the constrictive effect (impression at surgery and by virtue of the fact that the parietal layer had been held separate from the visceral layer by the effusion, which after drainage fell laxly from the visceral layer). The parietal layer was responsible for the compressive effect from the effusion.
- The signs that supported constriction remaining after pericardial fluid drainage were emergence of the *y* descent, which became dominant; ventricular interdependence seen on 2-dimensional echocardiography; typical catheterization findings (ventricular interdependence findings were not sought on the catheterization study); and obvious pericardial thickening and calcification detected by multiple imaging modalities.
- The hemodynamic parameters improved postoperatively but did not normalize for several months.

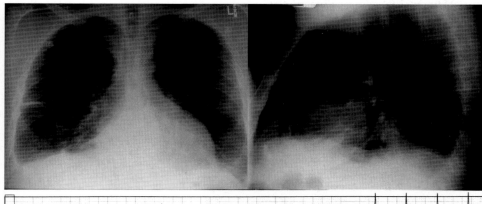

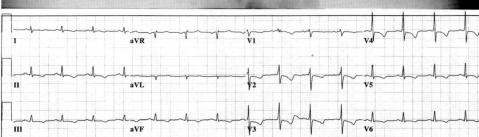

Figure 10-9. Chest radiography (TOP) demonstrates cardiomegaly (flask shaped), with lower lobe infiltrates and bilateral pleural effusions. Pericardial calcification can be appreciated retrosternally at the anterior aspect of the right ventricle on the lateral film. The ECG (BOTTOM) demonstrates sinus rhythm with nonspecific repolarization abnormalities and borderline low voltages due to the thickened and calcified pericardium impeding voltage recording at the surface.

10

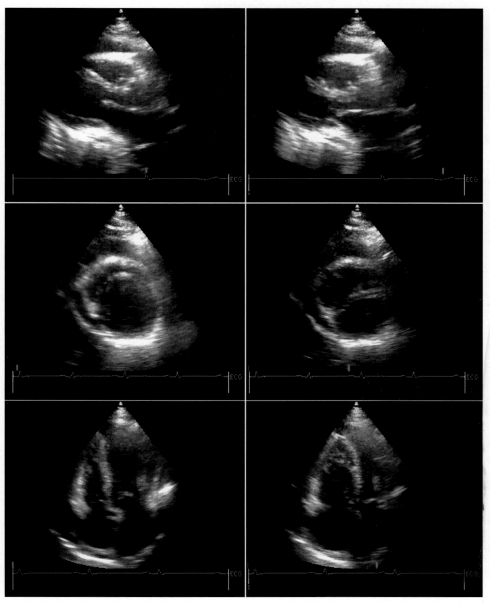

Figure 10-10. Transthoracic echocardiographic imaging of effuso-constrictive pericarditis. LEFT IMAGES, Expiration. RIGHT IMAGES, Inspiration. With inspiration, the right ventricle enlarges and the left ventricular dimension diminishes, a sign of ventricular interdependence. Inspiration is denoted by the upward deflection of the respirometry tracing.

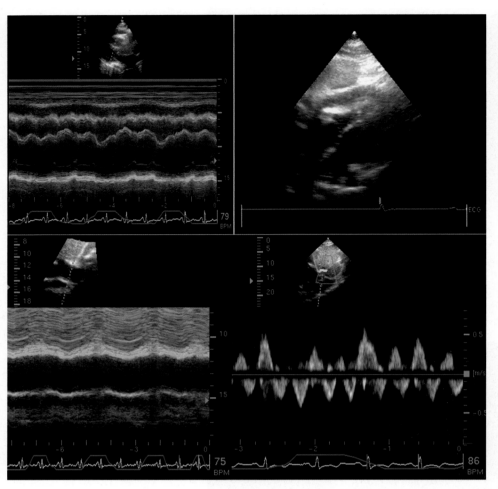

Figure 10-11. Transthoracic echocardiography. TOP LEFT, M-mode interrogation at the mid ventricle. Note the inspiratory increase of the right ventricular dimension and the reduction of the left ventricular dimension consistent with ventricular interdependence. (Inspiration is denoted by the upward deflection of the respirometry tracing.) TOP RIGHT, The subcostal view demonstrates the presence of some pericardial fluid. BOTTOM LEFT, The inferior vena cava is dilated and does not exhibit normal inspiratory collapse. BOTTOM RIGHT, Hepatic venous flow. There is an increase in diastolic flow reversal in expiration consistent with constrictive physiology.

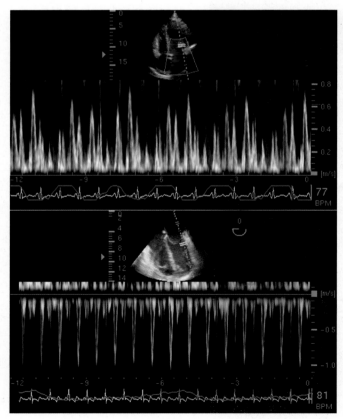

Figure 10-12. Mitral inflow. TOP, Transthoracic echocardiography. BOTTOM, Transesophageal echocardiography while ventilated. The transthoracic echocardiographic recording demonstrates prominent respiratory variations in early inflow velocity, consistent with constriction. On the transesophageal echocardiographic recording, the positive-pressure ventilation has nearly nullified the variation of inflow velocities.

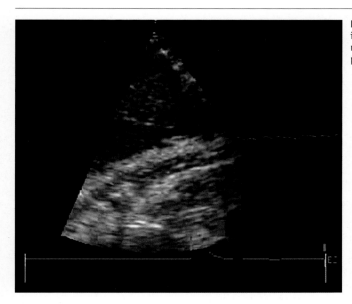

Figure 10-13. Transesophageal echocardiography, transgastric short-axis image. There is thickening of the pericardium (the lucent band) under the right ventricle, but the thickening is not precisely localized as the visceral or parietal layer, and confidently distinguishing it from a fat plane is difficult.

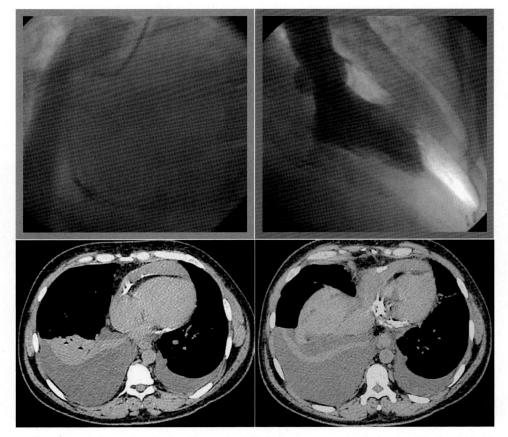

Figure 10-14. TOP IMAGES, Fluoroscopy during catheterization. There are calcified plaques seen under the heart and in the right atrioventricular groove (the right coronary artery has not yet been injected—the densities are calcium). BOTTOM IMAGES, Non–contrast-enhanced axial CT scans. Calcification is seen within the atrioventricular grooves and also along the right ventricle. Over the right side of the heart, the calcification appears to reside on both the epicardial and the parietal pericardial levels, which are separated presumably by effusion or other soft, noncalcified material. There is a pericardial effusion, and there are also pleural effusions.

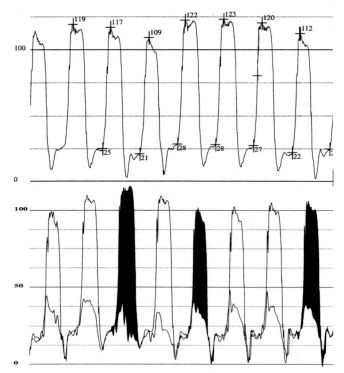

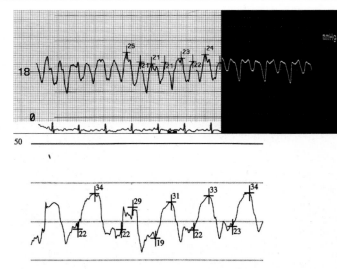

Figure 10-15. The left ventricular pressure waveform is notable for an elevated diastolic pressure with a dip-and-plateau pattern. Concurrent left and right ventricular recordings reveal directionally opposite variations of left and right ventricular systolic pressures—a sign of ventricular interdependence.

Figure 10-16. TOP, Right atrial pressure tracing during catheterization (LEFT) and after pericardial fluid drainage (RIGHT). Before pericardial fluid drainage, the mean right atrial pressure is elevated, and there is an M or W sign of prominent and equal *x* and *y* descents. After fluid drainage, the *y* descent predominates because residual constrictive physiology is present. BOTTOM, Right ventricular pressure tracings. Normal right ventricular systolic pressure. Elevated right ventricular diastolic pressure; right ventricular diastolic pressure $\geq 1/3$ right ventricular systolic pressure. Possible dip-and-plateau square-root pattern.

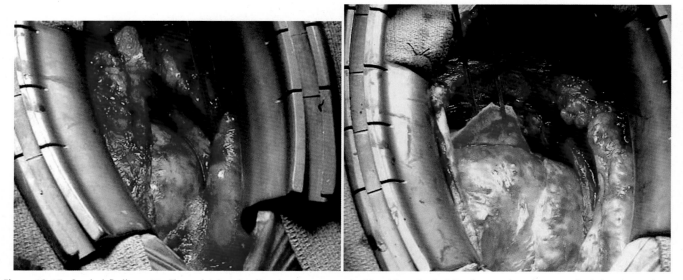

Figure 10-17. Surgical findings. TOP, The parietal pericardium has been opened with a triangular incision (apex up), and one can look down onto the visceral pericardium. Note the severely thickened *parietal* pericardium and the abnormal stiff and thick appearance of the visceral pericardium as well. BOTTOM, Note the severely thickened *visceral* pericardium held by forceps. Normally, the visceral pericardium is a microscopic monolayer of cells.

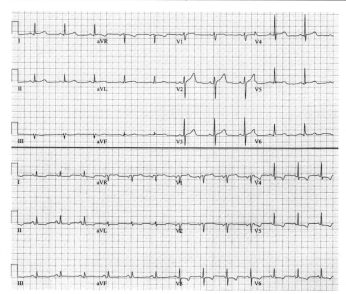

Figure 10-18. ECG on presentation with aortic dissection (TOP) showing sinus rhythm. ECG on presentation with edema and dyspnea (BOTTOM) showing sinus rhythm and nonspecific repolarization abnormalities. The voltages are less than they were previously because of the impedance to surface recording of the voltages by the pericardial thickening.

CASE 2

History

▸ 64-year-old man with a long history of untreated hypertension
▸ 3 months before presentation, experienced a type A aortic dissection requiring surgical repair with an ascending aortic composite graft
▸ Presented with 5-day history of limb swelling and dyspnea on exertion
▸ Left arm greater than right, right leg greater than left

Physical Examination

▸ BP 180/120 mm Hg, no pulsus paradoxus
▸ Elevated venous pressure with prominent y descent and presence of Kussmaul sign
▸ Normal heart sounds; no rub, knock, or gallop
▸ Asymmetric limb edema—left arm and right leg swelling
▸ Initial consideration of pulmonary thromboembolic disease as responsible for the edema and shortness of breath established that there was a right leg proximal deep venous thrombosis as well as a left subclavian deep venous thrombosis (related to prior catheterization) and an intermediate probability of pulmonary embolism by lung scan.
▸ Imaging findings are shown in Figures 10-18 to 10-20.

Evolution

▸ Pulmonary artery data: CVP 20 mm Hg, PCWP 21 mm Hg (Fig. 10-21)
▸ Because of the equilibrated compression in the context of pericardial fluid, the patient underwent percutaneous pericardial drainage, which yielded thick turbid fluid, but no organisms were identified or cultured. The right-sided heart catheterization data did not change significantly.

Management

▸ Surgical drainage of pericardial effusion was performed because of the suspicion of purulent pericarditis and evidence of systemic hypoperfusion. A modified partial pericardiectomy was performed.
▸ Pathologic examination showed thickened pericardium with focal inflammatory cells, occasional foreign body granulomas, and cartilage-like features. No organisms were identified by stains or culture. Hemodynamics showed slight improvement.

Outcome

▸ The symptoms improved during several months; the findings of elevated jugular venous pressure, exaggerated y descent, and inspiratory septal shift normalized.
▸ The patient was found to be lupus anticoagulant positive; he was already receiving warfarin anticoagulation for the mechanical aortic valve replacement.

Comments

▸ Early postoperative effuso-constrictive pericarditis
▸ Pericardial pathology noted cartilage-like changes, a plausible substrate for the clinically relevant stiffness of the pericardium.
▸ Partial resolution with surgical drainage, enough to increase urine output. Elevated central venous pressures persisted, with a y dominant descent.
▸ It was noted that positive-pressure ventilation obscured signs of ventricular interdependence.
▸ Tissue Doppler findings were abnormal, unusual for classic constriction but expected given the underlying heart abnormality (left ventricular hypertrophy from hypertension).
▸ Venous pressures and contours normalized during 4 months without pericardiectomy, making this a case of transient postoperative constriction.

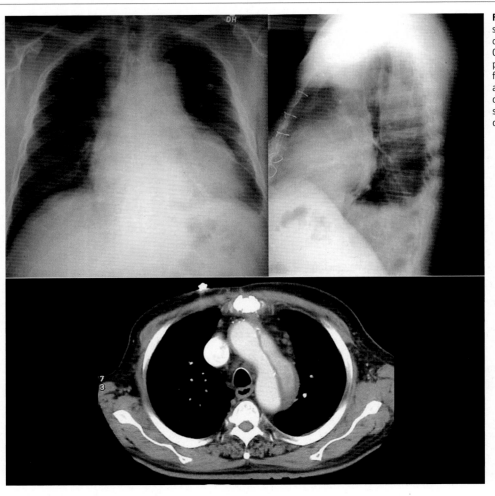

Figure 10-19. TOP, Chest radiographs show sternal wires and cardiomegaly without obvious chamber predominance. BOTTOM, Contrast-enhanced CT axial scan. Note the persistence of the intimal flap and the false lumen in the aortic arch. At this arch level, there is intimal displacement denoted by the intimal calcification—a specific chest radiograph sign of dissection.

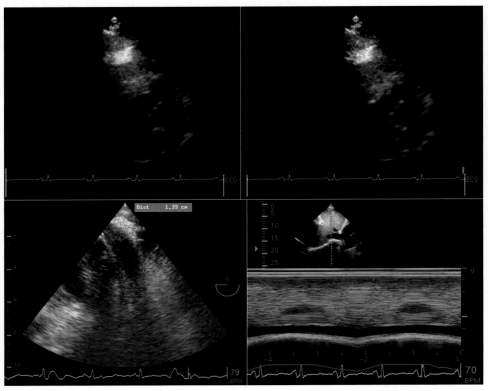

Figure 10-20. TOP, Transthoracic echocardiography, parasternal short-axis views. With inspiration (during the last cardiac cycle), the right ventricular size increases and the left ventricular size decreases—a sign of ventricular interaction or interdependence. BOTTOM LEFT, Transesophageal echocardiography after drainage and pericardial window. Note the thickening of the pericardium. BOTTOM RIGHT, The inferior vena cava is dilated, and there is failure of the inferior vena cava to collapse with inspiration consistent with physical diagnosis findings of elevated central venous pressure.

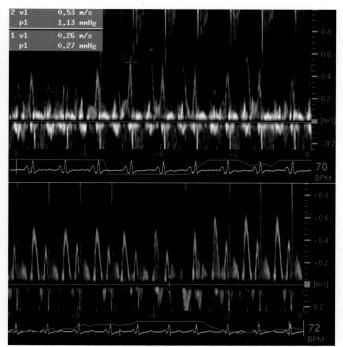

Figure 10-21. Left ventricular inflow, during spontaneous ventilation and with mechanical ventilation and positive end-expiratory pressure. TOP, The upper tracing depicts mitral inflow with normal spontaneous ventilation. The spectral profile is imperfect; sometimes the early inflow profile is faint. As an example of this, the first crosshair is placed on the correct profile, and the second is actually placed in error on the post–P wave profile, which is an A wave, not the E wave, which is pre–P wave. *Asterisks* mark the E-wave variation, consistent with ventricular interdependence. BOTTOM, The left ventricular inflow when the patient was undergoing surgical inspection; there is less respiratory variation of the E-wave profiles, an example of how mechanical ventilation obviates many signs of constriction.

CASE 3

History

- 76-year-old woman 6 weeks after aortic valve replacement and aortocoronary bypass for aortic stenosis and CAD
- Presented with edema and fatigue
- Had been in atrial fibrillation since the cardiac surgery

Physical Examination

- BP 110/70 mm Hg, no pulsus paradoxus; irregular pulse rhythm and volume
- Elevated venous pressure with prominent *y* descent and presence of Kussmaul sign
- Normal heart sounds
- No pericardial rub or knock
- Mild peripheral edema
- Imaging findings are shown in Figures 10-22 to 10-28.

Management and Outcome

- There was still clinical evidence of elevation of the right atrial pressure after drainage.
- The patient had clinically improved with diuretics, and although there was renal insufficiency, the renal function was sustained and then improved considerably.
- It was decided to observe her status to see the degree of improvement.

- Her findings (venous pressure and contour) normalized during 2 months. There was no need for diuretics after that time.

Comments

- Transient effuso-constrictive pericarditis after open heart surgery
- Drainage of the fluid and normalization of the intrapericardial pressure did not fully alleviate the clinical evidence of compression, and partial interdependence signs persisted initially.
- The left ventricular hypertrophy and bulk of the septum may have influenced the degree to which interdependence could be manifested. Left-sided heart catheterization across the mechanical aortic valve replacement could not be performed.
- Postoperative constriction cases often have structurally abnormal hearts underlying the constriction and influencing the findings (such as abnormal tissue Doppler findings).
- Atrial fibrillation is more common in early postoperative constriction cases and rendered some aspects of testing more difficult to assess.
- In this case, as with most postoperative cases of pericardial disease, physical examination and imaging findings are less typical because the underlying heart is abnormal, the pericardium is deformed by surgery, and there are coexisting pulmonary and other medical issues.

Text continued on p. 205.

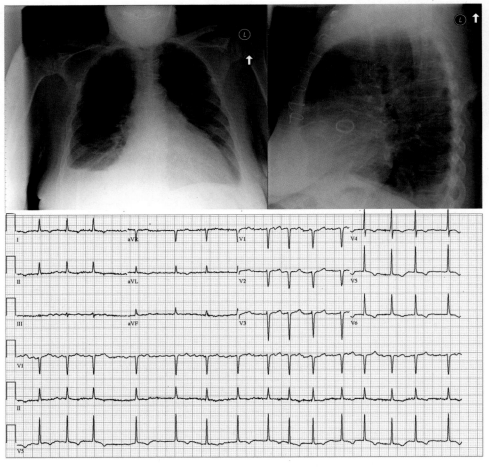

Figure 10-22. TOP, Chest radiographs show sternal wires, mechanical aortic valve replacement, and cardiomegaly. Posterior displacement of the left ventricular border and bilateral pleural effusions are seen on the lateral radiograph. BOTTOM, ECG shows atrial fibrillation, normal voltages, and no electrical alternans. Nonspecific repolarization abnormalities are not particularly suggestive of pericarditis.

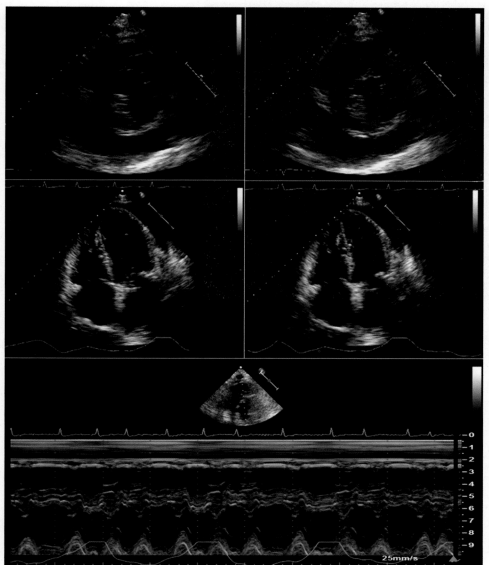

Figure 10-23. TOP FOUR IMAGES, Transthoracic echocardiography views show concentric left ventricular hypertrophy and a moderate-sized posterior pericardial effusion. The cardiac rhythm is irregular, but there may be an inspiratory septal shift. No early diastolic septal shift is seen. BOTTOM, M-mode study reveals an inspiratory increase in right ventricular dimension and a reduction in left ventricular dimension.

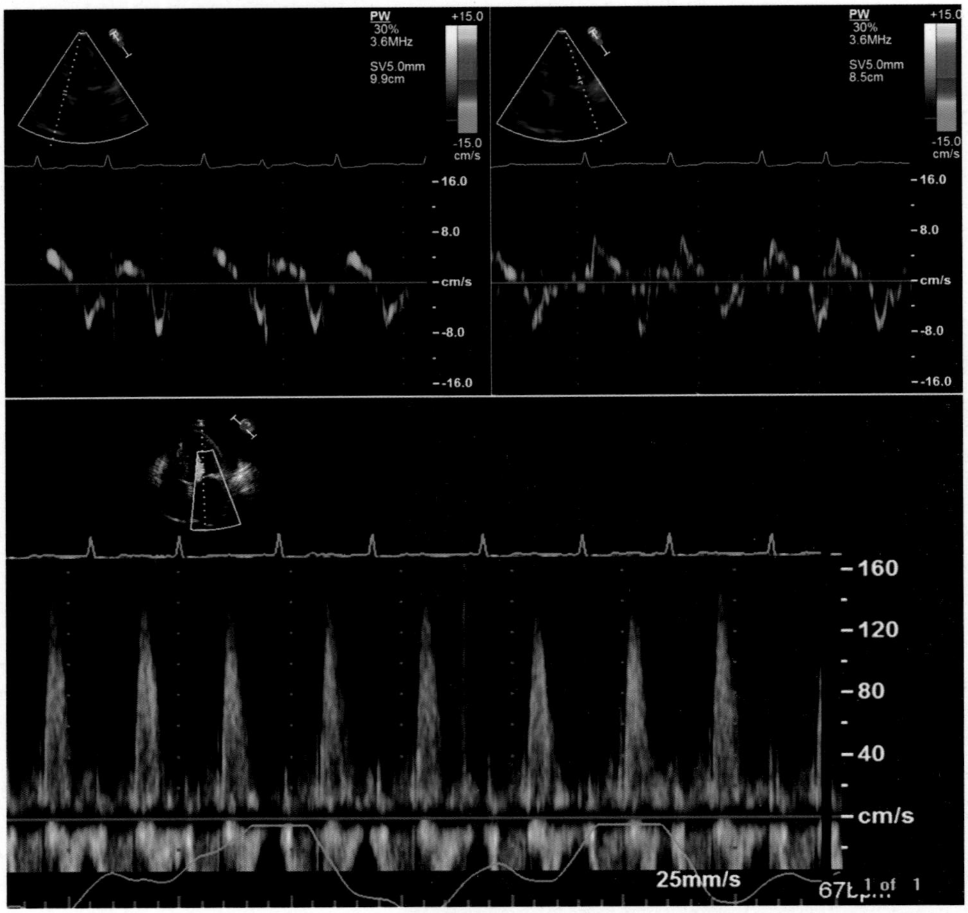

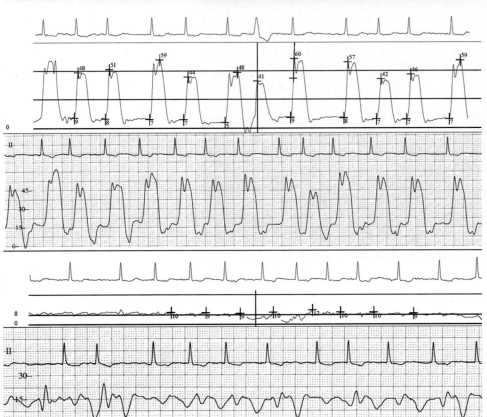

Figure 10-24. TOP, Tissue Doppler imaging. The septal and lateral annular E velocities are reduced. (This is consistent with the heart abnormality underlying the constrictive process—in this case, from the prior aortic stenosis.) BOTTOM, Left ventricular inflow. There is no decrease in the E-wave inflow in inspiration.

Figure 10-25. TOP TWO IMAGES, Right ventricular pressure before aortic valve replacement and at readmission. Before aortic valve replacement, the right ventricular systolic pressure is mildly elevated, and the diastolic pressure and waveform are unremarkable. At readmission, the right ventricular systolic pressure has not changed, but the right ventricular diastolic pressure is elevated to 15 mm Hg. The y descents are increased intermittently, presumably most obviously during inspiration. BOTTOM TWO IMAGES, Right atrial pressures before aortic valve replacement and at readmission. Before aortic valve replacement, the right atrial pressure is at the upper limit of normal, a possible reverse Bernstein effect of septal stiffness (from the left ventricular hypertrophy and aortic stenosis) reducing right ventricular compliance and raising the right atrial pressure. The contour is unrevealing. At readmission, the mean right atrial pressure is increased to 15 mm Hg and the y descent is exaggerated. There is inspiration-associated deepening of the y descent but not of the mean pressure (Kussmaul sign).

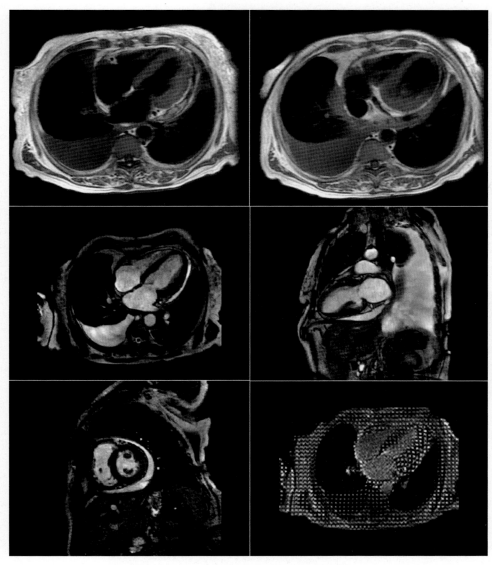

Figure 10-26. TOP, CMR T1-weighted spin echo black blood sequence. T1-weighted black blood sequences are usually the best to determine pericardial thickness. Neither image clearly shows pericardial thickening. TOP LEFT, There is normal pericardial thickness over the right ventricle and either an effusion or thickening at the base of the lateral left ventricle. TOP RIGHT, More extensive imaging of the parietal pericardium over the right ventricle. MIDDLE ROW AND BOTTOM LEFT, CMR SSFP sequences show left ventricular hypertrophy and normal systolic function. There is a small pericardial effusion located laterally to the mid left ventricular free wall. No definite pericardial thickening is seen. No early diastolic septal shift is seen. There are susceptibility or chemical shift artifacts lining the epicardial surface (fat:fluid interface especially) and the fluid:parietal pericardial interface, although there are artifacts along the fat:visceral and parietal pericardium interfaces as well. Because of the artifact, determination of pericardial thickness by SSFP is difficult. BOTTOM RIGHT, CMR tagging technique is used to determine slippage (sliding motion) of the pericardium over the heart or its absence, which is consistent with constriction. Although it is not well depicted here, there appears to be slippage where there is pericardial effusion but not where there is not.

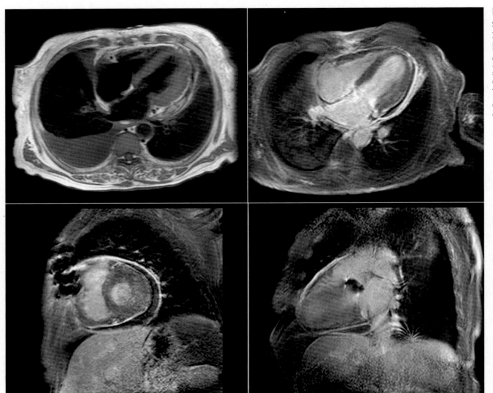

Figure 10-27. TOP LEFT, CMR T1-weighted spin echo black blood sequence. OTHER IMAGES, CMR T1-weighted spin echo black blood sequence and inversion recovery gradient echo (IRGRE) sequences. The IRGRE sequence depicts delayed gadolinium enhancement, consistent with pericarditis. There is enhancement of the pericardium, especially of the epicardium over the left ventricle.

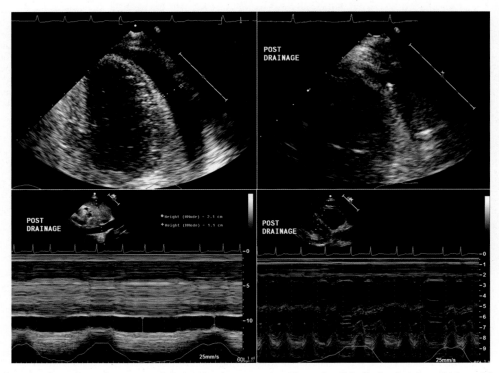

Figure 10-28. Transthoracic echocardiography. TOP LEFT, Apical 4-chamber zoom view. The pericardial effusion is 1.5 cm thick on this plane. Entry into the space is potentially possible only through a small apical window. TOP RIGHT, Pericardial fluid drainage. A small catheter has been introduced into the pericardial fluid, almost all of which has been drained to eliminate the effect of the fluid. The intrapericardial pressure was transduced and was 0 mm Hg after fluid evacuation. BOTTOM IMAGES, M-mode study of the interventricular septum after drainage. After drainage, the neck veins were clinically still elevated; the inferior vena cava remained dilated echocardiographically, and there was failure of the inferior vena cava to collapse with inspiration. There appears to be interdependence persisting after drainage.

CASE 4

History

▸ 75-year-old man 2 weeks after aortocoronary bypass
▸ Complaints include fatigue and orthopnea.

Physical Examination

▸ BP 110/70 mm Hg, 25 mm Hg pulsus paradoxus
▸ Elevated venous pressure with reduced *y* descent
▸ Kussmaul sign present
▸ Normal heart sounds; no pericardial rub or knock
▸ Imaging findings are shown in Figures 10-29 to 10-31.

Management

▸ The clinical picture was consistent with postoperative tamponade. The access to the fluid was relatively poor for percutaneous drainage, so the patient was referred for a pericardial window by the subcostal approach.
▸ However, as the right ventricle was adherent to the parietal pericardium along most of the diaphragmatic surface, the surgeon was careful to explore for apparent fluid before incising the parietal pericardium to avoid cutting the right ventricle. The procedure was uneventful and drained 600 mL of serosanguineous fluid. The echocardiographic view after drainage is shown in Figure 10-32.
▸ The arterial blood pressure and respiratory distress normalized, but the neck veins remained elevated.

Outcome

▸ The patient's exertional tolerance improved, and the elevation of the neck veins slowly normalized.
▸ Few abnormalities were found 6 weeks later.

Comments

▸ Tamponade and effuso-constrictive pericarditis. Initially, the tamponade was dominant because of a typically posterior localized pericardial effusion that presented drainage challenges.
▸ After complete drainage of the pericardial fluid and normalization of the intrapericardial pressure, there was still elevation of the right atrial pressure and findings of ventricular interdependence.
▸ Transient, self-limited course

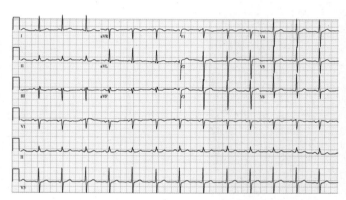

Figure 10-29. ECG shows sinus rhythm, normal voltages, and no electrical alternans. Nonspecific repolarization abnormalities are not particularly suggestive of pericarditis.

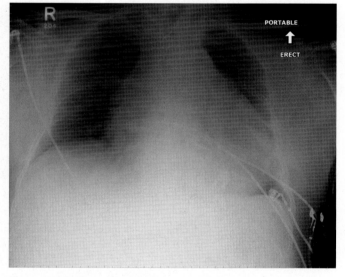

Figure 10-30. Chest radiograph shows sternal wires, cardiomegaly, and clear lung fields.

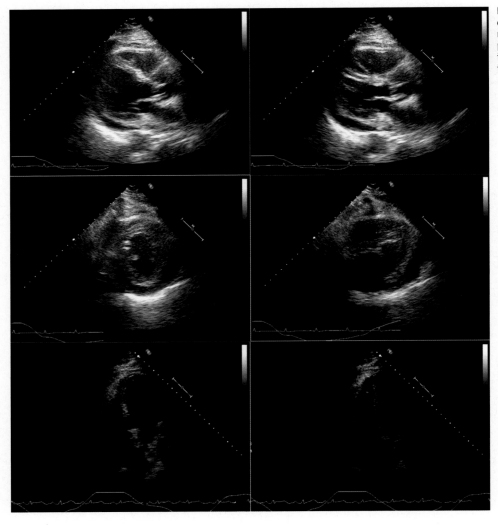

Figure 10-31. Transthoracic echocardiography views show a small to moderate-sized pericardial effusion, located posteriorly. There is a septal shift with inspiration consistent with ventricular interaction or interdependence.

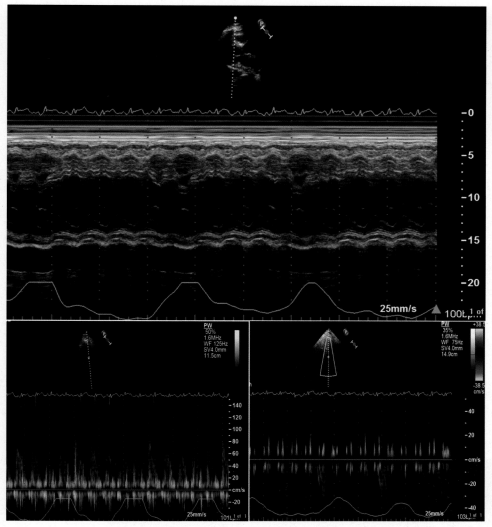

Figure 10-32. Transthoracic echocardiography after pericardial window and drainage. TOP, M-mode study of the septum; the inspiratory septal shift is still present. BOTTOM LEFT, Left ventricular inflow. The E and A waves are summated, confounding interpretation of E-wave height through the respiratory cycle. BOTTOM RIGHT, Hepatic venous Doppler study. There appears to be increased expiratory diastolic flow reversal, consistent with constrictive physiology.

CASE 5

History

▸ A 46-year-old man had increasing leg swelling during 18 months and gained 25 pounds during that period.
▸ There was no history of tuberculosis exposure, and there were no fevers or sweats.

Physical Examination

▸ Obese, BP 105/70 mm Hg, pulsus paradoxus of 20 mm Hg
▸ Markedly elevated venous pressure, with prominent y descent
▸ Presence of Kussmaul sign questionable
▸ Pericardial knock
▸ Poor air entry at both lung bases
▸ Ascites and pedal edema
▸ Imaging findings are shown in Figures 10-33 to 10-39.

Surgical and Pathologic Findings

▸ Total pericardiectomy off bypass found a minimally thickened but stiff pericardium.
▸ Fibrous thickening with focal calcification

▸ Nonspecific perivascular chronic inflammatory cell infiltrate
▸ Stains and cultures negative for tuberculosis

Outcome

▸ Postoperatively, there was resolution of the heart failure symptoms.
▸ The septal motion of interdependence improved during several months (but not immediately).

Comments

▸ Constrictive pericarditis with normal or nearly normal pericardial thickness, exemplifying the very poor correlation of pericardial thickness with constrictive effect.
▸ There was mild thickening noticed at surgery. No pericardial thickening was noticed by echocardiography (which is admittedly insensitive to thickening) or by CT scanning. CMR suggested mild thickening of the pericardium. Irrespective of the degree of thickening, the pericardium was clearly, in retrospect, responsible for the constrictive physiology.
▸ Most physiologic signs of constriction were present on examination, by imaging, and on hemodynamic study.

Text continued on p. 212.

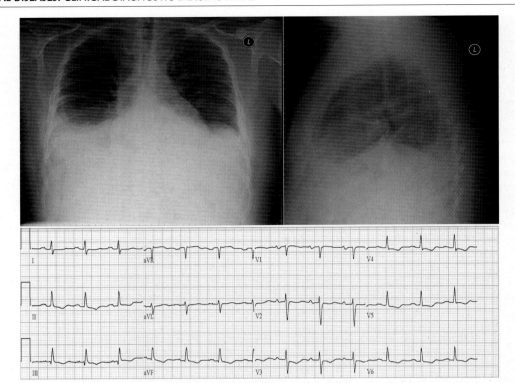

Figure 10-33. TOP, Chest radiographs show cardiomegaly, bilateral pleural effusions, clear lung fields, and possibly enlarged azygos vein. BOTTOM, ECG shows sinus rhythm, nonspecific repolarization abnormalities, and normal voltages.

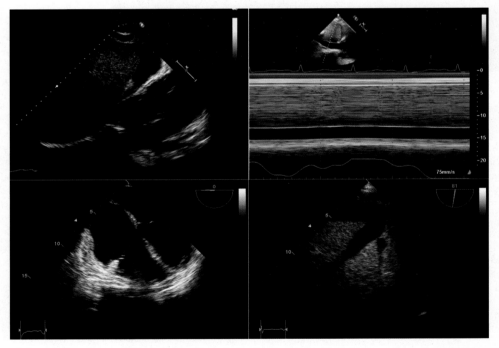

Figure 10-34. TOP LEFT, Subcostal view shows a thick rind of ascites over the liver. TOP RIGHT, The inferior vena cava is dilated through the respiratory cycle. BOTTOM LEFT, Transesophageal echocardiography image showing dilated right atrium and ventricle. The interatrial septum is shifted to the left side, suggesting right atrial > left atrial pressure. BOTTOM RIGHT, Transesophageal echocardiography view of the inferior vena cava and hepatic veins, which are dilated and full of spontaneous echo contrast, consistent with low flow.

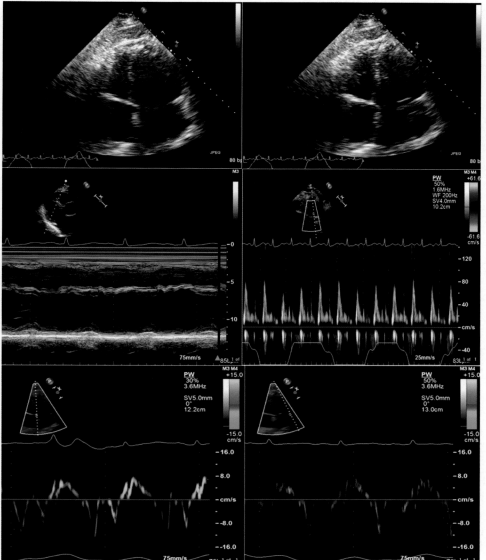

Figure 10-35. Transthoracic echocardiography. TOP IMAGES, Apical 4-chamber views revealing ventricular interaction or interdependence. With inspiration, the right ventricular dimension enlarges and the left ventricular dimension diminishes. MIDDLE LEFT, M-mode study of the septum. There is an early diastolic dip. MIDDLE RIGHT, Left ventricular inflow. Note the significant fall in left ventricular inflow velocity with inspiration (denoted by the upward deflection of the green respirometry tracing). Whether this is due to constrictive physiology or increased respiratory effort is unclear. BOTTOM IMAGES, Medial and lateral tissue Doppler studies of the mitral annulus. Normal early diastolic (E') velocities—normal myocardial relaxation.

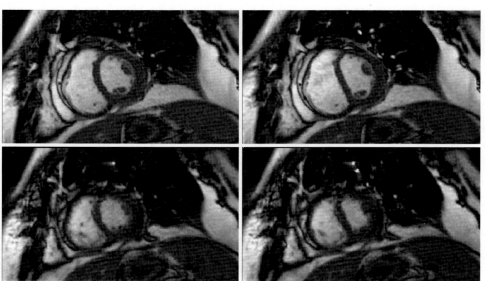

Figure 10-36. CMR SSFP short-axis views. LEFT IMAGES, End-diastole. RIGHT IMAGES, Early diastole. There is an early septal deviation—an early diastolic dip.

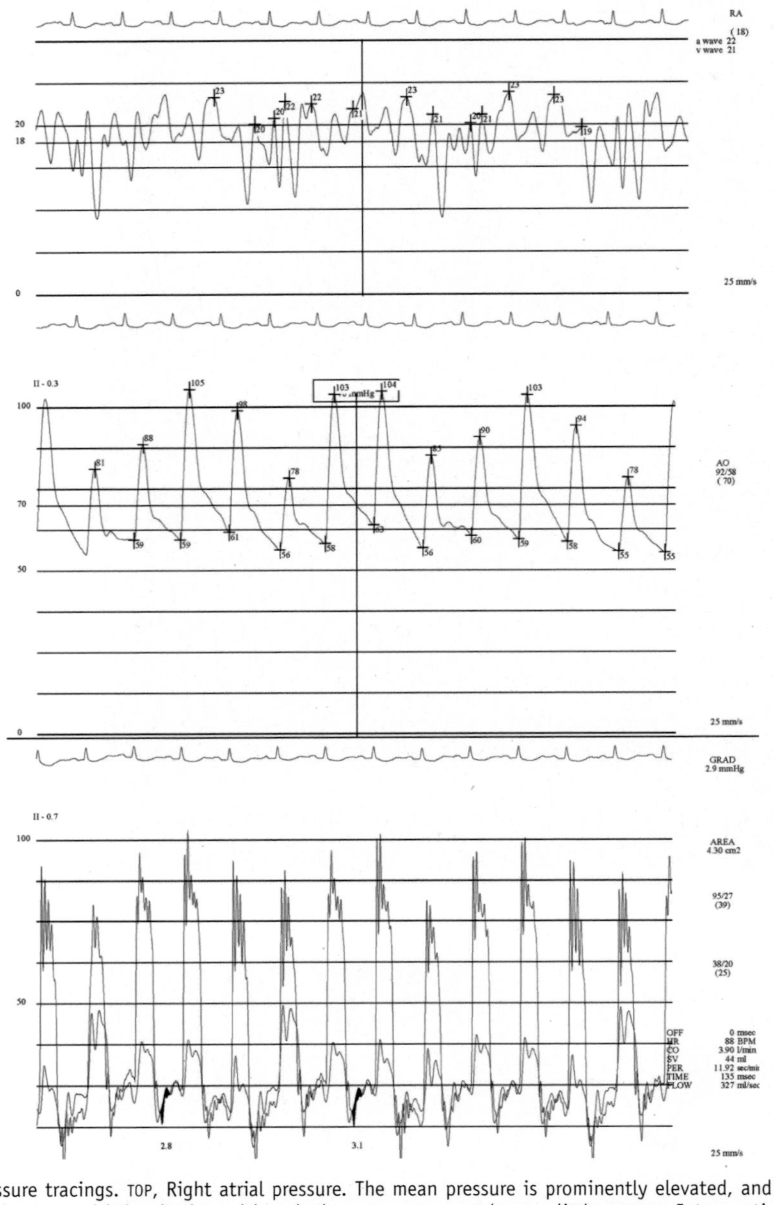

Figure 10-37. Hemodynamic pressure tracings. TOP, Right atrial pressure. The mean pressure is prominently elevated, and there are approximately equal *x* and *y* descents. These descents increase with inspiration, although the mean pressure changes little. MIDDLE, Intra-aortic pressure. There is a pulsus paradoxus—the systolic pressure and pulse pressure fall in inspiration. BOTTOM, Simultaneous left and right ventricular pressure tracings. Discordance of pressure changes is present, indicative of ventricular interdependence.

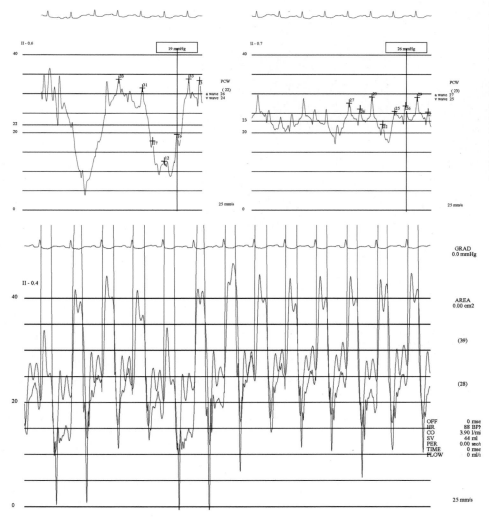

Figure 10-38. Hemodynamics. TOP, Pulmonary capillary wedge pressures with spontaneous inspirations (LEFT) and with breath-hold (RIGHT). The mean pressure is elevated, and there is a very prominent fall in pressure with inspiration. The inspiratory fall in pressure is due to an increase in pulmonary venous capacitance with inspiration. BOTTOM, Simultaneous pulmonary venous wedge pressure and left ventricular pressure tracings. With inspiration, both pressures fall, but the pulmonary capillary pressure falls more, resulting in an increase in the "wedge"–left ventricular gradient (>5 mm), a sign of constriction.

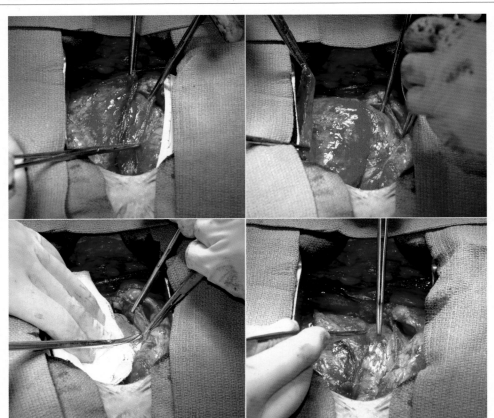

Figure 10-39. Surgical findings. TOP LEFT, The parietal pericardium has been incised and the free edges are being held upward; it is only minimally thickened. TOP RIGHT, The parietal pericardium has been mobilized without difficulty. It is about 2 mm thick. BOTTOM LEFT, The epicardial fat layer can be seen underneath the resected parietal pericardium, which is being dissected away from the underlying heart. BOTTOM RIGHT, The epicardial fat layer can be seen underneath the resected parietal pericardium.

CASE 6

History

A 22-year-old man presented with 10 weeks of leg swelling, worsening dyspnea, and intermittent fevers. He had a positive tuberculosis contact and pulmonary tuberculosis was initially suspected, but results of bronchoscopy proved negative for isolation of tuberculosis organisms.

Physical Examination

▸ Tachypneic, distressed, HR 120 bpm, BP 95/50 mm Hg, pulsus paradoxus of 25 mm Hg
▸ Markedly elevated venous pressure, with prominent *x* and *y* descents (Fig. 10-40)
▸ Presence of Kussmaul sign questionable
▸ No pericardial knock or rub
▸ Pedal edema, ascites, marked scrotal edema. Body weight was 18 kg higher than usual.
▸ Chest radiograph, ECG, and echocardiographic findings are shown in Figures 10-41 to 10-45.

Management

▸ Pericardial biopsy was performed through thoracotomy because results of bronchoscopy and other attempts to isolate tuberculosis

organisms were negative; pathologic findings are shown in Figure 10-46.
▸ At surgery, the pericardium was found to be more than 1 cm thick.

Management and Outcome

▸ A presumed diagnosis of tuberculous constrictive pericarditis (± pleurisy), given the granulomas but lack of acid-fast bacilli or culture positivity. He was started on antituberculous treatment.
▸ Diuresis was well tolerated; renal function improved with diuresis. Progressive and sustained improvement of dyspnea and functional tolerance
▸ The diuretic dose (initially 180 mg furosemide/day) was tapered to 0 mg. NYHA functional class became class I, and the patient resumed athletic activities, without impairment.

Comments

▸ Presumed tuberculous constrictive pericarditis in a young man
▸ Dramatic and progressive ongoing improvement in physical findings and functional class after institution of antituberculous antimicrobials and diuretics
▸ The clinical status continued to improve and fully normalize without surgery.
▸ Follow-up CT scanning showed that the pericardial thickness was virtually normalized.

Text continued on p. 217.

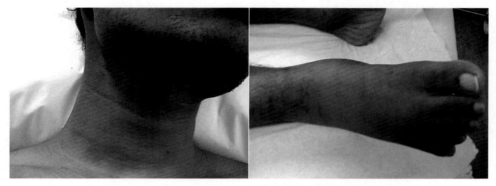

Figure 10-40. LEFT, Jugular venous distention to the angle of the jaw, with exaggerated and equal *x* and *y* descents. RIGHT, Foot and ankle swelling with pitting edema. The scrotum was enormously swollen as well.

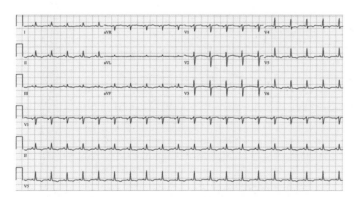

Figure 10-41. ECG shows sinus tachycardia, nonspecific repolarization abnormalities, borderline low limb lead voltages, and atrial abnormality.

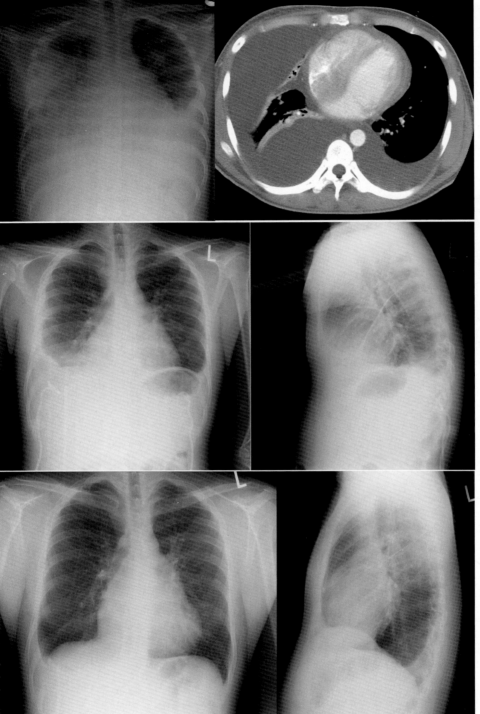

Figure 10-42. TOP LEFT, The chest radiograph at presentation shows cardiomegaly, bilateral pleural effusions, vascular engorgement, and left upper lobe airspace disease. TOP RIGHT, Cardiomegaly, pericardial thickening (versus fluid), and bilateral pleural effusions. The pericardial thickening probably explains the low voltages on the ECG. MIDDLE IMAGES, Chest drains inserted. LOWER IMAGES, After pleural drains and diuresis.

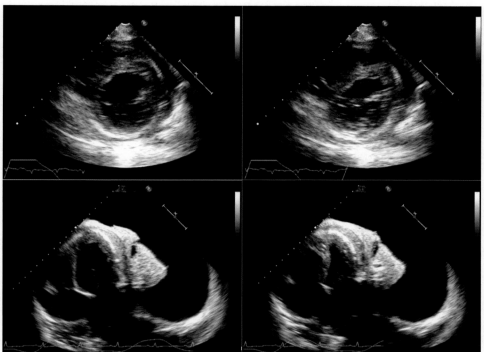

Figure 10-43. Transthoracic echocardiography images during expiration (LEFT IMAGES) and during inspiration (RIGHT IMAGES). There is a prominent inspiratory septal shift. The large left pleural effusion affords an unusual means to visualize the pericardial thickening, which is at least as great as the myocardial thickness. Atelectatic left lung is adjacent to the heart.

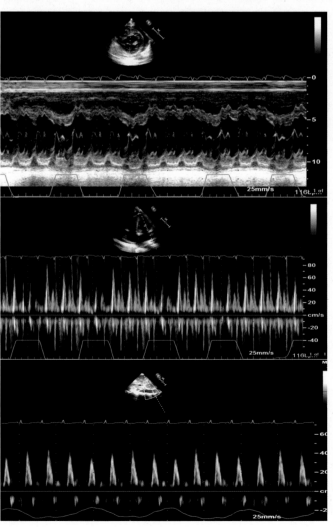

Figure 10-44. Transthoracic echocardiography. TOP, M-mode study of the interventricular septum. Early diastolic dip and septal bounce or shift with inspiration (note respirometry tracing) consistent with ventricular interaction or interdependence—increase in the right ventricular dimension and decrease in the left ventricular dimension at inspiration. MIDDLE, Left ventricular inflow. Significant fall in left ventricular inflow early diastolic velocity with inspiration (denoted by the upward deflection of the respirometry tracing). BOTTOM, Abdominal aortic flow spectral profiles. There are respiratory variations in the abdominal aortic peak velocity—the velocity falls with inspiration. This is likely to be the manifestation of ventricular interdependence rather than of increased respiratory effort.

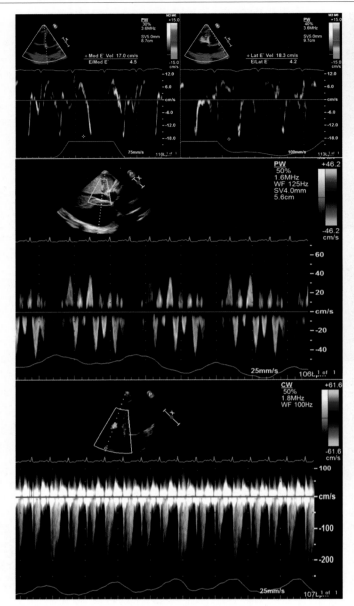

Figure 10-45. Transthoracic echocardiography. TOP, Mitral annular tissue Doppler study. Normal myocardial relaxation (E' velocity). MIDDLE, Hepatic venous flow spectral profiles. Note the augmented reversal of expiratory hepatic vein diastolic flow, consistent with constrictive physiology. BOTTOM, Tricuspid regurgitation spectral profiles. Note the significant increase in tricuspid regurgitation velocity with inspiration.

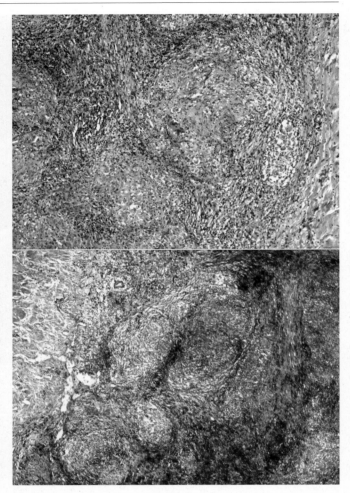

Figure 10-46. Pericardial histopathologic findings. TOP, Large granulomas with giant cells, central necrotic debris, and lymphocytic infiltration. BOTTOM, Higher magnification view: granuloma with giant cells, lymphocytic infiltration, and central necrotic debris. (Courtesy of Ashok Mukherjee, MD, Scarborough, Canada.)

CASE 7

History

A 50-year-old man with renal failure developed pericardial tamponade. There were no symptoms of pericarditis. Pericardial drainage was very difficult; although the introducer needle could be advanced into the pericardial space, the dilator could not be passed through the parietal pericardium over the guide wire, despite attempts from different puncture sites. Despite drainage of 650 mL through the introducer needle, the venous pressures remained elevated, with exaggerated descents. There was no pulsus paradoxus. Echocardiographic findings are shown in Figures 10-47 and 10-48.

Management

The patient underwent surgical resection of the parietal pericardium (pericardiectomy) and débridement of the thickened serosal pericardium.

10

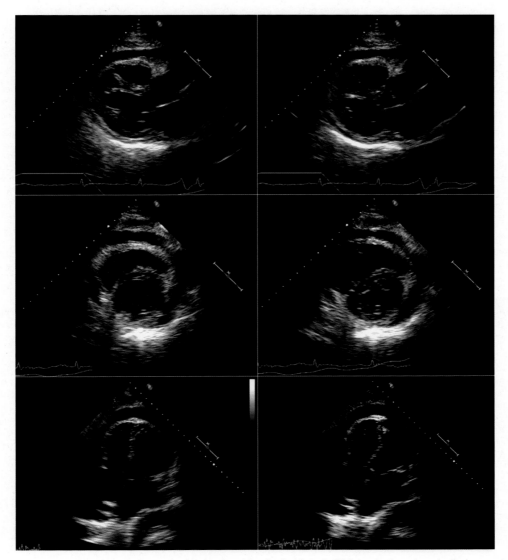

Figure 10-47. TOP, Parasternal long-axis views during expiration (LEFT) and inspiration (RIGHT). With inspiration, there is displacement of the interventricular septum toward the left side of the heart. MIDDLE, Parasternal short-axis views during expiration (LEFT) and inspiration (RIGHT). With inspiration, there is shift of the interventricular septum to the left side of the heart. BOTTOM, Apical 4-chamber views during expiration (LEFT) and inspiration (RIGHT). With inspiration, the interventricular septum shifts to the left side of the heart.

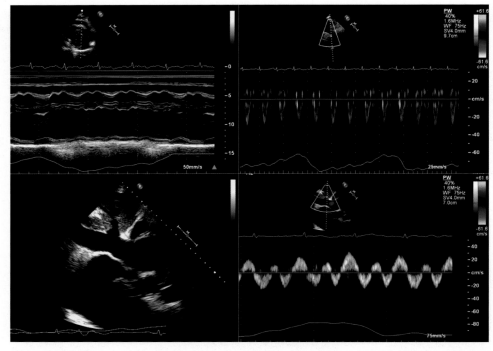

Figure 10-48. TOP LEFT, M-mode study through the interventricular septum. TOP RIGHT, Spectral profiles of descending aorta flow. There is little respiratory variation, akin to the lack of a recorded pulsus paradoxus. BOTTOM LEFT, Subcostal view. The inferior vena cava and hepatic veins are grossly dilated, consistent with elevated central venous pressure. BOTTOM RIGHT, Spectral display of pulsed wave recording of hepatic venous flow. With expiration (descent of respirometry tracing), there is augmentation of hepatic venous diastolic flow reversal.

CASE 8

History

An 18-year-old man was noted to have a large pericardial effusion on a chest CT scan. Three weeks previously, he had been stabbed in the chest and abdomen and undergone laparotomy and bilateral thoracotomies. The heart had been inspected and was not injured from the knife trauma. The CT scan had been ordered "pre-discharge."

Physical Examination

‣ BP 90/60 mm Hg, pulsus paradoxus of 20 mm Hg; HR 105 bpm
‣ Venous pressures were markedly elevated, with prominent descents, $y > x$.
‣ Kussmaul sign was present.
‣ There was edema to the knees.
‣ No pericardial knock or rub was present.
‣ Numerous parameters of hepatic dysfunction were present.
‣ His exertional tolerance was limited to walking 100 feet, and if rushing, he developed presyncope.

Management

‣ Given the clinical and echocardiographic signs of cardiac compression (Figs. 10-49 to 10-52) and secondary hepatic dysfunction (congestive), the patient was referred for surgical drainage of the pericardial fluid and resection of the pericardium (pericardiectomy) if the pericardium was found to be thickened.

‣ Surgical findings included 800 mL of red-black fluid under high pressure as well as a thickened and stiff (5 to 10 mm) parietal pericardium and thickened serosal pericardium.
‣ Pericardiectomy was performed (Fig. 10-53).

Outcome

‣ Rapid convalescence, large improvement in exertional tolerance within 3 days of the operation
‣ Despite the serosal pericardial thickening, the venous pressures were only mildly elevated, with equal and not prominent descents.
‣ The pulsus paradoxus and Kussmaul sign were eliminated by the pericardiectomy.

Comments

‣ Postpericardiotomy effuso-constrictive pericarditis developing within 3 weeks
‣ Clinical (Kussmaul sign and dominant y descent) and echocardiographic (early diastolic dip, prominent ventricular interdependence) signs pointed to a constriction component of the pathophysiologic process, in addition to the obvious tamponade compression.
‣ Transthoracic echocardiography did not give a hint of how thickened either layer of the pericardium actually was.
‣ Most of the compressive syndrome was caused by the parietal pericardium and pericardial fluid, as drainage and parietal pericardiectomy virtually normalized the filling pressures and pattern—effuso-constrictive pericarditis.

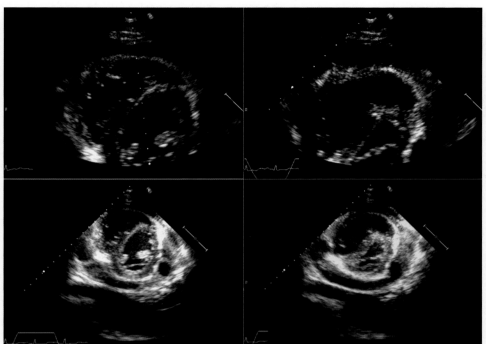

Figure 10-49. Transthoracic echocardiography. Parasternal short-axis views during expiration (LEFT IMAGES) and during the first cardiac cycle of inspiration (RIGHT IMAGES). A pericardial effusion of a moderate size is present. With inspiration (note respirometry tracing), there is obvious shift of the interventricular septum to the left side, consistent with ventricular interdependence. Neither the parietal nor serosal pericardium appears abnormal.

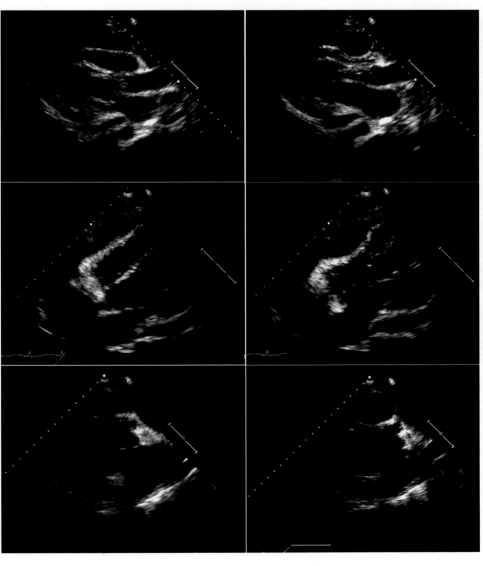

Figure 10-50. Transthoracic echocardiography. TOP, Parasternal long-axis views in systole (LEFT) and diastole (RIGHT). There is a pericardial effusion, more anteriorly than posteriorly located, with fibrinous strands. There is diastolic collapse of the right ventricular outflow tract. MIDDLE, Off-axis apical 4-chamber views in systole (LEFT) and diastole (RIGHT). There is prominent diastolic collapse of the lateral right ventricular free wall. BOTTOM, Right ventricular inflow views in systole (LEFT) and diastole (RIGHT). There is prominent diastolic collapse of the anterior right ventricular free wall.

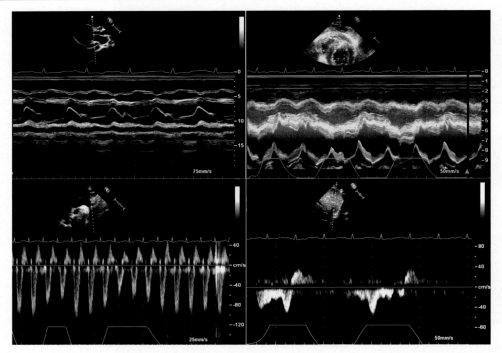

Figure 10-51. Transthoracic echocardiography. TOP LEFT, M-mode study through the septum, parasternal long-axis view. An anterior and posterior pericardial effusion is present, and there is right ventricular (outflow tract) diastolic collapse. TOP RIGHT, M-mode study through the septum, shallow parasternal short-axis view. Note the respirometry tracing. With inspiration, there is a prominent displacement of the interventricular septum posteriorly into the left ventricle, consistent with ventricular interdependence. As well, there is an "early diastolic dip" of the septum, consistent with briefly reversed early diastolic left and right ventricular pressures, a finding consistent with pericardial constriction. BOTTOM LEFT, Spectral Doppler display of flow in the descending aorta. Note the respirometry tracing. With inspiration, there is a nearly 50% fall in the flow velocity in the proximal descending aorta. BOTTOM RIGHT, Spectral Doppler display of hepatic venous flow. At end-inspiration–expiration, there is augmented diastolic flow reversal, a finding consistent with constriction.

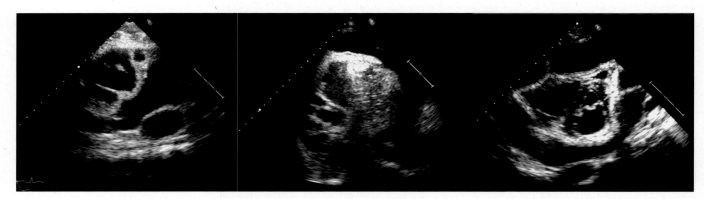

Figure 10-52. Transthoracic echocardiography. LEFT, High right parasternal view of the superior vena cava, which is compressed by pericardial fluid. There is loculation of the pericardial fluid. MIDDLE, Off-axis apical view of the pericardial fluid, revealing prominent stranding in some areas. RIGHT, Parasternal short-axis view demonstrating collapse of the right ventricular free wall and stranding or loculation.

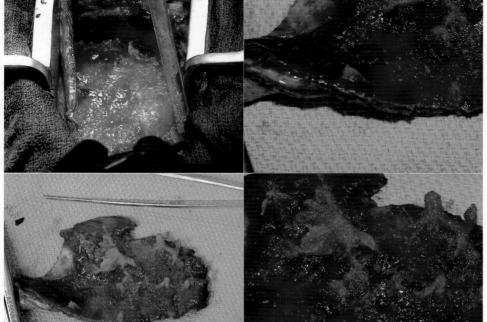

Figure 10-53. Surgical findings. TOP, View into the surgically opened chest. The anterior parietal pericardium has been resected; a free edge of it is seen on the left side of the images, retracted open. Its free edge is 7 mm thick. The serosal pericardium is thickened with stiff plastic-like fibrosis that has a highly irregular surface. OTHER IMAGES, The resected parietal pericardium is thick, is stiff (does not lie flat), and has the same irregular fibrotic surface on the underside. Despite the roughness of the layers of the pericardium, no "friction rub" was heard.

References

1. Talreja DR, Edwards WD, Danielson GK, et al: Constrictive pericarditis in 26 patients with histologically normal pericardial thickness. Circulation 2003;108:1852-1857.

2. Haley JH, Tajik AJ, Danielson GK: Transient constrictive pericarditis: causes and natural history. J Am Coll Cardiol 2004;43:271-275.

3. Tom CW, Oh JK: Images in cardiovascular medicine: a case of transient constrictive pericarditis. Circulation 2005;111:364.

4. Sagristà-Sauleda J, Angel J, Sánchez A, et al: Effusive-constrictive pericarditis. N Engl J Med 2004;350:469-475.

5. Thomas WJ, Steiman DM, Kovach JA, et al: Doppler echocardiography and hemodynamic findings in localized pericardial constriction. Am Heart J 1996;131:599-603.

6. Killian DM, Furiasse JG, Scanlon PJ: Constrictive pericarditis after cardiac surgery. Am Heart J 1989;118:563-568.

11

Congenital Absence of the Pericardium

Congenital absence of the parietal pericardium may be partial or complete absence of either the left or right side of the parietal pericardium. The most commonly described findings are representative of the most common form—partial left-sided absence. Other developmental abnormalities are associated in about a third of all cases, more likely in association with complete left-sided absence, and include patent ductus arteriosus, atrial septal defect, mitral stenosis, tetralogy of Fallot, bronchogenic cysts, pulmonary sequestration, and tricuspid insufficiency.[1] The incidence of congenital absence of the pericardium is approximately 0.01%.[1-4] The findings of congenital absence of the pericardium are naturally occurring examples of some of the anatomic features and functions of the pericardium.

The location of congenital absence has been variable in different series, but deficiency of the left side is most commonly described. Table 11-1 lists the percentages reported by the largest case series published to date (153 cases).[5]

Absence of the anterior pericardium and bilateral complete absence have also been described.[3] Most pericardial defects are pleuropericardial. Rarely, pericardial defects are pericardioperitoneal through the diaphragmatic pericardium and are always associated with other midline chest and abdominal malformations.[6]

The etiology of congenital absence of pericardium is unknown, but it is proposed to be premature involution of the left duct of Cuvier, compromising the blood supply to the developing pleuropericardial membrane and resulting in a defect.[1] There is male predominance (3:1 or 3:2).[3,6,7]

The particular findings will depend on the site of absence of the pericardium and the extent of absence of the pericardium. By any form of imaging, typical features of congenital absence of the pericardium (partial or complete left sided or complete) include levocardia (leftward displacement of the heart) without displacement of the trachea, a "tongue" of lung parenchyma interposed between the aorta and the main pulmonary artery where pericardium normally excludes lung parenchyma,[4] lung parenchyma interposed between the left inferior heart and the diaphragm (again where pericardium normally excludes lung parenchyma), and prominence of the main pulmonary artery.

CLINICAL PRESENTATION

Abnormal physical diagnostic findings include a systolic ejection murmur grade 1-2/6 at the left upper sternal border, sometimes leading to confusion with an atrial septal defect or pulmonic stenosis, and a systolic click and late systolic murmur, sometimes leading to confusion with mitral valve prolapse. Abnormalities may be detected on electrocardiography (ECG), chest radiography, echocardiography, computed tomography (CT), or cardiac magnetic resonance (CMR). It can also be an incidental finding at the time of sternotomy, thoracotomy, or necropsy. Chest pain may also be a presenting sign and is usually sharp, frequently positional, and seldom exertional. It is believed that lack of restraint of the heart's displacement in the chest underlies the pains, which are typically common and aggravated by certain body positions that result in displacement and possibly torsion.

Chest pain and death as complications of incarceration of the left atrial appendage or left ventricle through partial absence of the left pericardium have been reported.[8] Myocardial ischemia[7] and infarction[9] may occur secondary to compression of a coronary artery by the rim of the absent pericardium,[6] which may be provoked to demonstrate ischemia by postural body position changes,[7] or be due to frank torsion of a coronary artery within the incarcerated left side of the heart.

Commonly mistaken pathologic processes, on the basis of chest radiography, include pulmonic stenosis, idiopathic dilation of the pulmonary artery, atrial septal defect, cardiac tumor, mitral valve disease, left ventricular aneurysm, left hilar adenopathy, aneurysms of the left atrial appendage, mediastinal tumors, and bronchogenic carcinoma.[10]

DIAGNOSTIC TESTING

Absence of the pericardium typically confers abnormalities seen on most forms of imaging, although this is not to say that most imaging modalities can make the specific diagnosis with a high level of accuracy. Diagnostic testing is still incapable of confidently imaging the presence or absence of the pericardium throughout its complete normal anatomic extent; therefore, imaging seeks to identify findings that infer the absence of the pericardium rather than to identify the anatomic absence of pericardium. Adjacent fat planes are needed on both sides of the parietal pericardium to visually "offset" it from the myocardium.

Table 11-1. The Location of Congenital Absence of the Pericardium in a Series of 153 Cases

Type of Absence	Percentage
Total absence	9%
Left sided, partial	35%
Left sided, total	35%
Right sided, partial	4%
Right sided, total	0%
Diaphragmatic pericardial aplasia	17%

From Saint-Pierre A, Froment R: Total and partial absence of pericardium. Arch Mal Coeur Vaiss 1970;63:638-657. Copyright Elsevier, 1970.

The lack of sufficient fat over extensive areas of the left side of the heart renders identification of the parietal pericardium over the left side of the heart very challenging and often impossible. The parietal pericardium has an attenuation coefficient similar to that of myocardium on CT scanning and similar relaxation characteristics on CMR; therefore, the parietal pericardium cannot be distinguished from the myocardium where the two are directly adjacent.

ECG and echocardiography are generally abnormal in the presence of congenital absence of the pericardium, but with nonspecific findings. Apparent right ventricular volume overload findings are seen on echocardiography, which normalize with surgical repair. Whether there is right-sided heart volume overload is unclear; abnormal orientation of the heart may be responsible for the findings. The chest radiograph is very useful, and some findings, if present, appear to be accurate. CMR is also very useful but should not be held to image pericardial defects; rather, it identifies findings consistent with absence of the pericardium.

Chest Radiography

The chest radiograph is a very useful test to suggest absence of the pericardium (Figs. 11-1 to 11-3; Table 11-2).

Electrocardiography

ECG findings include right axis deviation (seen in 40%), right bundle branch block (seen in 60%), and leftward displacement of the R-wave transition in the precordial leads (seen in 40%).[4] None of these findings is specific for absence of the pericardium, alone or in combination, and their sensitivity is poor.

Echocardiography

Echocardiography findings include left lateral displacement of the heart/leftward acoustic "windows," apparent right ventricle dilation, and flat or paradoxical septal motion.[4,7] Echocardiography cannot delineate pericardium and therefore cannot establish

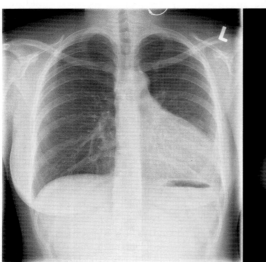
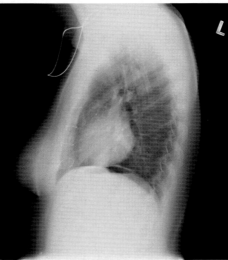

Figure 11-1. The levoposition of the heart, the absence of the right-sided heart border, and the lung tissue under the left ventricle and above the dome of the left hemidiaphragm are represented in this figure. Although there was a repair of the absence of the left pericardium, there is still a more prominent space between the main pulmonary artery and the aorta than is usual, and the levoposition has persisted. (Courtesy of Erwin Oechslin, MD, Toronto, Canada.)

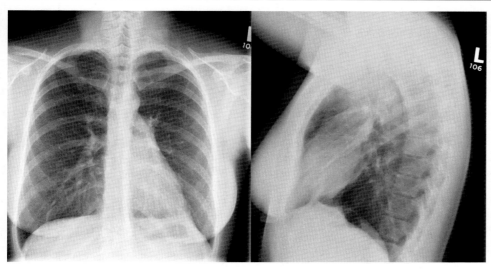

Figure 11-2. The slight levoposition of the heart, the absence of the right-sided heart border, and the lung tissue between the left ventricle and the left hemidiaphragmatic dome are represented in this figure. (Courtesy of Erwin Oechslin, MD, Toronto, Canada.)

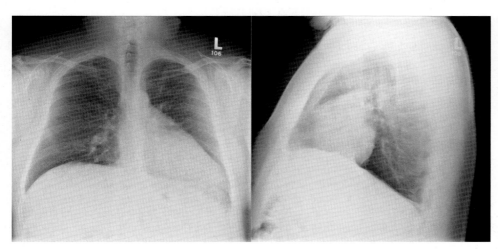

Figure 11-3. The levoposition of the heart, the absence of the right-sided heart border, and the prominence of the main pulmonary artery are represented in this figure. There is no lung parenchyma under the left ventricle and over the left dome of the diaphragm. (Courtesy of Erwin Oechslin, MD, Toronto, Canada.)

Table 11-2. Chest Radiography Findings of Congenital Absence of the Pericardium

Sign	Incidence	Notes
Levoposition of the heart	63%	Leftward displacement of the heart occurs because of absence of restraint from left-sided pericardium (partial left sided, complete left sided, or complete).
Loss of right-sided heart border	63%	Loss of the right-sided heart border occurs because it is superimposed on the shadow of the spine.
Irregular left-sided heart border	70%	
Prominence of main pulmonary artery	95%	The main pulmonary artery is more prominent on the posteroanterior film as it is displaced to the left side of the chest and demarcated by the tongue of air between it and the aorta.
A protruding left atrial appendage	33%	This suggests left atrial extrusion through a defect but is not specific and may be seen with aneurysmal left atrial appendage.
Lung interposed between the main pulmonary artery and aorta	78%	A tongue of lung parenchyma is interposed between the aortic arch and the main pulmonary artery—an illustration of how this anatomic recess is normally intrapericardial and excluding of lung tissue.
Lung interposed between heart and diaphragm	43%	Lung tissue is interposed between the left hemidiaphragmatic dome and the diaphragmatic surface of the heart—another example of how this anatomic recess is normally intrapericardial and excluding of lung tissue.

absence of pericardium. Echocardiography may identify findings consistent with absence of the pericardium, but such findings are neither sensitive nor specific. The actual contribution of echocardiography is not to identify absence of the pericardium but to identify or to exclude other lesions that may be responsible for the physical diagnosis findings.

Computed Tomography

CT scanning is useful to determine the presence of aerated lung tissue between the main pulmonary artery and the aorta and what would otherwise be the pericardial space between the left ventricle and the diaphragm (Fig. 11-4). It has not yet been established whether gated cardiac CT can determine the completeness or incompleteness of pericardial continuity.

Cardiac Magnetic Resonance

Useful CMR sequences include ECG-gated T1-weighted spin echo "black blood" sequences and ECG-gated steady-state free precession (SSFP) cine CMR imaging. CMR, as the preeminent form of cardiac imaging, is actually limited in its ability to depict the pericardium in its entire extent around the heart. Therefore, imaging absence of the pericardium, particularly over the left side of the heart where sufficient fat to offset the parietal pericardium is often absent, is at the least challenging and often realistically impossible. Hence, CMR uses many indirect findings to infer the absence of pericardium rather than to image the absence of pericardium. T1-weighted imaging depicts the parietal pericardium as a dark stripe between high signal fat layers. SSFP imaging is an excellent means to depict chamber shape, size, and function. CMR findings consistent with absence of the pericardium are listed in Table 11-3.[4]

TREATMENT

The treatment of absence of the pericardium is discretionary and based on assessment of the risk and perceived benefit. Asymptomatic cases are left as is. Severely symptomatic cases have undergone surgical treatment with good outcome and follow-up. Rare cases of believed true atrial appendage incarceration typically undergo surgery, although not all cases are found to be absence of the pericardium at the time of surgery.

Complete absence of the pericardium seldom requires treatment because there is no risk of incarceration. Surgical pericardiectomy establishes that complete absence of the pericardium is physiologically viable. Positional pains that are attributable to undue motion of the heart within the chest may prompt surgery to attach the heart more securely to the chest wall. Surgical options include reconstruction (porcine or Gore-Tex) to reduce the motion of the heart and to obviate the risk of incarceration and pericardiectomy to obviate the risk of incarceration.

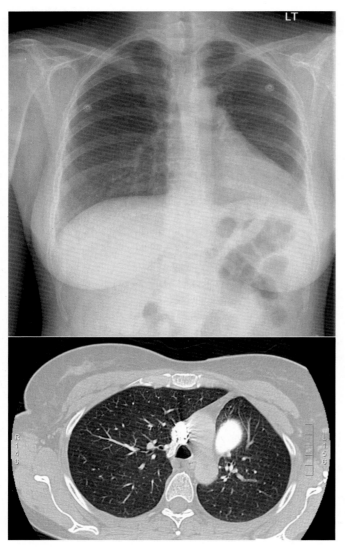

Figure 11-4. A chest radiograph (TOP) and a CT image (BOTTOM) showing congenital absence of the pericardium. (Courtesy of Rachel Wald, MD, Toronto, Canada.)

Table 11-3. Cardiac Magnetic Resonance Findings Consistent with Absence of the Pericardium

Displacement ("falling") of the heart into the left hemithorax

Displacement of the main pulmonary artery and left atrial appendage beyond the margins of the mediastinum

A tongue of lung parenchyma interposed between the aortic arch and the main pulmonary artery (an example and an illustration of how this anatomic recess is normally intrapericardial and excluding of lung tissue)

An irregular left-sided heart border, a protruding left atrial appendage

Interposed lung tissue between the left hemidiaphragmatic dome and the diaphragmatic surface of the heart (again, an example and an illustration of how this anatomic recess is normally intrapericardial and excluding of lung tissue)

An elevated apex

Left myocardial crease

From Gatzoulis MA, Munk MD, Merchant N, et al: Isolated congenital absence of the pericardium: clinical presentation, diagnosis, and management. Ann Thorac Surg 2000;69:1209-1215. Copyright Elsevier, 2000.

References

1. Nasser WK, Helmen C, Tavel ME, et al: Congenital absence of the left pericardium: clinical, electrocardiographic, radiographic, hemodynamic, and angiographic findings in six cases. Circulation 1970;41:469-478.

2. Southworth H, Stevenson CS: Congenital defects of the pericardium. Arch Intern Med 1938;61:223-240.

3. Van Son JA, Danielson GK, Schaff HV, et al: Congenital partial and complete absence of the pericardium. Mayo Clin Proc 1993;68:743-747.

4. Gatzoulis MA, Munk MD, Merchant N, et al: Isolated congenital absence of the pericardium: clinical presentation, diagnosis, and management. Ann Thorac Surg 2000;69:1209-1215.

5. Saint-Pierre A, Froment R: Total and partial absence of pericardium. Arch Mal Coeur Vaiss 1970;63:638-657.

6. Nasser WK: Congenital diseases of the pericardium. Cardiovasc Clin 1976;7:271-286.

7. Larsen RL, Behar VS, Brazer SR, et al: Chest pain presenting as ischemic heart disease: congenital absence of the pericardium. N C Med J 1994;55:306-308.

8. Robin E, Ganguly SN, Fowler MS: Strangulation of the left atrial appendage through a congenital partial pericardial defect. Chest 1975;67:354-355.

9. Saito R, Hotta F: Congenital pericardial defect associated with cardiac incarceration: case report. Am Heart J 1980;100:866-870.

10. Payvandi MN, Kerber RE: Echocardiography in congenital and acquired absence of the pericardium. An echocardiographic mimic of right ventricular volume overload. Circulation 1976;53:86-92.

11

Pericardial Cysts

KEY POINTS

▸ Pericardial cysts represent approximately 5% of thoracic cysts.

▸ Pericardial cysts are located at the right cardiophrenic angle in 70% of cases, at the left cardiophrenic angle in 20%, in the superior mediastinum in 5%, and in the posterior mediastinum in 5%.

▸ Pericardial cysts are often first detected as incidental findings on chest radiography or CT.

▸ Transthoracic echocardiography, although able to detect fluid in cysts, is limited in its value for cyst imaging because not all cysts abut the chest wall, and interposed lungs obscure visualization.

▸ CMR is a far more robust modality to image cysts irrespective of their location and to establish their fluid-filled nature.

▸ CT is a critical component of evaluation to exclude signs of potential malignancy or infection elsewhere.

▸ Treatment is individualized and discretionary.

Pericardial cysts are uncommon mass lesions located beside midline structures in the chest. In 70% of cases, pericardial cysts are located at the right cardiophrenic angle; in 20% of cases, at the left cardiophrenic angle; in 5% of cases, in the superior mediastinum; and in another 5% of cases, in the posterior mediastinum.[1] The predominance of right versus left cardiophrenic angle pericardial cysts is 3 or 4:1. Absence of contact with the pericardium and diaphragm is uncommon.[2] There is a male:female predominance of 3:2. Most pericardial cysts are detected in the fourth decade of life.[3]

The etiology of pericardial cysts is unknown but presumed to be defective embryologic development of the pericardium. Hence, pericardial cysts are said to be congenital; however, rarely they may be acquired, and they have been observed to grow.[2] During embryologic development, the pericardial cavity occupies a large extent of the thorax; hence, residual pericardial tissue that may result in cysts may be found away from the usual position of the heart.

Pericardial cysts are thin walled and lined by a monolayer of serosal cells and contain a notably clear fluid.[4] Other names for pericardial cysts reflect the embryology, similarities, and fluid characteristics of pericardial cysts. These include hydrocele of the mediastinum, serosal cyst, "spring water" cyst, "clear water" cyst, pleuropericardial cyst, pericardial coelomic cysts, mesothelial mediastinal cysts,[4] and pericardial diverticulum.[3] Confusion arises with the term and entity of pericardial diverticulum, which is held to be a different lesion.[3]

The large majority of pericardial cysts are unilocular. Imaging of an incomplete septum may confer the appearance of complete septation if the septum is not well detailed. Similarly, imaging of a fold may engender the appearance of septation. Rarely, pericardial cysts are truly multilocular or multiple (Fig. 12-1).

The initial differential diagnosis of a pericardial cyst includes the many forms of solid tissue mass lesions, but echocardiographic and cardiac magnetic resonance (CMR) imaging are useful to establish that the lesion is fluid filled or cystic rather than benign solid tissue and limits the differential to that of cystic lesions of the chest. Before echocardiography and CMR, many cysts directly underwent attempted aspiration or surgical exploration. Pericardial cysts represent approximately 5% of thoracic cysts.[4,5]

Most primary cystic tumors within the heart are pericardial cysts (McAllister/Armed Forces Institute of Pathology: pericardial cysts, 15.4% of primary cardiac and pericardial tumors, versus bronchogenic cysts, 1.3%).[1] Pancreatic pseudocysts may extend into the thorax beside the heart. A Morgagni-type hernia may easily be confused with a pericardial cyst as it lies at the diaphragm. Some malignant tumors are cystic or may generate contained effusion.

Because most pericardial cysts are located at the cardiodiaphragmatic angle, adjacent to the heart, and few other cystic lesions commonly are, the diagnosis of a pericardial cyst is easiest when masses are evaluated in this location. Conversely, because pericardial cysts are located only 10% of the time in the mediastinum and many other cystic lesions may be located there, the diagnosis of a pericardial cyst is more demanding when it is in the mediastinum. Pericardial cysts are usually located in the

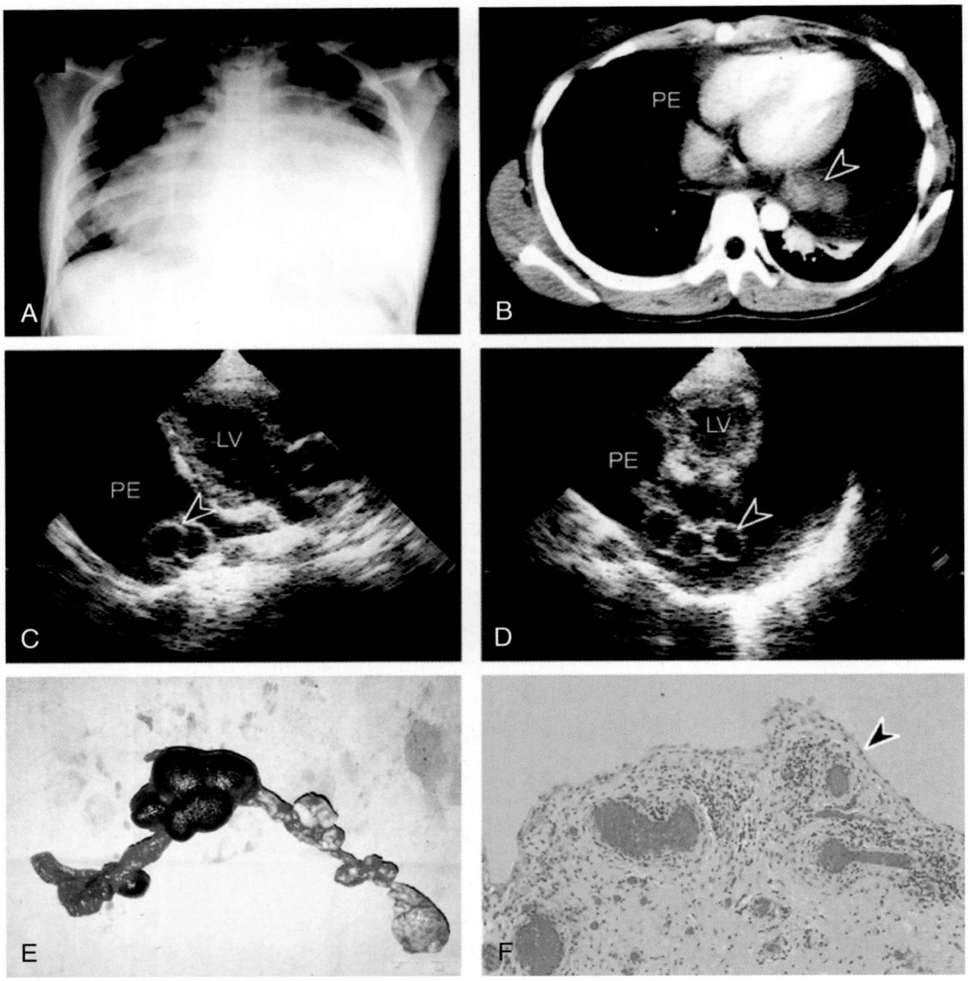

Figure 12-1. The chest radiograph (**A**) demonstrates gross cardiomegaly with a globular, pericardial fluid suggesting shape. The older generation CT scan (**B**) suggests mass lesions posterior to the left ventricle; current generation CT scanning would achieve better imaging. Echocardiography establishes that there is a left pleural effusion (PE) and cystic-appearing lesions (arrows) within it (**C** and **D**). These transthoracic echocardiographic images are unusually good for depicting cysts because one of them has ruptured into the pericardium, producing a large reactive pericardial effusion that has greatly facilitated visualization. Gross pathology (**E**) specimens reveal the multiple lobulated natures of the lesions. Microscopy (**F**) establishes that that the lesions are lined by a single serosal layer of cells. LV, left ventricle. (From Shiraishi I, Yamagishi M, Kawakita A, et al: Acute cardiac tamponade caused by massive hemorrhage from pericardial cyst. Circulation 2000;101: e196-197.)

middle mediastinum.[6] Malignant tumors are often higher in the mediastinum, particularly in the posterior mediastinum.[3,6] Thyroid and thymic cysts are located in the anterior superior mediastinum.[3] Congenital foregut cysts (epithelium lined) are the most common mediastinal cysts and account for 20% of mediastinal masses.[6] Bronchogenic cysts are lined by tracheal or bronchial mucosa and contain the glands and smooth muscle typical of bronchi. Enterogenous cysts are lined by alimentary (squamous or enteric) epithelium or pancreatic tissue. Bronchogenic cysts are 5 to 10 times more common than enterogenous cysts (Table 12-1).[6]

Confusion occurs in distinguishing the entity of the cystic hygroma from pericardial (coelomic) cysts.[2] The typical cystic hygroma is multilocular, whereas the typical coelomic pericardial cyst is unilocular. The typical cystic hygroma receives blood supply from adjacent tissues and is incorporated into adjacent tissues, whereas the typical coelomic pericardial cyst is easily "shelled out" at surgery without needing to isolate and ligate its blood supply.[2] The distinction of the two is achieved by surgical and pathologic findings.

Cardiac hydatid cysts are a very uncommon (1% to 2%) form of echinococcal disease and represent a stage in the life cycle of *Echinococcus granulosus* and *Taenia echinococcus*. Echinococcal cysts that involve the heart generally reside within the most vascular part of the heart (the left ventricular walls) rather than in the pericardial space. Commonly, the sheer bulk of the myocardial hydatid cysts bulges into the pericardial cavity. Rupture into the pericardial cavity may occur, resulting in acute pericarditis, which may become chronic and organizing. Actual pericardial involvement is exceedingly rare, but the topic arises more often in discussion of pericardial cysts. Hydatid cysts are usually single and univesicular, although more than one cyst may occur.

Pericardial cysts are, with rare exceptions, first detected as incidental imaging findings, usually on chest radiography or computed tomography (CT). They uncommonly develop complications or plausibly attributable symptoms (less than one third).

IMAGING FEATURES OF PERICARDIAL CYSTS

Chest Radiography

A pericardial cyst appears on the chest radiograph as a rounded mass, usually at either cardiodiaphragmatic angle and less commonly in the mediastinum. The fluid-filled nature (versus soft

Table 12-1. Differential Diagnosis of Pericardial Cysts

Thyroid cyst

Thymic cyst

Cystic hygroma

Congenital foregut cysts

  Bronchogenic

  Enterogenous

  Esophageal

  Stomach

  Pancreatic

Indeterminate, nonspecific

  Esophageal duplication cysts

  Neurenteric cysts

Cyst of lymph tissue

Mediastinal duct cysts

  Mediastinal thoracic duct cyst

  Cisterna chyli cyst

Mediastinal tumors

  Hemangioma

  Lymphangioma

Hernia of Morgagni, of a viscus or peritoneal fat

Eventration of the diaphragm

Intrathoracic meningocele

Mediastinal pancreatic pseudocyst

Hydatid (echinococcal) cyst

Neoplasms (benign or malignant) of the heart, pleura, or lung

tissue nature) of the cyst is not discernible by chest radiography. There is no air-fluid level within the cyst because there is not normally air within the cyst (Fig. 12-2).

Echocardiography

Ultrasound imaging of pericardial cysts reveals the cyst as thin walled and fluid filled and without flow inside it (excluded by Doppler interrogation). Ultrasonography is one of two modalities (CMR being the other) that can determine that the mass is fluid filled and hence likely to be a cyst (Fig. 12-3). Importantly, many cysts, particularly if they are not large, do not obligingly abut the chest wall to enable imaging by transthoracic echocardiography. Transesophageal echocardiography[7] and superiorly oriented transthoracic subcostal views may depict cysts that are not appreciated by transthoracic echocardiography.

Computed Tomography

CT scanning reliably depicts the size, shape, location, and thin-walled nature of pericardial cysts and the absence of other masses within the chest or pleural effusions. Pericardial cysts are non–contrast-enhancing, excluding continuity with the vascular space. Although the attenuation coefficient of the fluid within a pericardial cyst is typical of water, CT does not reliably establish that the lesion is fluid containing (ultrasonography and CMR are superior). CT scanning, like CMR, is able to image a cyst whether or not it abuts the chest wall (Figs. 12-4 and 12-5). The thinness of the wall of the pericardial cyst and its similar attenuation coefficient to the fluid within render the wall difficult to image. The rare occurrence of mural calcification of a pericardial cyst is readily detected by CT scanning.[6]

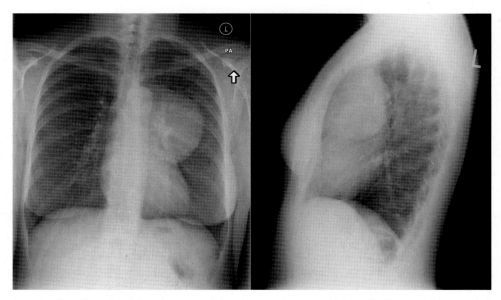

Figure 12-2. Chest radiography. The silhouette of the large pericardial cyst arising from the middle mediastinum–left hilum is obvious. The fluid-filled nature of the cyst is not apparent. Most pericardial cysts are located lower in the chest, at the diaphragmatic level, and are more commonly on the right side.

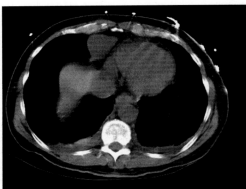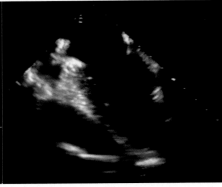

Figure 12-3. LEFT, Transthoracic echocardiographic image showing a large pericardial cyst that has contact with the anterior chest wall, allowing visualization by this modality, by which it is seen to be thin walled and fluid containing. RIGHT, Transesophageal echocardiography (in another patient) reveals a fluid-filled cyst anterior to the left ventricle. The thickness of the wall of the cyst is not discernible, nor is the pericardial tissue plane there or elsewhere. As the cyst had not abutted the chest wall, it was not apparent by transthoracic echocardiography.

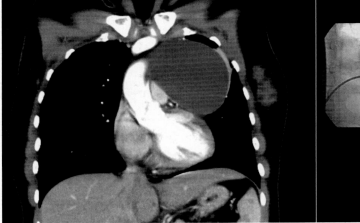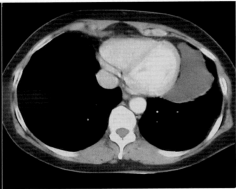

Figure 12-4. Pericardial cysts appear as thin-walled, fluid- or soft tissue–filled bodies that do not enhance by contrast CT and are generally located at the cardiodiaphragmatic angle. Usually, they are located on the patient's right side (LEFT); less commonly, they are located on the patient's left side (RIGHT). CT scanning is limited in its ability to conclusively establish the content of the cyst as fluid and may not exclude soft tissue. Echocardiography and CMR are far better suited to establish the fluid-filled nature of cysts.

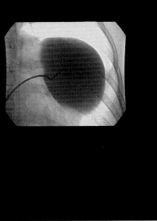

Figure 12-5. LEFT, Contrast-enhanced coronal CT image showing a low-attenuation, thin-walled mass over the left hilum, seemingly compressing the main pulmonary artery. RIGHT, Fluoroscopic image of the injection of a contrast agent into the same lesion through a pigtail catheter.

Cardiac Magnetic Resonance

CMR is an excellent modality for imaging the size, shape, location, and thin-walled and fluid-filled nature of pericardial cysts. The fluid content of the pericardial cyst has low T1 signal intensity on T1-weighted images and high T2 signal intensity on T2-weighted images. Pericardial cysts are nonenhancing after intravenous injection of gadolinium contrast material, excluding continuity with the vascular space.

A combination of imaging tests should be used to delineate the margins of the cyst (CT scanning and CMR; Fig. 12-6), to determine that the lesion is fluid containing (echocardiography and CMR), and to determine that there is no suggestion of malignant mass lesion characteristics or infections elsewhere (CT scanning).[8] Before modern imaging, at least half of suspected pericardial cyst cases that underwent thoracotomy were found not to be pericardial cysts.[2]

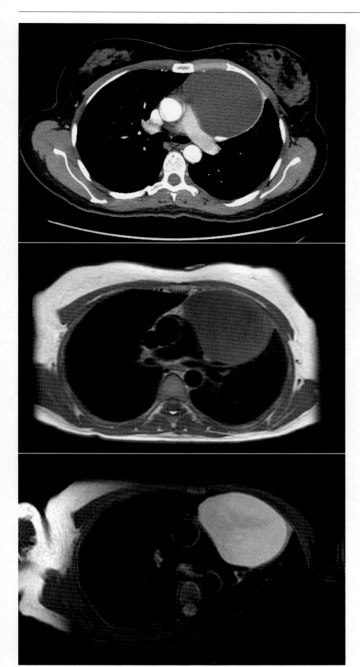

Figure 12-6. TOP, Contrast-enhanced CT image showing a large, thin-walled, low-attenuation, probably fluid-containing mass. MIDDLE, CMR T1-weighted image is commensurate with the CT image. BOTTOM, CMR T2-weighted image detects the high signal of the high proton (fluid) content.

TREATMENT

The optimal treatment of a pericardial cyst is unknown and probably best discretionary. Surgical removal should be considered for symptomatic cysts and when there is concern about possible malignancy of a cyst, as one of the undeniable benefits of surgery is that malignancy is excluded when the lesion is simply a pericardial cyst. Surveillance is reasonable for presumed cysts of typical appearance that are stable in size. Resection may be performed, depending on site and available expertise, through sternotomy, thoracotomy, or thoracoscopy. Resection is definitive for pericardial cysts. Approximately one third of bronchogenic cysts, a possible differential diagnosis of cystic lesions located in the mediastinum, will recur after surgical resection.

CASE 1

History

▸ 52-year-old woman with no chest or cardiovascular complaints
▸ While the patient was undergoing an imaging work-up for abdominal surgery, abnormal findings on a chest radiograph prompted a CT scan.

Management and Outcome

▸ Although she was asymptomatic, excision was undertaken to exclude the possibility of malignant disease.
▸ The lesion was removed uneventfully under general anesthesia by thorascopic technique. It was well tolerated, and the incision scars were small. The mass lifted out easily.
▸ The result of pathologic examination was benign and consistent with a pericardial cyst.
▸ There was no recurrence.

Comments

▸ Cyst location at the left costophrenic angle is less common than at the right costophrenic angle (20% of cysts).
▸ The cyst was asymptomatic, as most are believed to be, and an incidental finding on imaging.
▸ CT demonstrated the position well but could not conclusively establish that the cyst was fluid filled and not a soft tissue mass.

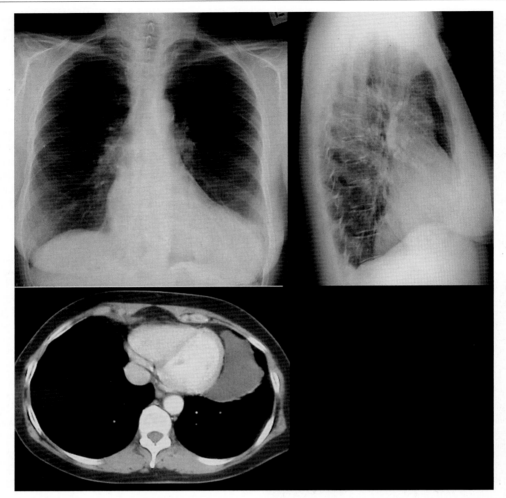

Figure 12-7. TOP, Chest radiography. The left-sided heart border silhouette is elongated on the posteroanterior film, and the lateral film demonstrates an inferoposteriorly bulging curvature of the cardiopericardial silhouette at the level of the diaphragm. BOTTOM, Contrast-enhanced axial CT image shows a large mass with a thin rim attached to the left pericardium. The mass does not opacify with intravenous administration of contrast material, establishing either that it is fluid filled but not in communication with the blood space or that it is soft tissue. There are no pericardial effusions or other abnormalities seen. The location of the mass corresponds to the abnormal contour on the chest film.

CASE 2

History

▸ A 58-year-old man with no history of hypertension presented with a distal aortic dissection that was managed conservatively.
▸ Chest radiograph and CT scan for the evaluation of the dissection revealed a right-sided, rounded paracardiac mass resembling a cyst.
▸ The patient had not had a chest radiograph for many years and no comparison of films was possible.

Outcome

▸ The lesion has been stable during the 4 years of follow-up and has been left in situ.

Comments

▸ The cyst was an incidental finding on chest radiography and CT scan.
▸ This cyst was difficult to image by echocardiography because of a partial pectus excavatum; consequently, determination that the lesion was fluid filled was difficult and speculative. Claustrophobia precluded CMR.
▸ The shape and position of the cyst were typical for a pericardial cyst, but imaging does not conclusively establish the cause of a cyst.

12

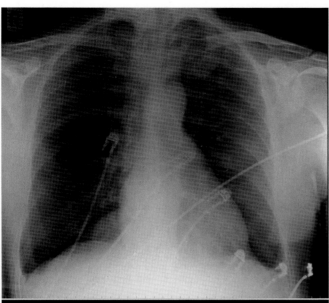

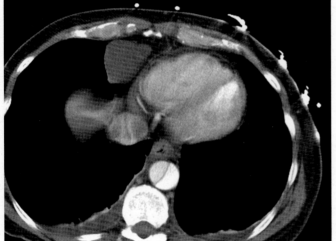

Figure 12-8. TOP, Chest radiograph shows a rounded right paracardiac mass at the level of the diaphragm. BOTTOM, Contrast-enhanced axial CT image shows a triangular right anterior paracardiac mass beside the heart at the level of the diaphragm. Its attenuation coefficient is ambiguous with respect to fluid or soft tissue. The dome of the diaphragm is apparent lateral to the posterior right atrium. The location on the CT scan matches that of the mass seen on the chest radiograph and is typical of a cyst. The actual wall, though, is not visualized, as is often difficult to do by CT scanning. The paracardiac mass does not enhance by contrast. The true and false lumens of the dissection are apparent by differential dye opacification.

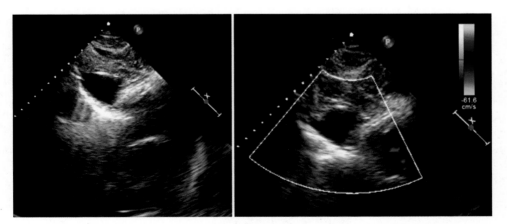

Figure 12-9. Transabdominal echocardiography, subcostal views oriented steeply superiorly into the chest. LEFT, A fluid-filled cyst is visible. RIGHT, Color Doppler flow mapping demonstrates that there is no flow in the cyst. The shape is similar to that seen on CT scanning.

CASE 3

History

▸ A 78-year-old woman undergoing a routine cardiovascular assessment was found to have an abnormal chest radiograph.
▸ She was asymptomatic, and her past history was unremarkable other than for hypertension.
▸ Her physical examination findings were normal.

Outcome

▸ Ultrasonography and CMR were able to characterize the lesion as fluid filled.
▸ The lesion has been stable during 2 years of follow-up and is being observed.

Comments

▸ Superior mediastinal location accounts for 5% of pericardial cysts.

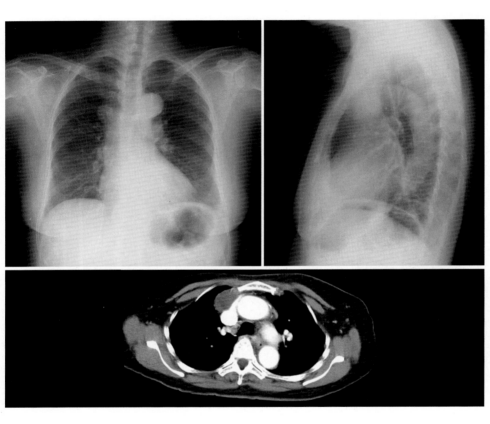

Figure 12-10. TOP, Chest radiographs. Other than mild cardiomegaly, the cardiopericardial silhouette is normal. There is a rounded mass arising from the right superior mediastinum. There are no pleural effusions. BOTTOM, Contrast-enhanced axial CT image. Immediately anterior to the innominate vein, seen entering the superior vena cava, there is a non–contrast-enhancing round or triangular lesion.

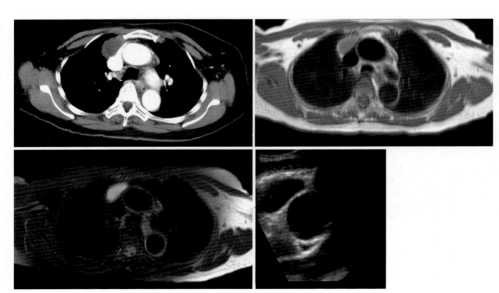

Figure 12-11. TOP LEFT, Contrast-enhanced axial CT image depicts a thin-walled mass that is non–contrast-enhancing, but the nature of its content (fluid versus soft tissue) is ambiguous. TOP RIGHT, CMR mixed T1- and T2-weighted spin echo image shows the same lesion, but without further characterization. BITTOM LEFT, CMR T2-weighted spin echo image shows both the lesion and the high signal consistent with high water content. BOTTOM RIGHT, Transthoracic echocardiography can image this mass because there is no interposed air between it and the chest wall. Echolucency of the mass confirms that it contains fluid. There was no Doppler evidence of flow within it.

CASE 4

History

▸ A 40-year-old woman undergoing a routine evaluation was discovered to have an abnormal chest radiograph. A chest radiograph performed a few years before was normal.

▸ She was without cardiovascular symptoms, significant past medical history, infectious exposures, or physical examination abnormalities. She did note a sensation of dysphagia, new during approximately a year.

Management and Outcome

▸ It was decided to percutaneously drain the presumed cyst.

▸ Complete recurrence and resumption of symptoms developed.

▸ Because of this, the patient was referred for surgical removal of the presumed cyst, which was removed off pump, easily, with some of the attached pericardium. The cyst was thin walled and had one distinct feeder vessel. It contained brown fluid; the percutaneous drainage had removed "clear water" fluid.

▸ The symptom of dysphagia improved, and there was a sense of breathing more easily, presumably because of removal of the 300-g mass.

Comments

▸ This cyst was notable for its mediastinal location (far less common than cardiodiaphragmatic location), large size, relatively recent development, prompt recurrence (which may have been due to hemorrhage from the rapidity of reaccumulation), and distinctly brown tinge of the fluid once the cyst was removed weeks later at surgery.

▸ Surgical removal was straightforward, without attachment to any adjacent structures.

12

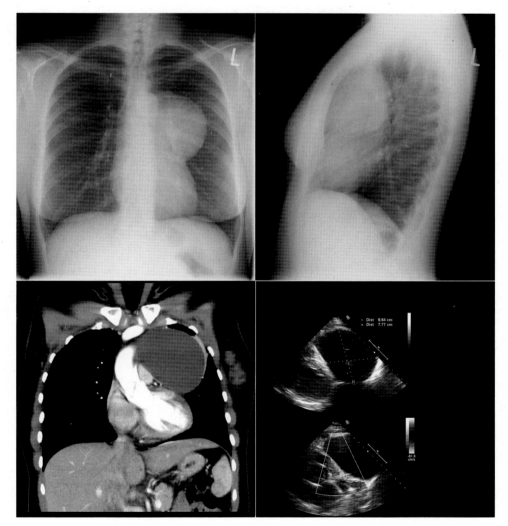

Figure 12-12. TOP LEFT AND RIGHT, Chest radiographs show a huge round mass arising from the left hilar area. There are no other masses or pleural effusions, and the heart is otherwise normal. BOTTOM LEFT, Contrast-enhanced axial CT image shows a large round mass at the level of the ascending aorta and pulmonary artery that does not enhance with contrast material. There is no pleural effusion. BOTTOM RIGHT, By transthoracic echocardiography (and other modalities), the lesion measures 8 × 9 cm. The fluid-containing nature of the cyst is evident by its echolucency. The walls appear thin, and the right ventricular outflow tract and pulmonary artery pulsate against it. No flow is seen within the mass.

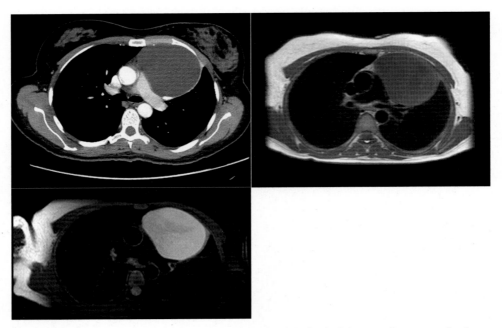

Figure 12-13. TOP LEFT, Contrast-enhanced axial CT scan shows a large round mass at the level of the ascending aorta and pulmonary artery that does not enhance with contrast material. There is no pleural effusion. The nature of the mass content (fluid versus soft tissue) is ambiguous. TOP RIGHT, CMR mixed T1- and T2-weighted spin echo image also shows a rounded mass extending along the main pulmonary artery and left pulmonary artery. The content of the mass is ambiguous. BOTTOM LEFT, CMR T2-weighted spin echo image demonstrates fluid content within the mass.

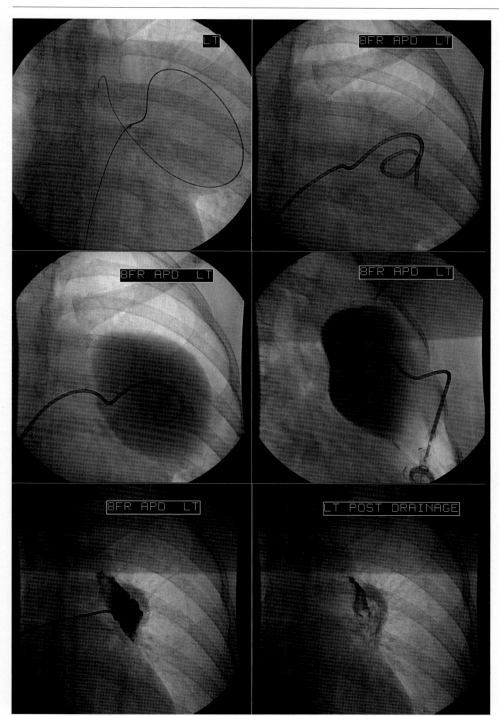

Figure 12-14. Pericardial cyst drainage by ultrasound guidance. TOP LEFT, The wire is inserted. TOP RIGHT, The drainage catheter is inserted. MIDDLE LEFT, Injected dye outlines the cyst. MIDDLE RIGHT, Fluid is withdrawn. BOTTOM LEFT, The cyst has collapsed. BOTTOM RIGHT, The cyst is virtually empty.

12

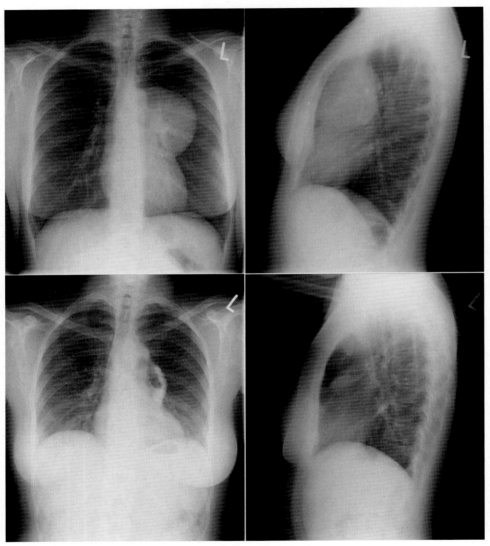

Figure 12-15. TOP, Before drainage. BOTTOM, Immediately after drainage, there is a small amount of air in the residua of the cyst.

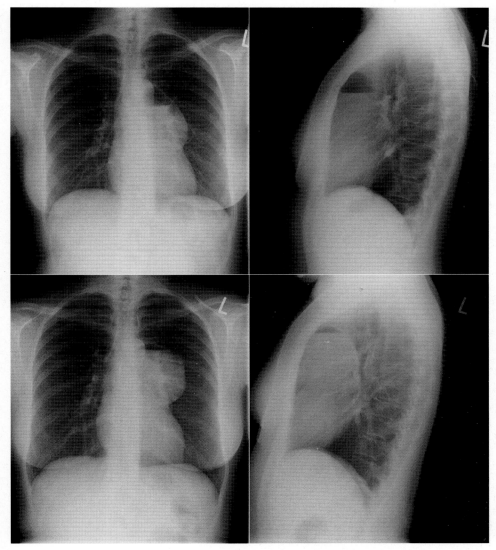

Figure 12-16. TOP, One week after drainage, the fluid is reaccumulating. There is a well-formed air-fluid level. BOTTOM, Two weeks after drainage, the cyst has nearly completely recurred. By a week later, it had fully reestablished its former size and shape, and the air-fluid level had disappeared.

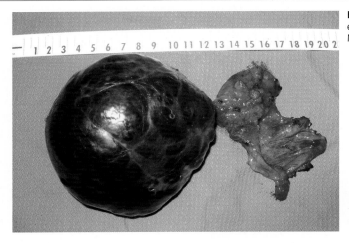

Figure 12-17. Excised surgical specimen, 11 cm in diameter, smoothly encapsulated and attached to the pericardium. (Courtesy of Daniel Bonneau, MD, and Robert Chisholm, MD, both of Toronto, Canada.)

CASE 5

History

▸ A 40-year-old man was referred for evaluation of an abnormal chest radiograph that he had undergone because of a chest infection.
▸ He was without cardiovascular complaints, and his physical examination findings were normal.

Outcome

▸ The referring physician and the patient opted for a strategy of observation, which has been uneventful thus far.

Comments

▸ Incidental detection of a presumed pericardial cyst in the fourth decade of life
▸ The patient is asymptomatic, and the cyst is being observed.

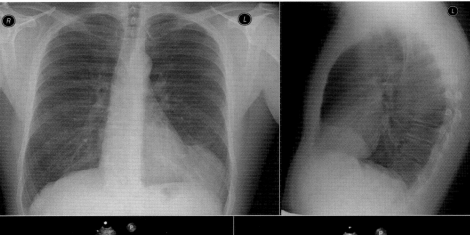

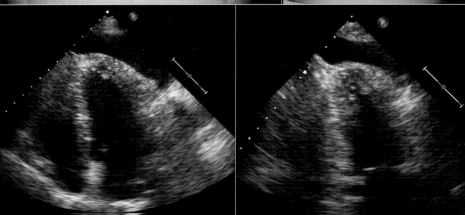

Figure 12-18. TOP, Chest radiographs show a rounded mass at the left cardiodiaphragmatic angle and no apparent pleural effusion. BOTTOM, Transthoracic echocardiographic apical images show an echolucent, fluid-filled cavity located apically, extending over the apicolateral wall of the heart.

References

1. McAllister HA Jr, Fenoglio JJ Jr: Tumors of the cardiovascular system. Atlas of Tumor Pathology, 2nd Series, Fascicle 15. Washington, DC, Armed Forces Institute of Pathology, 1978.
2. Le Roux BT, Kallichurum S, Shama DM: Mediastinal cysts and tumors. Curr Probl Surg 1984;21:1-77.
3. Nasser WK: Congenital diseases of the pericardium. Cardiovasc Clin 1976;7:271-286.
4. Butany J, Woo A: The pericardium and its diseases. In Silver M, Gotlieb AI, Schoen FJ, eds: Cardiovascular Pathology, 3rd ed. New York, Churchill Livingstone, 2001.
5. Basso C, Valente M, Poletti A, et al: Surgical pathology of primary cardiac and pericardial tumors. Eur J Cardiothorac Surg 1997;12:730-737.
6. Strollo DC, Rosado-de-Christenso ML, Jett JR: Primary mediastinal tumors: tumors of the middle and posterior mediastinum. Chest 1997;112:1344-1357.
7. Hutchison SJ, Smalling RG, Albornoz M, et al: Comparison of transthoracic and transesophageal echocardiography in clinically overt or suspected pericardial heart disease. Am J Cardiol 1994;74:962-965.
8. Altbach MI, Squire SW, Kudithipudi V, et al: Cardiac MR is complementary to echocardiography in the assessment of cardiac masses. Echocardiography 2007;24:286-300.

Pericardial Masses, Tumors, and Pericardial Encasement

▸ Pericardial masses are usually due to malignant involvement of the heart. In some cases, this occurs without pericardial effusion.

▸ Pericardial thrombus is another common cause of pericardial "soft tissue."

▸ Rare benign pericardial tumors occur.

▸ Most intrapericardial masses are without physiologic effect; but if they are associated with effusion of

sufficient size or if they are massive, they can compress the heart (encasement).

▸ Echocardiography is somewhat useful, but CT scanning is more useful, particularly as it is likely to assess other relevant aspects of intrathoracic disease. Ultimately, the combination of echocardiography and CT scanning is the most comprehensive imaging strategy, supplemented when needed with CMR.

Soft tissue masses may arise on the visceral pericardium or on either side of the parietal pericardium, and they may occur with or without associated pericardial effusion. Pericardial soft tissue masses may be solitary or multiple or even fill the pericardial space. When pericardial tumor bulk competes with the heart for intrapericardial space, the compressive syndrome of encasement develops. Most pericardial tumor masses are metastatic extension of common bulky intrathoracic malignant disease (bronchogenic carcinoma, breast carcinoma, lymphomas, and thymomas) rather than uncommon tumors of primary cardiac origin (Table 13-1).

Some intrapericardial masses represent widely disseminated malignant disease, such as melanoma or leukemia. Typically, such lesions tend to be diffuse and with little bulk. Malignant involvement of the pericardium is 30 times more likely to be metastatic than to result from a primary cardiac malignant neoplasm. As with most advanced malignant disease states, accompanying effusions (pericardial and pleural) are common. Nonmalignant masses, such as thrombi, and foreign bodies may also occur within the pericardial space. There are rare benign pericardial tumors.[1]

Although there are usually no apparent physiologic consequences of most pericardial masses, compressive syndromes due to either tamponade or encasement (restricted filling by mass effect) may develop.[2]

Cardiac and vascular compression from pericardial masses may occur from pericardial effusion; encasement of the great vessels by large bulk of material, leading to superior vena cava (SVC) syndrome; pulmonary artery compression or pulmonary

venous compression, which may produce asymmetric pulmonary edema; or encasement of the heart by large bulk of material within the pericardial space or chest, producing a compressive constriction-like syndrome. Encasement, often insidious in onset in an ill patient, may be a subtle and confusing diagnosis, leading to delayed recognition. Although echocardiography is a reliable test to recognize tamponade, the diagnosis of encasement is more difficult because the obvious presence of fluid and the usual range of dynamic signs of tamponade physiology are uncommonly present. Distinguishing fluid from tumor by older generation echocardiographic[3] or computed tomographic (CT)[4] scanning systems has not always proven successful.

IMAGING

Optimal imaging of pericardial masses includes imaging of the heart to assess for signs of compression and also detailed tomographic imaging of the entire chest (± abdomen) for the many potentially relevant intrathoracic disease details that would be inapparent by echocardiography, such as bronchial narrowing, SVC or pulmonary vein narrowing, intrapulmonary masses, pleural masses, mediastinal masses, and bone metastases. The combination of echocardiography for the heart and CT scanning for the chest is robust, to be supplemented with cardiac magnetic resonance (CMR) when needed. CT and CMR modalities are particularly important as they are superior means to ascertain and to delineate other intrathoracic complications of disease.

Table 13-1. Pericardial Tumors

Metastatic malignant neoplasms

  Lymphoma (very common involvement of the pericardium)

  Bronchogenic carcinoma (very common involvement of the pericardium)

  Breast carcinoma (very common involvement of the pericardium)

Other carcinomas

  Melanoma (highest incidence of metastases to the heart but uncommon)

  Leukemia (very high incidence of metastases to the heart but uncommon)

  Sarcomas

  Malignant thymomas

  Malignant mesothelioma of the lung

  Nerve sheath tumors

Primary pericardial malignant neoplasms

  Mesotheliomas

  Lymphangiomas

  Paragangliomas

  Neurofibromas

  Sarcomas (angiosarcoma, Kaposi sarcoma, rhabdomyosarcoma, fibrosarcomas, leimyosarcomas)

  Malignant teratomas

  Primary lymphomas

Benign pericardial tumors

  Fibromas

  Teratomas

  Hemangiomas

  Bronchogenic cysts

  Thymomas

PERICARDIAL EFFUSIONS IN PATIENTS WITH MALIGNANT DISEASE

Not all pericardial effusions in patients with malignant disease are due to malignant involvement. Bloody effusions are commonly due to erosive malignant involvement but may also be due to aggressive chemotherapy (e.g., cyclophosphamide at more than 1 g/m², which may cause hemorrhagic pericarditis and tamponade) or radiotherapy. Serous effusions may also be due to malignant involvement, caused by treatment, and seen in advanced malignant disease–related cachexia.

PERICARDIAL PSEUDOTUMORS

Although pericardial masses are all too commonly a manifestation of advanced malignant disease, fresh thrombus and organized thrombus or scar tissue (typically sequelae from prior bleeding into the pericardium, such as after open heart surgery) may also result in intrapericardial masses. Some chronic organized intrapericardial thrombi may resemble intrapericardial tumors (pericardial pseudotumor) by their mass effect and complex appearance and imaging features on echocardiography, CT scanning, and CMR.[5] Obtaining a careful history is therefore crucial in making a correct diagnosis.

CASE 1

History

▸ 65-year-old man with new-onset atrial fibrillation

▸ Remote pericardiectomy for tuberculous constrictive pericarditis at 15 years of age. Incredibly, the records could be obtained as microfiche. Operative notes described that part of the pericardium could not be excised; as well, there was myocardial laceration and bleeding during the procedure.

Physical Examination

▸ Normal BP, no pulsus paradoxus
▸ Normal venous pressure and contours
▸ Normal heart sounds;, no "knock"
▸ No pericardial rub
▸ Abnormally prominent precordial impulse

Outcome

▸ The patient remained well, other than atrial fibrillation.

Comments

▸ The mass is believed to be a calcified organized intrapericardial or paracardiac hematoma beside the left ventricle and atrium. Understanding the exact location of the mass is a conundrum, given that pericardiectomy would leave only recesses within which a clot could reside and organize, and seldom in constriction (unless it is effuso-constriction) could a clot accumulate in the pericardial space, which is actually obliterated in true constriction.

▸ The mass appears to have some "mass effect" as the heart is displaced away from it in diastole, but there are no features of constriction or compression.

▸ Although it does deform the heart, surgical excision did not seem warranted for lack of hemodynamic disturbances or attributable symptoms.

13

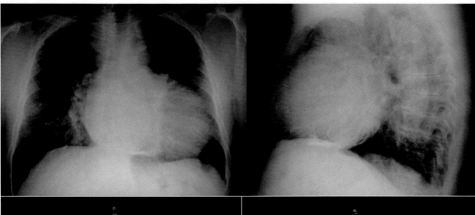

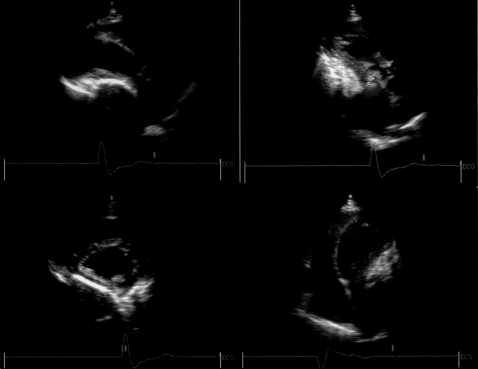

Figure 13-1. TOP, Chest radiographs. There is cardiomegaly with a globular shape of the cardiopericardial silhouette. Probable calcification on the diaphragmatic aspect of the heart. MIDDLE AND BOTTOM, Transthoracic echocardiography. There is an unusual and large mass posterior and lateral to the left ventricle. The anterior aspect of the mass is very echogenic, and it flattens the posterior and lateral aspects of the left ventricle. There appears to be shadowing, suggesting calcification of the mass. There is no pericardial effusion or left pleural effusion.

CASE 2

History

▸ 61-year-old man, smoker, with a 3-month history of hemoptysis and shortness of breath and type 2 diabetes mellitus

Physical Examination

▸ BP 120/70 mm Hg, pulsus paradoxus of 15 mm Hg, HR 90 bpm
▸ Elevated neck veins, $x > y$ descents
▸ Peripheral edema

Outcome

▸ Mild to moderate tamponade from suspected metastatic disease. Plans were made for surgical drainage, but the patient died suddenly of refractory ventricular arrhythmias.
▸ Autopsy findings:
   ▸ Widely metastatic melanoma of unknown primary, with extensive cardiac and pulmonary involvement

▸ 700 mL of pericardial fluid
▸ Many pericardial melanoma masses
▸ A mass of melanoma had extensively involved the myocardium, which was not identified ante mortem on echocardiography.
▸ The right atrial mass arising off the interatrial septum was a benign myxoma.
▸ Encasement of the great vessels in the chest by lymph nodes

Comments

▸ Although malignant involvement of the heart by melanoma is less often encountered than by lymphoma or breast or lung carcinoma, when melanoma is widely metastatic, it is particularly likely to involve the heart.
▸ The cause of the sudden arrhythmic death was not determined with certainty, but myocardial infiltration by the tumor was suspected.

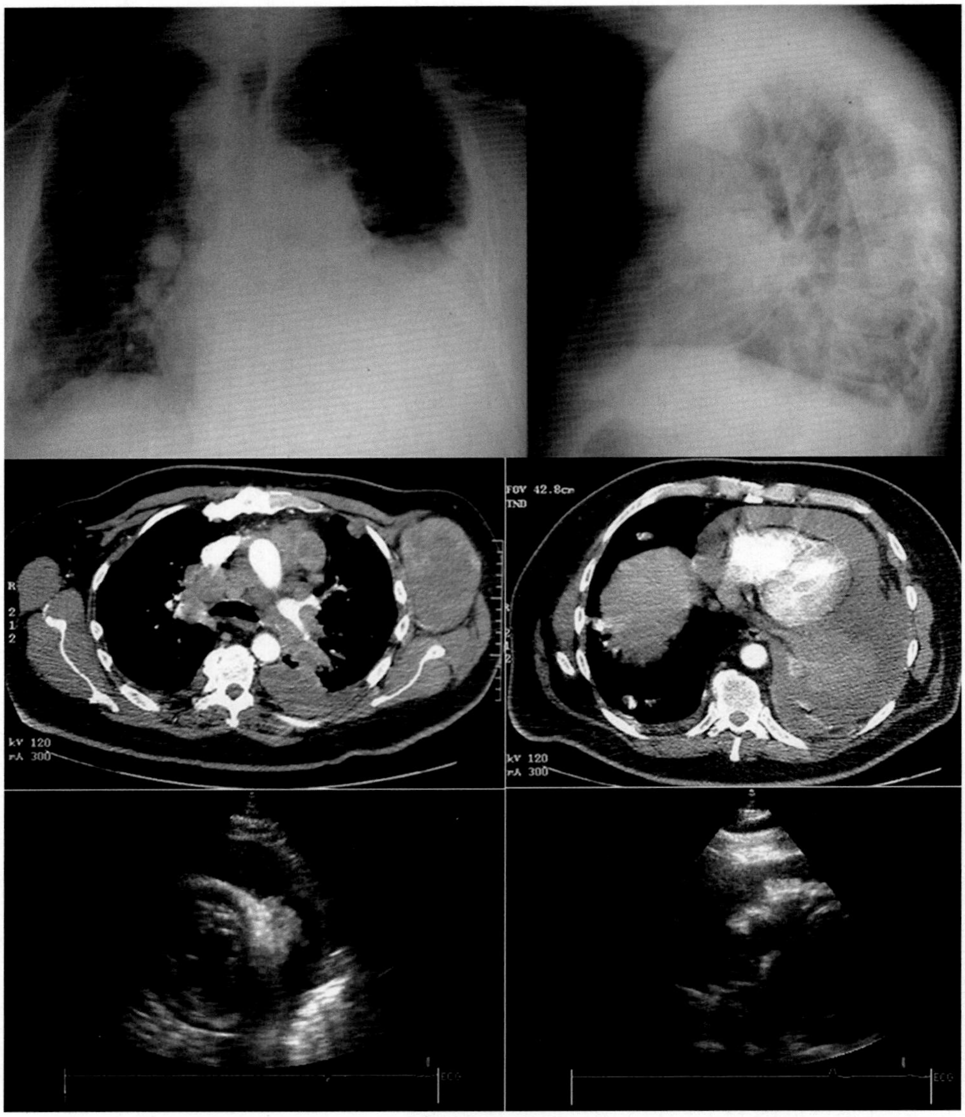

Figure 13-2. TOP, Chest radiographs show cardiomegaly, a left pleural effusion, hilar and mediastinal widening, and multiple lesions in the lungs. MIDDLE, Contrast-enhanced CT scans depict many hilar and mediastinal lymph nodes, a left axillary mass, a pericardial effusion, and a left pleural effusion. BOTTOM, Transthoracic echocardiographic images show a medium-sized pericardial effusion and masses on the epicardial surface of the heart.

CASE 3

History

▸ 75-year-old man with previous three-vessel aortocoronary bypass 15 years previously
▸ 6 years previously, an intracardiac mass impinging on the right ventricle was discovered. Although no direct details were available, it was the patient's understanding that the mass was believed to be a residual and organized intrapericardial hematoma.
▸ He presented with low-threshold angina and underwent angiography, which showed advanced saphenous graft and native vessel disease.

Outcome

▸ The mass remained stable for years and is presumed to represent an organized hematoma from the prior cardiac surgery, as had been thought.

Comments

▸ The mass distorted the cardiopericardial silhouette of the chest radiograph, resulting in bulging and displacement of the left ventricle posteriorly.
▸ There was no significant functional disturbance (tricuspid stenosis) from the mass.
▸ The CT scan established the relation of the localized mass to the cardiac chambers but was not entirely definitive in determining that the mass was intrapericardial or whether it was fluid filled.
▸ Echocardiography established that the mass was soft tissue and without fluid but could not appreciate whether it was calcified.

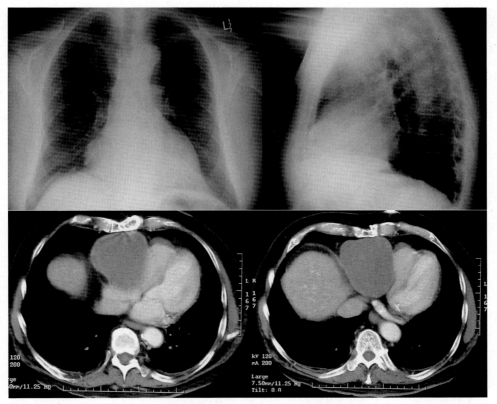

Figure 13-3. TOP, Chest radiographs. Clear lung fields and no pleural effusions. There is cardiomegaly with unusual contours—there is a bulge of the lower anterior heart on the lateral chest radiograph as well as a bulge on the lower right border. The left ventricular posterior border projects more posteriorly than usual. BOTTOM, Contrast-enhanced axial CT scans. There is a large mass indenting the right ventricle and atrium. It appears to account for the abnormal radiographic findings. It is difficult to appreciate whether the mass is intrapericardial or paracardiac, but there appears to be parietal pericardium extending over it anteriorly. There is no apparent calcification within the mass.

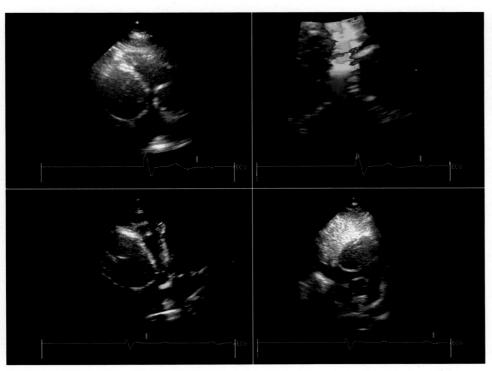

Figure 13-4. Transthoracic echocardiographic images show a large rounded mass, of similar shape to what was seen on the CT scan, again seen principally lateral to the right ventricle. There is no pericardial effusion. The mass narrows the right ventricular inflow, resulting in some flow acceleration at the tricuspid level.

CASE 4

History

- 44-year-old man with HIV infection
- Presented with ocular symptoms and skin lesions
- Biopsy specimens of skin lesions were obtained and established to be lymphomatous.
- He underwent a CT scan, which unexpectedly showed cardiac involvement.

Outcome

- The patient underwent chemotherapy for the lymphoma.
- Follow-up CT scanning showed disappearance of the mass over the ventricles and from the right ventricular cavity.
- He survived 2 more years.

Comments

- The elevated right atrial pressure and central venous pressure were due to diastolic failure from the tumor's encasing the right ventricle.
- The mass encased the right ventricle, resulting in elevation of the venous pressures but not frank constriction.
- Despite the extensive involvement of the heart, the tumor lysis did not result in rupture of the heart or tamponade.

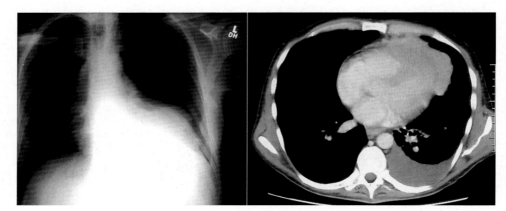

Figure 13-5. Chest radiograph (LEFT) and contrast-enhanced axial CT scan (RIGHT). The cardiopericardial silhouette is abnormal with a bulge over the apex. There is no right pleural effusion. The CT scan shows poor contrast enhancement. There is a large mass around the distal half of both ventricles and appearing to infiltrate and obliterate the right ventricular apex. There is no pericardial effusion, but there is a left pleural effusion.

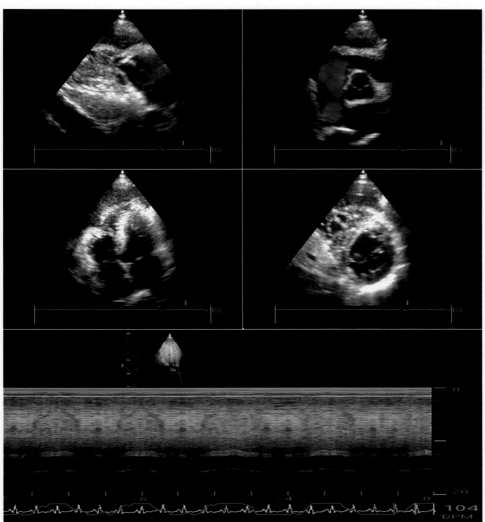

Figure 13-6. Transthoracic echocardiography. Best seen on the right ventricular inflow view (TOP), there is a large mass of soft tissue around the right ventricle, and the right ventricular cavity is very small; it appears obliterated in its distal half. The pericardium is difficult to see. MIDDLE LEFT, The apical 4-chamber view suggests a thick rind of soft tissue over the apices of the ventricles. MIDDLE RIGHT, The short-axis view supports abnormal soft tissue present over the right ventricular anterior wall. BOTTOM, The inferior vena cava is dilated and without respiratory collapse, indicating elevated central venous pressure.

CASE 5

History

▸ 60-year-old man undergoing aortocoronary bypass

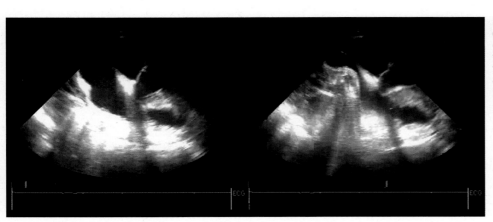

Figure 13-7. Transesophageal echocardiography, lower esophageal views oriented to the right side. (The "mass" indenting the heart on the right image at the right atrial level is a surgeon's finger as the atrium is being manipulated in preparation for insertion of the efferent bypass cannula.)

CASE 6

History

▸ 58-year-old woman presented with 2-month history of biventricular failure
▸ Past medical history is significant for hypertension and sarcoma excised from the lower leg 5 years previously, with no local recurrences.

Imaging

▸ Cardiomegaly was noted on the chest radiograph.
▸ Echocardiography was not able to clearly image the heart. There was additional soft tissue anterior and lateral to the heart, which impaired the imaging of the heart itself. The cavities appeared very small. The mass appeared to be soft tissue, not fluid.

Outcome

▸ CT suggested fluid in the mass, whereas echocardiography suggested soft tissue mass.

▸ Needle aspiration was dry.
▸ She deteriorated and was in obvious low output (central venous pressure was 38 mm Hg).
▸ She was referred for exploratory surgery and died during surgery when anesthesia was induced because of loss of arterial and venous constriction as compensation for the cardiac compression.

Comments

▸ Extensive malignant involvement within the pericardial space by an enormous myxoid sarcoma had led to severe compression of the heart.
▸ The consistency of the tumor was gelatinous, explaining its misleading imaging qualities.
▸ Severe compressive syndrome from the bulk of the mass within the pericardial space

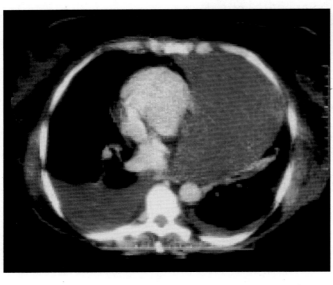

Figure 13-8. Contrast-enhanced axial CT scan. There is a very large mass next to the heart. It is difficult to determine whether it is within the pericardial space or on the outside of the pericardium. The heart cavities are extremely small and severely displaced to the right side.

CASE 7

History

▸ 72-year-old man with palpitations
▸ He underwent echocardiography, which detected a "myxoma," and he was referred for surgery.

Physical Examination

▸ Normal vitals, no pulsus paradoxus
▸ Mild venous distention, no rub
▸ Small supraclavicular and asymmetric axillary adenopathy

Outcome

▸ B-cell lymphoma was diagnosed from lymph node biopsy.
▸ The patient underwent chemotherapy that was well tolerated.
▸ Complete remission and cure were achieved.

Comments

▸ Encasement of the atria by tumor
▸ Normalization of venous pressures after chemotherapy
▸ Chest radiograph showed unilateral pulmonary edema from pulmonary vein compression, which also normalized after chemotherapy.
▸ Despite the massive involvement of the tumor through the atria, lysis of the tumor did not cause tamponade.

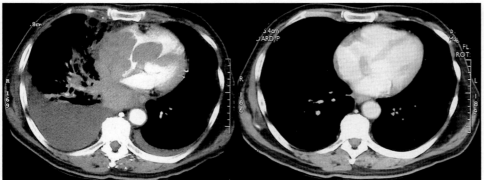

Figure 13-9. LEFT, Contrast-enhanced axial CT scan before treatment shows large masses within the right and left atria, also around the right ventricle, cava, and pulmonary veins. There are bilateral pleural effusions. RIGHT, Contrast-enhanced axial CT scan after treatment demonstrates a near-complete dissolution of the masses around and in the atria and right ventricle and resolution of the pleural effusions. Small mass still remains at the interatrial septum.

CASE 8

History

▸ A 68-year-old woman presented with fatigue and shortness of breath but no chest pain.
▸ The patient became distressed with shortness of breath and was intubated and transferred.

Physical Examination

▸ BP 100/60 mm Hg, tachycardic, no pulsus paradoxus
▸ Facial plethora, distended neck and hand veins
▸ Distant heart sounds, no rub
▸ Wheezes

Outcome

▸ Bronchial compression rendered ventilation difficult.
▸ Adenocarcinoma was found on biopsy.
▸ The patient died on the third day in the hospital.

Comments

▸ Encasement of the heart and great vessels, infiltration of the left ventricle, and severe SVC syndrome (internal jugular vein pressure, 45 mm Hg; femoral vein pressure, 15 mm Hg)
▸ The large discrepancy between the upper and lower venous pressures means that the SVC syndrome was a worse problem than the encasement of the heart.

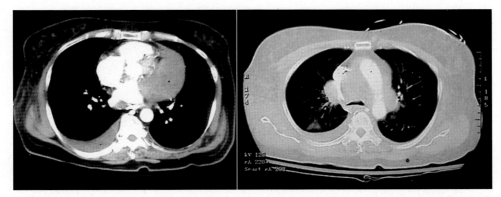

Figure 13-10. Contrast-enhanced axial CT scans. There is a large soft tissue mass within the pericardial space surrounding the apex and compressing and infiltrating the left ventricle. There is a right pleural effusion. There is also a large mass of soft tissue around the aorta, compressing the pulmonary artery, the right mainstem bronchus, and the SVC. A right peripheral lung lesion is present, and there is a right pleural effusion.

CASE 9

History

▸ 30-year-old woman with malignant lymphoma poorly responsive to chemotherapy
▸ Pericardial tamponade 5 months previously treated with surgical drainage and a pericardial window
▸ Progressive fatigue and generalized weakness

Physical Examination

▸ BP 85/50 mm Hg, pulsus paradoxus of 20 mm Hg, HR 130 bpm
▸ Venous distention, distant heart sounds, no rub

Outcome

▸ Protracted terminal state, followed by death

Comments

▸ True encasement of the heart by tumor around the heart and within the pericardial space, with constriction-like cardiac compression physiology, resulting in hypotension and tachycardia and low output
▸ The basis of the distant heart sounds and low voltages on the electrocardiogram was the interposed soft tissue of the tumor.

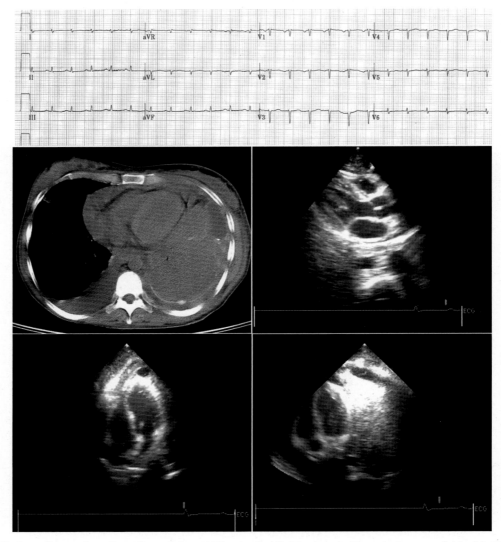

Figure 13-11. TOP, Electrocardiogram shows low voltages (<5 mm in the standard limb leads and <10 mm in the precordial leads). MIDDLE LEFT, Non–contrast-enhanced axial CT scan demonstrates enormous soft tissue mass within the pericardial space and extending into the left hemithorax. Tumor-related calcification and a loculated anterior right pleural effusion are evident. Distinguishing the soft tissue from fluid is ambiguous in some areas. MIDDLE RIGHT AND BOTTOM, Transthoracic echocardiographic views show an extensive amount of soft tissue surrounding the heart and involving the left hemithorax. There is only a small anterior pleural effusion.

References

1. Dias BD, Yau T, Sasson Z, et al: Right atrial mass. Can J Cardiol 2001;17: 1299-1300.
2. Lagrotteria DD, Tsang B, Elavathil LJ, Tomlinson CW: A case of primary malignant pericardial mesothelioma. Can J Cardiol 2005;21:185-187.
3. Foote WC, Jeffferson CM, Price HL: False-positive echocardiographic diagnosis of pericardial effusion: result of tumor encasement of the heart simulating constrictive pericarditis. Chest 1977;71:546-549.
4. Lee DS, Barnard M, Freeman MR, et al: Cardiac encasement by metastatic myxoid liposarcoma. Cardiovasc Pathol 2002;11:322-325.
5. Moon JC, Sheppard MN, Lloyd G, et al: Cardiac pseudotumor: tissue characterization by cardiovascular magnetic resonance. J Cardiovasc Magn Reson 2003;5:497-500.

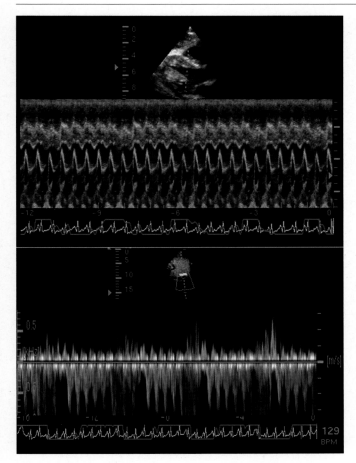

Figure 13-12. TOP, Transthoracic echocardiographic M-mode study across the interventricular septum shows signs of ventricular interdependence. There is an increase in right ventricular volume (dimension) and a fall in left ventricular volume (dimension) with inspiration, which is denoted by the upward deflection of the red respirometry tracing. BOTTOM, Lower tracing denotes hepatic venous flow pattern. There is an increase in diastolic flow reversal in expiration, a finding of constriction-like physiology.

Pneumopericardium

KEY POINTS

▸ Pneumopericardium is often well depicted on a chest radiograph, but the lateral film is important to exclude the common entity of a hiatus hernia, whose supradiaphragmatic air may be superimposed onto the heart shadow on a frontal chest film.

▸ There is generally little risk to the pneumopericardium itself; risk more likely relates to the underlying cause,

the development of pneumopyopericardium, and the rare development of tension pneumopericardium.

▸ Pneumomediastinum can extend by pulmonary venous perivascular sheaths into the pericardium through pericardial reflections at the pulmonary veins.

ETIOLOGY

Pneumopericardium (air within the pericardial space) may result from the following:

- Trauma: blunt force trauma, penetrating trauma, or barotrauma from positive-pressure ventilation. Pneumopericardium occurs most commonly in premature infants on positive-pressure ventilation and in adults with asthma or COPD on positive-pressure ventilation.
- Fistulization of air from the trachea or bronchus, the transverse colon (from inflammatory bowel disease or carcinoma), the stomach (from inflammatory bowel disease, peptic ulcer disease,[1-3] or carcinoma), or the esophagus (from carcinoma, after esophageal dilation,[4] secondary to reflux disease, after lye ingestion, after esophageal surgery[5])
- Tracking of air along the pulmonary venous perivascular sheath from pneumomediastinum through the pulmonary venous pericardial reflection, into the pericardial space
- Gas-forming bacterial infection
- Congenital pericardial or diaphragmatic absence may allow air within the peritoneum to track into the pericardium.

The risk of pneumopericardium principally relates to the cause (e.g., cancer), the development of bacterial superinfection (pneumopyopericardium) of the pericardial space from fistulization, and the rare occurrence of compression of the heart by tension pneumopericardium.[6,7]

The potential air channels from alveoli along peribronchial and perivascular pathways to the mediastinum have been well described.[7] Air in the hilum may gain entry into the pericardial space at the pericardial reflections along the pulmonary veins, where the fibrous reflection of the pericardium is not continuous (see Figure 1-17).[6]

Tension pneumopericardium may occur with pressurization of the pericardial space to greater than 145 cm H_2O.[8] Hemodynamic instability is usual. The mortality of tension pneumopericardium exceeds 50%.[9] The constellation of physical diagnosis findings of tension pneumopericardium may not be typical of tamponade due to fluid.[6] The bruit de moulin (mill wheel sound), a combination of a rub and a splashing sound, may be heard in pneumopericardium.

DIAGNOSIS

Chest Radiography

Although the diagnosis of pneumopericardium may be obvious on a posteroanterior or anteroposterior film alone, it is wise to obtain the lateral chest radiograph to ensure that the air resides within the heart rather than being retrocardiac (from a hiatus hernia or achalasia). Radiographic signs include an air collection, an air-fluid level (if there is associated fluid), and a stripe of pericardium seen on a tangential view of the parietal pericardium. Cases of tension pneumopericardium reveal air extensively surrounding a heart diminished in size or compressed (Figs. 14-1 to 14-5).

Computed Tomography

Computed tomographic (CT) scanning is an excellent means to localize air to within the pericardial space and also to seek for structural diseases that may be responsible for pneumopericardium (Figs. 14-6 and 14-7).

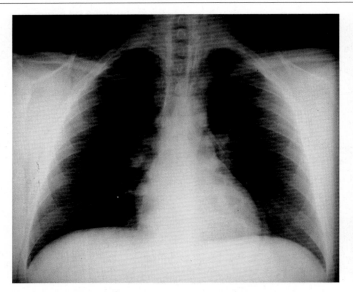

Figure 14-1. A 42-year-old man after bronchoscopy and transbronchial biopsy. There is subcutaneous emphysema and an obvious thin stripe of air on the lateral aspect of the heart and also of parietal pericardium, seen tangentially on the lateral border of the heart. The thicker diaphragmatic aspect of the stripe is due to the fat pad at the pericardiodiaphragmatic angle. Note how the parietal pericardium extends superiorly over the main pulmonary artery.

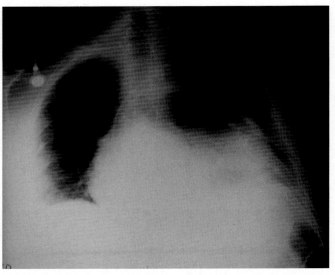

Figure 14-2. A 58-year-old man with carcinoma of the transverse colon that eroded through the diaphragm into the pericardial space, causing purulent pericarditis and sepsis. The large collection of air in the pericardial space, the pericardium seen as a tangential stripe in silhouette, and the air-fluid level within the pericardial space are seen in this image.

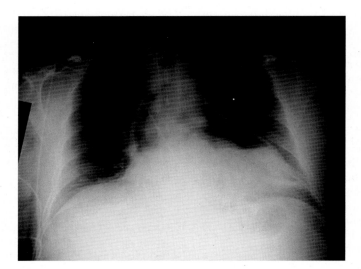

Figure 14-3. A 62-year-old man with esophageal cancer that eroded into the pericardial space, causing purulent pericarditis. The air-fluid level, the air pocket on both sides of the heart, the pericardium seen tangentially as a stripe on both sides of the heart, and the outline of the ascending aorta within the pericardial space are represented in this image. Note how far superiorly the pericardium extends along the ascending aorta.

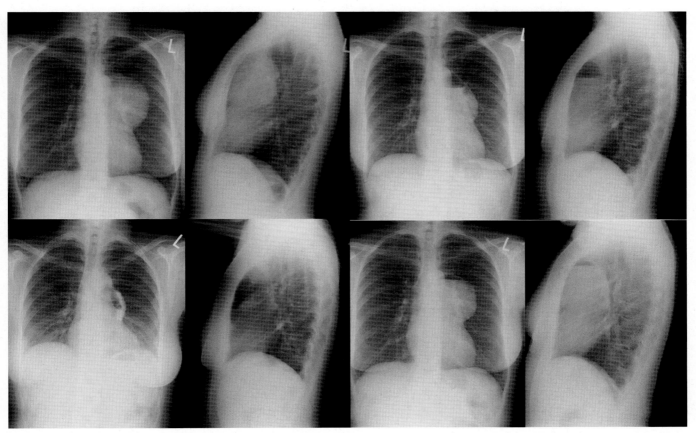

Figure 14-4. Large anterior pericardial cyst undergoing drainage. TOP LEFT, Before percutaneous drainage. BOTTOM LEFT, After removal of 700 mL of light yellow, clear fluid. The cyst has collapsed. There is a small amount of air now within the cyst, which presumably entered by the drainage procedure, as the fall in intrapleural pressure during inspiration would be exerted on the body of the cyst, facilitating entry of exterior air through the needle and drain, unless it were sealed to air. TOP RIGHT, During the next weeks, the cyst reaccumulated fluid. BOTTOM RIGHT, The cyst returned to its baseline state, the air was resorbed, and the air-fluid level disappeared by 3 weeks after drainage.

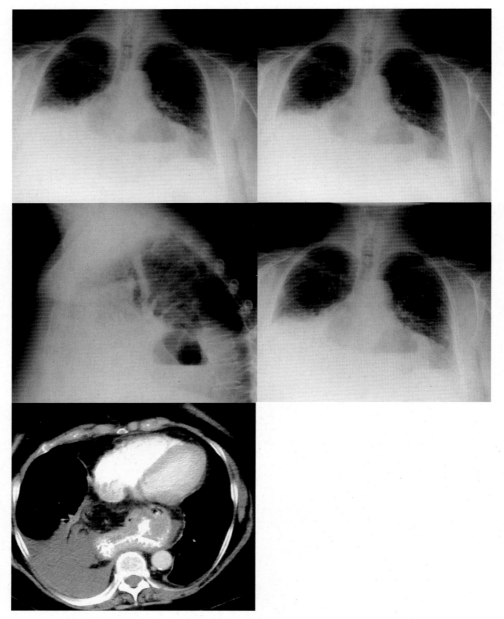

Figure 14-5. A 78-year-old woman with 3 weeks of dyspnea. A large right pleural effusion was the cause of the shortness of breath. TOP LEFT, The air collection and air-fluid level that appear to be within the heart are not associated with a stripe of pericardium seen tangentially. TOP RIGHT AND MIDDLE LEFT, The air collection that appears to be within the heart is really retrocardiac, within a large hiatus hernia, and is not pneumopericardium. The lateral chest radiograph is needed to establish the location of the air along the anteroposterior axis. MIDDLE RIGHT AND BOTTOM, The air collection that appears to be within the heart is easily appreciated on the confirmatory CT scan to be retrocardiac, within a large hiatus hernia, and is not pneumopericardium. The pleural effusion was determined by cytology to be malignant of ovarian origin.

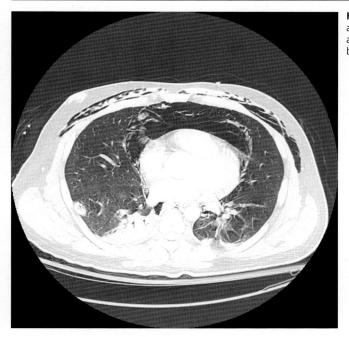

Figure 14-6. Contrast-enhanced axial CT scan. There appears to be air anteriorly in the pericardial space. It is actually air in the mediastinum, associated with subcutaneous emphysema and bilateral pneumothoraces—barotrauma from positive-pressure ventilation.

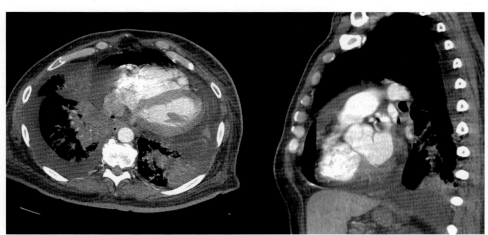

Figure 14-7. Contrast-enhanced axial CT scans. An air-fluid level is present within the pericardial space. It is located anteriorly, as the patient is supine during CT scanning, whereas air and air-fluid levels on chest radiography are located superiorly when the patient had been sitting for the film exposure. The patient had undergone pericardial drainage for relief of malignant tamponade due to lung carcinoma; the pericardial air entered through the drain because of lack of seal.

Echocardiography

Transthoracic echocardiography is confounded by air within the pericardial space. Ultrasound waves poorly penetrate air, and echocardiographic imaging is therefore at a disadvantage. In some cases, transesophageal echocardiography may be able to assess the heart in the presence of pneumopericardium when the air is distributed anteriorly. The esophagus, residing posterior and between the pulmonary veins, generally permits visualization from a posterior perspective.[6]

References

1. West AB, Nolan N, O'Briain DS: Benign peptic ulcers penetrating pericardium and heart: clinicopathological features and factors favoring survival. Gastroenterology 1988;94:1478-1487.

2. Romhilt DW, Alexander JW: Pneumopyopericardium secondary to perforation of benign gastric ulcer. JAMA 1965;191:140-142.

3. Matsubara T: Purulent pneumopericarditis due to ulcer of the retrosternal stomach roll after esophagectomy. Eur J Cardiothorac Surg 2002;22:1007.

4. Lehmann KG, Blair DN, Siskind BN, Wohlgelernter D: Right atrial–esophageal fistula and hydropneumopericardium after esophageal dilation. J Am Coll Cardiol 1987;9:969-972.

5. Susarla S, Khouzam RN, Lowell D, Marshall T: Gastropericardial fistula presenting 22 years after lye ingestion. Can J Cardiol 2005;21:371-372.

6. Levin S, Maldonado I, Rehm C, et al: Cardiac tamponade without pericardial effusion after blunt chest trauma. Am Heart J 1996;131:198-200.

7. Macklin CC: Transport of air along sheaths of pulmonic blood vessels from alveoli to mediastinum. Arch Intern Med 1939;64:913-921.

8. Adcock JD, Lyons RH, Barnwell JB: The circulatory effects produced in a patient with pneumopericardium by artificially varying the intrapericardial pressure. Am Heart J 1940;19:283-291.

9. Cummings RG, Wesley RL, Adams DH, et al: Pneumopericardium resulting in cardiac tamponade. Ann Thorac Surg 1984;37:511-518.

Index

Note: Page numbers followed by f indicate figures; those followed by t indicate tables.